FRONTIERS IN ATHEROSCLEROSIS RESEARCH

FRONTIERS IN ATHEROSCLEROSIS RESEARCH

KARIN F. KEPPER
EDITOR

Nova Science Publishers, Inc.
New York

For permission to use material from this book please contact us:
Telephone 631-231-7269; Fax 631-231-8175
Web Site: http://www.novapublishers.com

Library of Congress Cataloging-in-Publication Data

Frontiers in atherosclerosis research / Karin F. Kepper (editor).
p. ; cm.
Includes bibliographical references and index.
ISBN 13 978-1-60021-371-7
ISBN 10 1-60021-371-5
1. Atherosclerosis. I. Kepper, Karin F.
[DNLM: 1. Atherosclerosis--drug therapy. 2. Atherosclerosis--physiopathology. WG 550 F935 2006]
RC692.F762 2006
616.1'36--dc22 2006022799

Published by Nova Science Publishers, Inc. ✢ New York

CONTENTS

PREFACE

Atherosclerosis is a degenerative condition in which arteries build up deposits called plaques (atheromas) which consist of lipids (mainly cholesterol), connective tissue and smooth muscle cells originating from the arterial wall. Plaques develop quietly over a period of years and are unnoticeable until there is an interruption in the normal flow of blood. Plaques may partially or totally block the blood's flow through an artery. Two things that can happen where plaques occur are: bleeding (hemorrhage) into the plaque; and formation of a blood clot (thrombus) on the plaque's surface. Atherosclerosis affects large and medium-sized arteries. The type of artery and where the plaque develops varies with each person. Atherosclerosis research has witnessed startling progress in recent years, partially due to new drugs as well as to breakthroughs in molecular medicine.

Polyunsaturated fatty acids (PUFAs) are necessary for normal cellular function. However PUFAs are prone to peroxidation, which can cause cell death including apoptosis. Susceptibility to peroxidation increases with the degree of unsaturation, i.e. with greater numbers of carbon-carbon double bonds per fatty acid molecule. Studies of human cancer cell lines treated with PUFAs in vitro demonstrated that apoptosis increased with degree of fatty acid unsaturation. This suggests that apoptosis can be induced by a peroxidative mechanism. This might translate into an atherosclerosis-modulating effect of PUFAs in vivo. Atherosclerosis is a chronic inflammatory disease. The lipid-rich foam cells of human atherosclerotic lesions are predominantly monocyte-derived macrophages (HMM), and their death contributes to the lipid cores of plaques (advanced lesions). HMM death is implicated in destabilisation of advanced atherosclerotic lesions, leading to plaque rupture with thrombogenic consequences, including cardiovascular events and strokes. In vitro, HMM treated with PUFAs showed a general trend for increasing apoptosis with increasing degree of fatty acid unsaturation, although arachidonic acid (AA; 20:4, n-6) stood out above the trend (in contrast to its behaviour in cancer cell lines) as it induced apoptosis more strongly than both the more highly unsaturated (and more peroxidisable) EPA and DHA. In HMM in vitro, AA-induced apoptosis was diminished by the cyclo-oxygenase inhibitor indomethacin and by the lipoxygenase inhibitor nordihydroguaiaretic acid, suggesting roles for these enzymes in the induction of apoptosis by AA. Moreover 15(S)-hydroperoxy-5,8,11,13-eicosatetraenoic acid was a very strong inducer of apoptosis in HMM, whereas 15(S)-hydroxy-5,8,11,13-eicosatetraenoic acid was innocuous. A major source of PUFAs in atherosclerosis is plasma low-density lipoprotein (LDL). Much evidence implicates oxidation of LDL in atherogenesis, including the apoptosis-inducing effect of oxidised LDL (oxLDL) on HMM in vitro. LDL oxidation involves peroxidation of the PUFA chains of LDL lipids, which are predominantly esters. Various LDL oxidation products can induce death in HMM in vitro, and radical scavengers such as alpha-tocopherol and BO-653 can prevent both LDL oxidation and the ensuing HMM death. Evidence from an oral alpha-tocopherol supplementation study in carotid endarterectomy patients suggests that within LDL and atherosclerotic lesions, alpha-tocopherol can inhibit lipid peroxidation. Lipoprotein-associated phospholipase A_2 (Lp-PLA_2) is a naturally present LDL-borne enzyme that hydrolyses oxidised phospholipids (but not non-oxidised phospholipids) forming lysophosphatidylcholine and oxidised, non-esterified fatty acids. Treatment of LDL with inhibitors of Lp-PLA_2, especially the highly specific inhibitor SB222657, diminished the ensuing HMM death including apoptosis, when the LDL was oxidised and added to HMM in vitro, even though the Lp-PLA_2 inhibitors did not diminish LDL oxidation. These findings in chapter 1, may be relevant to potential mechanisms of fatty acid influences on atherosclerosis and cancer and may suggest strategies for combating these diseases.

The mortality rate resulting from atherosclerosis is a large enough incentive to continue research efforts toward disease prevention and treatment. But the stakes are raised when one considers the enormous burden placed on society as a result of lost productivity and health care expenditure. The complexities of atherosclerosis pathophysiology are numerous and new facets continue to unfold at a rapid pace. Following the completion of several landmark trials over the past decades, the importance of altering lipid metabolism through the inhibition of HMG-CoA reductase has been demonstrated. The role of cholesterol absorption, has also led to the development of cholesterol absorption inhibitors which add to the portfolio of effective medications in the fight against coronary artery disease. Other metabolic pathways and factors are currently being explored which include cholesterol ester transfer protein (CETP), microsomal transfer protein (MTP), peroxisome proliferator-activated receptor (PPAR), and Acyl coenzymeA: cholesterol acyltransferase (ACAT). Excess cholesterol is stored as cholesteryl ester (CE) through an esterification process regulated in part by ACAT. The ACAT enzyme is found in many tissues types which require the storage of cholesterol. Since cholesterol is both an essential building block, but also a risk factor for cardiovascular a clear understanding of the role of ACAT in human metabolism is important. While cholesterol is an essential component of steroid, hormones, bile acids, and cellular membranes, high levels of serum cholesterol increases the deposition in the arterial wall. Most notably for cardiovascular disease ACAT activity is significant in intestinal and hepatic tissue and arterial macrophages. ACAT has been evaluated in cell cultures, experimental animal models and clinical trials for several decades. Much information has been gained in chapter 2, regarding the contribution of this enzyme and it continues to be evaluated as a potential target for therapeutic intervention. Several ACAT inhibitors have been investigated for their potential to favorably alter serum lipoprotein levels by blocking intestinal absorption, hepatic inhibition and/or slow the progression of atherosclerosis through a non-lipid arterial inhibition. However, no ACAT inhibitor to date has proven to be a safe and effective therapy for the management of patients with atherosclerotic disease or at risk for cardiovascular events. Recent evaluations of ACAT and ACAT inhibitors have provided some insight into the therapeutic potential and risks of ACAT inhibition as a means of treating atherosclerosis.

The fundamental principle of radiotherapy is to destroy malignant cells while minimizing damage to normal tissues. Almost all patients who receive radiotherapy to the head and neck area develop some grade of acute mucositis, which is not only painful, but may compromise tumor control by determining decrease in dose intensity and interruptions of the treatment. The term 'oral mucositis' describes the adverse effect of chemotherapy or radiation induced inflammation of the oral mucosa. Symptoms of mucositis vary from pain and discomfort to an inability to tolerate food or fluids. The degree and duration of mucositis in patients receiving radiotherapy are related to radiation source, cumulative dose, dose intensity, volume of irradiated mucosa, smoking/alcohol consumption and oral hygiene conditions. To the authors' knowledge in chapter 3, there is no other controlled study which has evaluated vitamin E as a single radioprotective agent in patients with head and neck tumors treated with radiation therapy alone or post-operative. For this reason, they conducted a double-blind, randomized trial with the objective to investigate the potential mucosal protection of vitamin E in irradiated patients with head and neck cancer, motivated by its simplicity of administration, no severe toxicity in conventional doses, low cost and easy availability.

Recent research on Vitamin E (vit E) has pointed out novel mechanisms of action in addition to its well-known antioxidant activity. One of the main non-antioxidant actions of vit E is the modulation of intracellular signaling cascades. Vit E has been reported to directly or indirectly modulate different kinases such as protein kinase C (PKC), phosphatidylinositol-3-phosphate kinase (PI3K), glycogen syntase kinase-3β (GSK-3ß), phosphatases such as protein phosphatase type 2A (PP2A), and key regulatory enzymes such as phospholipase A2 (PLA2) and cyclooxygenase-2 (COX-2). The neuroprotective effects attributed to vit E show complex mechanisms of action, in which its non-antioxidant activities are also playing a key role. In chapter 4, the authors have reviewed the effects of vit E in the intracellular signaling pathways in brain, focusing on its modulation of neuronal survival and growth, glial inflammatory response and vascular function. The authors will conclude with a note on the putative protective role of vit E in neurodegenerative processes.

Coronary artery disease events have a circadian rhythmicity, clustering more in the second quartile of the day. n-3 fatty acid supplementation reduces the rate of cardiac events, but its effect on their circadian rhythmicity has not been tested. The Indo-Mediterranean Diet Heart Study discussed in chapter 5, was a single blind randomized study that assessed the effect of a diet rich in alpha-linolenic acid, the parent n-3 fatty acid, on the occurrence of myocardial infarction and sudden cardiac death. One thousand subjects of the Indo-Mediterranean Diet Heart Study, focusing on the 115 patients from both control and intervention groups in which cardiac events occurred. The timing of cardiac events throughout the day was compared between the intervention and control groups. The distribution of cardiac events along the four quartiles of the day was compared between groups as well as against equal distribution.

A circadian cell cycle resides in every cell, and peripheral timing mechanisms are documented in molecular biologic terms at about 24-hour (circadian) and higher (ultradian) frequencies with coordination in mammals by the adrenal and the pineal-hypothalamic-pituitary network. The suprachiasmatic nuclei (SCN) and clock gene contribute to the coordination of the circadian rhythms' phase and amplitude in everyday life. The SCN are influenced by the daily alternation between light and darkness directly via the eyes and by plasma melatonin concentrations secreted by the pineal gland, which is a window to both light and geomagnetics. A clinical event occurs when the neuroendocrine time structures (chronomes) are not able to cope with the adverse effects of stimuli acting from within or from without, e. g., via the sympathetic nervous system. Triggering of the neuroendocrines by environmental factors may activate the pineal gland, pituitary functions and adrenal secretions, resulting in adverse effects on circadian variations, heart rate variability (HRV) and blood pressure variability (BPV). Circadian rhythm has been known to ancient man from the time of Homoerectus and Homosapiens who used to have intercourse in the early morning hours, prior to going hunting in the forests, causing increased secretion of testosterone in the morning. The role of time-adjusted drug intake, especially in the early morning, was also known to ancient Indian physicians. In the Ayurveda, drinking of large amounts of water in the early morning is advised, which appears to be in an attempt to increase vagal tone due to gastric distention. Frey considered the mean distribution of deaths along the scales of the day and the year. In one industrial population, Pell and D'Allonzo, discussed time-macroscopically the occurrence of a peak in the morning hours in a study of acute myocardial infarction (AMI), a proposition also ascertained and extended to the yearly pattern time-microscopically. The subsequent reports from other countries, the Soviet Union and the extensive data by WHO in the report of myocardial infarction Community Registers from 19 European centers demonstrated a peak incidence of onset of chest pain due to AMI from 8.00 to 11.00 AM with a ratio of approximately 2 In one study from India, in 605 AMI patients, 39% of those who had Q wave infarction (n=174) had the onset between 6. 00 AM to 12. 00 noon. In a more recent Mechanism of Acute Myocardial Infarction (MAMI) study by Singh et al, among 202 AMI patients, the incidence of onset of chest pain was highest in the second quarter of the day (41. 0%), mainly between 4-8 AM, followed by the 4th quarter, usually after large meals (28. 2%). Emotion was the second most common trigger (43. 5%), which was the most common in the patients with onset of chest pain in the second quarter of the day (51. 8%). Cold weather was a predisposing factor in 29. 2% and hot temperatures (40°C) was common in 24. 7% of the patients. A large meal, especially a large breakfast in the morning was an important trigger of AMI in this study in chapter 6, which poses the intriguing possibility that some heart attacks could be prevented by not eating breakfast or by eating a small superfood breakfast containing walnuts, almonds, raisins and yogurt which are known to be protective against cardiovascular disease. Blood pressure is usually lower during the night, starts increasing before awakening, and remains high during the day-time, mostly in the second quarter of the day. Circadian rhythms of triggers and cardiac events and their mechanisms have been described by various workers. It is possible that circadian rhythm could be a new target for treatment with lifestyle changes, nutrient, nutraceuiticals such as w-3 fatty acids and coenzyme Q10, prayer and drug therapy in the management of cardiovascular disease.

It has been repeatedly shown in chapter 7, that statins (3-hydroxy-3-methylglutaryl coenzyme A reductase inhibitors) are very effective in primary and secondary prevention of ischemic heart disease. In the settings of acute coronary syndrome (ACS), different pathological pathways are triggered that are known to be inhibited by statins, including endothelial dysfunction and activation of inflammation and coagulation; the idea to use these drugs also under conditions of ACS seems to be, therefore, fully justified. Recently, several prospective controlled clinical trials have been presented, showing safety and in some points also efficacy of statins, when administered early after ACS. An increasing number of publications demonstrates, however, that statins may express a positive effect not only in the early secondary prevention but also directly in the therapy of ACS, i.e. when statin treatment is started as a first-line care in clinically unstable patients. This therapeutic option is supported by (i) experimental studies, showing a protective effect of statins under the condition of acute ischemia, (ii) analysis of different registers and trials, demonstrating better prognosis of statin-treated patients, and (iii) small clinical trials, describing a lower peri-procedural infarction rate during coronary intervention or lower level of C-reactive protein and other inflammatory markers as a result of statin therapy. Nevertheless, confirmation of this hypothesis by large prospective controlled clinical trials will be necessary before introduction of statins as the first line therapy in unstable patients with ACS, even without knowledge of the blood cholesterol level.

The objective of the present investigation in chapter 8, was to find out whether the addition of fenofibrate to statin monotherapy produced any synergistic or additive beneficial effects in reducing risk factors, especially plasma fibrinogen, in patients of Acute Coronary Syndromes (ACS) requiring Percutaneous Coronary Interventions (PCI). This was a randomized, non-blind, prospective study with parallel group design, conducted in 102 patients who had angiographically documented Coronary Artery Disease (CAD). All had undergone angioplasty. The patients were randomized to atorvastatin (20mg/day, n=25), simvastatin (40mg/day, n=27), atorvastatin(10mg/day)-fenofibrate (200mg/day) combination (n=25) and simvastatin (20mg/day)-fenofibrate(200mg/day) combination (n=25). The serum lipid profile and plasma fibrinogen were recorded before initiation of therapy and after 3 months of the respective treatments. All the patients already had desirable lipid levels as per the NCEP ATP III guidelines. The addition of fenofibrate to statin monotherapy produced additional benefits on reduction in triglyceride (TG) and very low density lipoprotein (VLDL) levels, and an increase in high density lipoprotein (HDL) levels. All the treatment groups showed a significant decrease in the plasma fibrinogen levels. This did not correlate with any of the study parameters like age, body weight, hemodynamic characteristics and lipoprotein levels. Statin monotherapy produced a significant decrease in the fibrinogen levels and the addition of fenofibrate further enhanced the reduction. Addition of fenofibrate to statins seems to be beneficial in patients with ACS. Statins, contrary to various reports, were found to decrease plasma fibrinogen significantly.Further, in combination with fenofibrate there was enhanced reduction of the novel risk factor, fibrinogen.

Functional recovery of ischemic cardiomyopathy depends on accurate identification of viable myocardium. The authors in chapter 9 evaluated the value of delayed contrast-enhanced magnetic resonance imaging (MRI) in the assessment of myocardial viability. Forty patients with significant coronary artery disease and severe left ventricular (LV) dysfunction received delayed contrast-enhanced MRI and ^{201}Tl single-photon emission computed tomography (SPECT) within one month. Ten of them received simultaneous ^{201}Tl SPECT and dobutamine stress echocardiography (DSE). Three imaging modalities were compared based on a standardized 17-segment model. Improved regional wall thickening on follow-up MRI was used as an index of functional recovery in patients received revascularization. Of 680 segments, MRI hyperenhancement showed positive correlation with ^{201}Tl reduction (r =0.61, $p < 0.0001$). The viability concordance was 75.3% between DSE and MRI, 80.5% between ^{201}Tl SPECT and MRI, and 66.5% among all tests. Contrast-enhanced MRI detected more myocardial viability than ^{201}Tl SPECT, especially in the inferior wall and apex ($p < 0.0001$). Eight patients underwent revascularization. Comparing with functional recovery in the follow-up results, the diagnostic accuracy, sensitivity, specificity, positive predictive value, and negative predictive value of delayed contrast-enhanced MRI were 64%, 95%, 24%, 62% and 77%, respectively. For ^{201}Tl SPECT, these values were 55%, 75%, 29%, 58% and 54%, respectively. Areas under the ROC curves by MRI and ^{201}Tl SPECT were 0.59 ± 0.04, $0.52 \pm$

0.05, respectively (p=0.07). Of 16 segments viable on MRI but nonviable on ^{201}Tl SPECT, 12 (75%) recovered function after revascularization, while only one of 3 segments classified as nonviable on MRI but viable on ^{201}Tl SPECT recovered function ($p < 0.05$). Of 10 segments classified as scar by both tests, none recovered function after revascularization. Delayed contrast-enhanced MRI detects viability better than ^{201}Tl SPECT, especially in the inferior wall and apex. Myocardial viability detected by MRI may predict functional recovery after revascularization in ischemic cardiomyopathy, even in patients with severe LV dysfunction

Aspirin as a therapeutic drug has been in use for over hundred years. Its use as an anti-platelet drug was recognized in the early 70s. For secondary prophylaxis of vascular disease, it is the most useful and cost-effective drug. Large number of clinical trials using aspirin has concluded that at any given vascular risk, low to medium dose of aspirin (80-160mg), is as effective as any other drug of choice. However, in recent years, there are several studies, in which aspirin resistance in patients with various vascular diseases have been demonstrated. Furthermore, some studies have suggested worst outcome in aspirin non-responders. Variety of methods has been used in these studies in chapter 10, to determine "non-responders" to the action of aspirin .The definition of "aspirin resistant" individuals is those whose platelet cyclooxygenase are not inhibitable by aspirin. Methods used for monitoring aspirin resistance in these studies are non-specific platelet function tests. Differences in the definition of aspirin resistance, variations in the methods used to detect "non-responders", inter-individual variations in the response of platelets to the action of different agonists, and lack of data from large clinical trials have hampered the advancement of knowledge in this area. Therefore, there is a great need to develop specific and rapid Point-of-Care assays that could detect the prevalence of aspirin resistance in patient populations, so that those found to be non-responders to the action of aspirin might be provided alternate treatment regimen.

Recent studies in chapter 11, indicate that sildenafil is cardioprotective by preconditioning of the myocardial and endothelial cells. In the present review, the authors examine the available evidence regarding this beneficial effect. Experimental studies indicate that sildenafil can provide beneficial effects to the myocardium and endothelium by enhancing preconditioning. There are a few clinical studies among healthy subjects and a few observational studies indicating that sildenafil is useful in patients with poor endothelial function and in those with myocardial ischaemia. They found among 6 volunteer patients with nonST-elevation myocardial infarction that treatment with sildenafil was protective in limiting infarct size. They also observed that sildenafil can decrease blood pressure among hypertensives and provide benefits against heart failure in patients with acute left ventricular failure. Experimental and clinical experiences support the usefulness of sildenafil in patients with acute myocardial infarction, heart failure and hypertension. Randomized, controlled trials and long-term follow-up are necessary to confirm these observations.

In: Frontiers in Atherosclerosis Research
Editor: Karin F. Kepper, pp. 1-28
ISBN 1-60021-371-5

Chapter 1

THE ROLES OF POLYUNSATURATED FATTY ACIDS, LIPID PEROXIDATION AND CELL DEATH IN ATHEROSCLEROSIS

Keri L. H. Carpenter [a*], ***Karin Müller*** [a], ***Balaji Muralidhar*** [a], ***Iain R. Challis*** [a], ***Jeremy N. Skepper*** [b] ***and Mark J. Arends*** [a]

[a]University of Cambridge, Department of Pathology, Cambridge UK
[b]University of Cambridge, Multi-Imaging Centre, Cambridge, UK

ABSTRACT

Polyunsaturated fatty acids (PUFAs) are necessary for normal cellular function. However PUFAs are prone to peroxidation, which can cause cell death including apoptosis. Susceptibility to peroxidation increases with the degree of unsaturation, i.e. with greater numbers of carbon-carbon double bonds per fatty acid molecule.

Studies of human cancer cell lines treated with PUFAs in vitro demonstrated that apoptosis increased with degree of fatty acid unsaturation. This suggests that apoptosis can be induced by a peroxidative mechanism. This might translate into an atherosclerosis-modulating effect of PUFAs in vivo.

Atherosclerosis is a chronic inflammatory disease. The lipid-rich foam cells of human atherosclerotic lesions are predominantly monocyte-derived macrophages (HMM), and their death contributes to the lipid cores of plaques (advanced lesions). HMM death is implicated in destabilisation of advanced atherosclerotic lesions, leading to plaque rupture with thrombogenic consequences, including cardiovascular events and strokes. In vitro, HMM treated with PUFAs showed a general trend for increasing apoptosis with increasing degree of fatty acid unsaturation, although arachidonic acid (AA; 20:4, n-6) stood out above the trend (in contrast to its behaviour in cancer cell lines) as it induced apoptosis more strongly than both the more highly unsaturated (and more peroxidisable) EPA and DHA. In HMM in vitro, AA-induced apoptosis was diminished by the cyclo-oxygenase inhibitor indomethacin and by the lipoxygenase inhibitor nordihydroguaiaretic acid, suggesting roles for these enzymes in the induction of apoptosis by AA. Moreover 15(S)-hydroperoxy-5,8,11,13-eicosatetraenoic

* Corresponding author. Address for correspondence: University of Cambridge, Academic Unit of Neurosurgery, Box 167, Addenbrooke's Hospital, Hills Road, Cambridge CB2 2QQ, UK. Tel: +44 1223 336933; Fax: +44 1223 216926; Email: klc1000@wbic.cam.ac.uk

acid was a very strong inducer of apoptosis in HMM, whereas 15(S)-hydroxy-5,8,11,13-eicosatetraenoic acid was innocuous.

A major source of PUFAs in atherosclerosis is plasma low-density lipoprotein (LDL). Much evidence implicates oxidation of LDL in atherogenesis, including the apoptosis-inducing effect of oxidised LDL (oxLDL) on HMM in vitro. LDL oxidation involves peroxidation of the PUFA chains of LDL lipids, which are predominantly esters. Various LDL oxidation products can induce death in HMM in vitro, and radical scavengers such as alpha-tocopherol and BO-653 can prevent both LDL oxidation and the ensuing HMM death.

Evidence from an oral alpha-tocopherol supplementation study in carotid endarterectomy patients suggests that within LDL and atherosclerotic lesions, alpha-tocopherol can inhibit lipid peroxidation.

Lipoprotein-associated phospholipase A_2 (Lp-PLA$_2$) is a naturally present LDL-borne enzyme that hydrolyses oxidised phospholipids (but not non-oxidised phospholipids) forming lysophosphatidylcholine and oxidised, non-esterified fatty acids. Treatment of LDL with inhibitors of Lp-PLA$_2$, especially the highly specific inhibitor SB222657, diminished the ensuing HMM death including apoptosis, when the LDL was oxidised and added to HMM in vitro, even though the Lp-PLA$_2$ inhibitors did not diminish LDL oxidation.

These findings may be relevant to potential mechanisms of fatty acid influences on atherosclerosis and cancer and may suggest strategies for combating these diseases.

INTRODUCTION

Cell death, including apoptosis, is an important process in atherosclerosis, and it also plays an important role in diabetes and a number of obesity-related health problems leading to cardiovascular complications. Whether apoptosis is beneficial or detrimental in atherosclerosis is still debated. In diabetes, the death of pancreatic beta-cells is thought to lie at the centre of organ failure. Epidemiological evidence shows that diets rich in polyunsaturated fatty acids (PUFAs), especially eicosapentaenoic acid (EPA) and docosahexaenoic acid (DHA) can protect against cardiovascular risk, although the mechanisms are often unclear. In contrast, high plasma levels of saturated fatty acids can be toxic, leading to the phenomenon of lipoapoptosis in diabetes and some obesity-related illnesses, which have high risk of cardiovascular complications. Monounsaturated fatty acids (e.g. oleic acid) can in some cases modulate the pro-apoptotic effect of other fatty acids. This article will highlight some of the mechanisms by which PUFAs and saturated fatty acids can induce cell death, including apoptosis, and how this could translate into effects on atherosclerosis, discussing some of the authors' own work as well as that of other researchers.

DIETARY PUFAS: EPIDEMIOLOGICAL EVIDENCE

Polyunsaturated fatty acids (PUFAs) are necessary for normal cellular functions, such as maintaining correct membrane fluidity, cell signalling, and energy storage. However PUFAs are prone to peroxidation, which can cause cell death including apoptosis. Susceptibility to peroxidation increases with the degree of unsaturation, i.e. with greater numbers of carbon-carbon double bonds per fatty acid molecule. Monounsaturates are relatively resistant to peroxidation. PUFAs therefore possess the potential to do harm as well as good in biological systems.

Dietary eicosapentaenoic (EPA; 20:5, n-3) and docosahexaenoic (DHA; 22:6, n-3) have long been considered protective against cardiovascular disease, supported recently by evidence from a patient supplementation study [GISSI-Prevenzione Investigators, 1999], though the mechanisms are not fully understood. Fish oil is a rich source of EPA and DHA. "Mediterranean diets" are also considered to protect against cardiovascular disease. This cuisine traditionally contains olive oil, rich in the monounsaturate oleic acid (OA; 18:1, n-9). Such diets are also rich in natural antioxidants, including vitamin E. Another PUFA component of at least some Mediterranean diets is α-linolenic acid (18:3, n-3), which has been reported to confer protection against cardiovascular disease [de Lorgeril et al. 1994]. Part of α-linolenic acid's effect might be due to its ability to act as a precursor to the longer chain, more highly unsaturated n-3 fatty acids EPA and DHA.

Fish oil fatty acids appear also to protect against colorectal, breast and prostate cancer [Bartsch et al. 1999]. Dietary modification to include oily fish, PUFA supplements or functional foods might promote apoptosis of cancer cells or their precursors and prevent tumour development at an early stage. Moreover raising intake of fish oil fatty acids appears beneficial, not only against heart disease and cancer, but also against inflammatory bowel disease and rheumatoid arthritis, with little evidence of adverse side-effects [Connor 2000]. In dietary oils and fats, PUFAs are present predominantly in the form of triglycerides, also termed triacylglycerols. In vivo, PUFAs are found in many forms, including phospholipids, triacylglycerols (and to a lesser extent di- and mono- acylglycerols), cholesterol esters, and non-esterified fatty acids (NEFA), also termed free fatty acids (FFA).

PUFAs (n-3 and n-6) in human plasma and tissues are derived from diet, as mammals cannot synthesise them de novo. In mammals, linoleic acid (LIN; 18:2, n-6) comes from diet, and arachidonic acid (AA; 20:4, n-6) is synthesised by elongation and desaturation of linoleic acid. EPA (20:5, n-3) and DHA (22:6, n-3) can be synthesised from dietary α-linolenic acid (18:3, n-3), and they can also come directly from diet (e.g. oily fish). Plasma fatty acid concentrations are rather variable, depending on diet and the individual fatty acid species in question. For example, in a group of apparently healthy postmenopausal women in the USA, the average plasma level (free plus esterified) of EPA was 110 μM and that of DHA was 283 μM [Wander and Du 2000]. However, in a group of patients in the UK (male and female, average age 69 y) awaiting carotid endarterectomy, the average plasma level of DHA was only a quarter of that of the above-mentioned "healthy" group of USA women (K.L.H. Carpenter and I.R. Challis, unpublished observation). On dietary supplementation with fish oil, at a level equivalent to consumption of ca. 400 g salmon per day (for the particular type of fish oil used in this study, EPA > DHA), the EPA and DHA concentrations (free plus esterified) in plasma of the USA women after 5 weeks rose to 734 μM and 515 μM respectively [Wander and Du 2000].

Understanding the mechanisms by which PUFAs and their products and metabolites induce apoptosis may provide important information relevant to optimising their beneficial effects, and to minimising any adverse effects, in vivo within the general population and possibly also in high-risk subjects and patients.

Cell Death and Atherosclerotic Plaque Destabilisation

Atherosclerosis is a chronic inflammatory disease. Early lesions, termed fatty streaks, consist of clusters of lipid-filled macrophage "foam cells" directly beneath the endothelial surface of the artery wall. In the intermediate stage a fibrous cap consisting of smooth muscle cells and connective tissue starts to develop under the endothelium and over the macrophage foam cells, and some extracellular lipid starts to appear in the core of the lesion. By the advanced stage (plaque) the lesion has a distinct fibrous cap and an acellular lipid core (gruel). Macrophage foam cells at the shoulders of the lesion appear to be dying and spilling their contents into the core. The relative proportions of cap and core vary. Fatty streaks and intermediate lesions are asymptomatic. Advanced lesions are often "silent" also, but in some cases they can be sufficiently large to impede blood flow. Moreover, some advanced plaques are prone to rupture, with serious clinical consequences. Advanced lesions are mostly found at sites of branches (e.g. carotid artery; abdominal aorta) or bends (e.g. coronary arteries) suggesting that haemodynamic stress plays an important role in lesion development.

A major cause of heart attacks and strokes is thrombo-embolism from ruptured atherosclerotic plaques, which exposes highly thrombogenic contents. Plaques with proportionally large lipid cores and thin fibrous caps are unstable and prone to rupture. Conversely, plaques with relatively thick fibrous caps and small lipid cores are more stable. Rupture-prone, unstable plaques contain large lipid deposits within a macrophage infiltrate, which enters from the bloodstream (monocytes) and accumulates at the plaque "shoulder." Macrophages accumulate lipid, forming "foam cells" which die spilling their contents into the core of the lesion, enlarging the lipid pool of the core, and predisposing to haemorrhage and an increase in intra-plaque pressure. Death of smooth muscle cells (SMC) attenuates the fibrous cap, which also contributes to plaque destabilisation. Moreover macrophages can secrete enzymes such as matrix metalloproteinases that can degrade the fibrous cap. Plaques tend to rupture at the shoulder. In cases of sudden coronary death, apoptotic macrophages were found localised at the site of plaque rupture [Kolodgie et al. 2000].

Among the evidence implicating oxidative stress and cell death in atherosclerosis is that oxidised LDL (oxLDL) and lipid oxidation products occur in atherosclerotic lesions [Yla-Herttuala et al. 1989 and 1990; Carpenter et al. 1995; Waddington et al. 2001], and that some of these substances induce death, including apoptosis, in macrophages and SMC [Guyton et al. 1995; Marchant et al. 1995; Hardwick et al. 1996; Siow et al. 1999; Müller et al. 1998; Carpenter et al. 2001 and 2003; Clare et al. 1995; Müller et al. 1996].

PUFAs and Atherosclerosis

Recently, fish-oil (rich in EPA and DHA) supplementation of patients awaiting carotid endarterectomy lowered the number of macrophages within the excised advanced atherosclerotic plaques, relative to plaques from patients supplemented with sunflower oil (rich in LIN) or with control oil (rich in OA and palmitic acid) [Thies et al. 2003]. Also, more of the patients in the fish-oil supplemented group had plaques with thick fibrous caps, and fewer had thin fibrous caps, than the patients in the sunflower and control oil groups. Since macrophages appear to be major contributors to plaque instability, by degrading the fibrous cap, Thies and colleagues [2003] suggested that macrophage death induced by EPA and DHA might be responsible for the lowering in number of macrophages in plaques and hence to a lower proportion of patients with plaques possessing thin fibrous caps. However they also acknowledged that actual mechanisms by which EPA and DHA supplementation might lead to the suggested rise in plaque stability need to be established. Fish-oil supplementation of mildly hypertriacylglycerolaemic men increased the susceptibility of their LDL to ex vivo oxidation [Leigh-Firbank et al. 2002], whilst lowering their plasma concentrations of triacylglycerol (fasting and postprandial) and NEFA (postprandial), raising platelet EPA and DHA content, and decreasing platelet AA content. Whether the effect of EPA and DHA on LDL oxidisability would translate into increased cell-death in atherosclerotic lesions is unknown. Within this context, the balance between PUFAs and natural antioxidants such as tocopherols is likely to be important.

The idea of Thies and colleagues [2003] that macrophage death might be beneficial in advanced lesions is debatable. Above, we have mentioned that apoptotic macrophages have been found at the shoulders of "culprit" ruptured plaques in cases of sudden coronary death [Kolodgie et al. 2000]. Macrophages that die in advanced plaques are incompletely scavenged, evidenced by the detection of apoptotic bodies, which are highly condensed remnants of apoptotic cells [Hegyi et al. 2001]. Moreover the lipid contents of macrophages appear to be spilled to contribute to the acellular "lipid core" (gruel) of the plaque. The unscavenged apoptotic bodies and the extracellular lipid in plaques may constitute inflammatory stimuli that help propagate the chronic inflammatory state of lesions, by activating live macrophages that are in lesions and causing recruitment of monocytes from the bloodstream that once inside the lesion mature into macrophages, accumulate lipid and die, in a vicious cycle.

An alternative explanation for the macrophage-lowering effect of EPA and DHA in lesions is monocyte recruitment to the plaque. 4-Hydroxyhexenal (HHE), produced by peroxidation of n-3 PUFAs, is a weaker chemoattractant for monocytes than is HNE, a peroxidation product of n-6 PUFAs [Müller et al. 1996]. Therefore, although being more peroxidisable, oxidation of EPA-/DHA-rich LDL may produce less chemotactic degradation products than LDL rich in n-6 PUFAs, resulting in decreased monocyte infiltration.

Lipoprotein-Associated Phospholipase A_2 and Death of Monocyte-Macrophages

A major source of PUFAs in atherosclerosis is plasma low-density lipoprotein (LDL). Much evidence implicates oxidation of LDL in atherogenesis, including the apoptosis-inducing effect of oxidised LDL (oxLDL) on HMM in vitro. LDL oxidation involves peroxidation of the PUFA chains of LDL lipids, which are predominantly esters. Various LDL oxidation products such as 4-hydroxynonenal (HNE) [Müller et al. 1996], oxysterols [Clare et al. 1995], and lipid hydroperoxides [Muralidhar et al. 2004] can induce death in HMM in vitro. Radical scavengers such as alpha-tocopherol and BO-653 can prevent both LDL oxidation and the ensuing HMM death [Marchant et al. 1995; Müller et al. 1999]. Lipoprotein-associated phospholipase A_2 (Lp-PLA_2) is a naturally present LDL-borne enzyme that hydrolyses oxidised phospholipids (but not non-oxidised phospholipids) forming lysophosphatidylcholine and oxidised, non-esterified fatty acids (oxNEFA).

Treatment of LDL with inhibitors of Lp-PLA_2 diminished the ensuing toxicity when the LDL was oxidised and added to HMM in vitro, even though the Lp-PLA_2 inhibitors did not diminish LDL oxidation [Carpenter et al. 2001]. The inhibitors of Lp-PLA_2 were the highly specific SB222657 and the broad-spectrum serine esterase/protease inhibitors Pefabloc and diisopropyl fluorophosphate (DFP), and all of them inhibited the rise in lysophosphatidylcholine levels that occurred when LDL was oxidised in the inhibitors' absence. SB222657 treatment of LDL also diminished oxLDL-induced apoptosis in HMM. In the same study, we also compared the toxicities of lysophosphatidylcholine and a phosphatidylcholine that we chemically synthesised to contain an oxidatively fragmented chain (1-palmitoyl-2-(9-oxononanoyl)-*sn*-glycero-3-phosphocholine), and found that lysophosphatidylcholine was appreciably the more toxic of the two species for HMM. Thus all the evidence suggests that by preserving oxidised phospholipids from hydrolysis, the death-inducing effect of oxidised LDL can be diminished.

We found that a mildly oxidised form of LDL was a stronger death inducer in HMM than a moderately oxidised form of LDL [Carpenter et al. 2003a]. This was true for toxicity, measured by lactate dehydrogenase (LDH) release, and also true for apoptosis induction (nucleosome ELISA). The mildly oxidised LDL had a higher hydroperoxide content (FOX assay) than the moderately oxidised LDL, whilst the latter had higher levels of later-stage lipid oxidation products (malondialdehyde and 7-oxysterols) and more negative charge (indicating modification of LDL protein by aldehydes). Inhibition of Lp-PLA_2 by the specific inhibitor SB222657 diminished both the LDH release and apoptosis for both the mildly and moderately oxidised LDLs. This observation was consistent with evidence from different experiments [Macphee et al. 1999] that Lp-PLA_2 can hydrolyse phospholipids with full-length PUFA-hydroperoxide chains as well as those with oxidatively fragmented PUFA chains. The oxidised non-esterified fatty acid (oxNEFA) fraction arising from Lp-PLA_2-mediated hydrolysis of oxLDL has been shown to possess chemoattractant activity for human monocytes, and pretreatment of LDL with SB222657 before oxidation inhibited the subsequent chemoattractant production [Macphee et al. 1999]. The same study established that the oxNEFA fraction was the main chemoattractant (for monocytes) within oxLDL lipids.

Lp-PLA_2 has rather permissive substrate requirements [Min et al. 1999 and 2001], so besides hydrolysing oxidised phosphatidylcholine it might also hydrolyse oxidised forms of the less abundant LDL phospholipid classes, and maybe also hydrolyse oxidised tri- and di-acylglycerols.

Experiments with the PPARγ antagonist GW9662, the PPARγ agonist ciglitazone and the Lp-PLA_2 inhibitor SB222657 suggested non-hydrolysed, oxidised phospholipids in oxLDL activate PPARγ as a cellular defence mechanism in HMM [Carpenter et al. 2003a]. The significance of PPARγ is discussed in more detail below, in the section entitled "PUFAs and activation of peroxisome proliferator activated receptors".

Elevation of plasma Lp-PLA_2 has emerged as a novel inflammatory marker for cardiovascular risk, independent of various established risk factors and other markers of inflammation, in several recent studies, reviewed by Macphee et al. [2005 and 2006]. Also reviewed were some apparent exceptions to this, notably a genetic variant with reduced Lp-PLA_2 activity, which may or may not be associated with increased atherosclerosis within the

Japanese population. Mature macrophages and to a lesser degree freshly isolated monocytes secrete Lp-PLA_2 identical to LDL associated Lp-PLA_2 found in plasma [Stafforini et al. 1990; Tjoelker et al. 1995; Hakkinen et al. 1999]. Lp-PLA_2 mRNA and protein occur in macrophages in rabbit and human atherosclerotic lesions [Hakkinen et al. 1999]. Moreover, Lp-PLA_2 is highly expressed in rupture-prone lesions [Macphee et al. 2005]. Administration of Lp-PLA_2 inhibitors to healthy volunteers dose-dependently reduced plasma Lp-PLA_2 activity by up to 95 %. Initial clinical studies in patients undergoing carotid endarterectomy suggest that Lp-PLA_2 inhibitors (administered for 14 d prior to surgery) can inhibit activity of this enzyme in atherosclerotic lesions and in plasma [Macphee et al. 2005]. Whether Lp-PLA_2 inhibitors can confer clinical benefit on cardiovascular outcomes will require further studies, of longer duration.

PUFAs and Death of Monocyte-Macrophages

The pro-apoptotic activity of PUFAs cannot entirely be explained in all cases by peroxidation, formation of reactive oxygen species (ROS) and degradation products. In vitro, HMM treated with PUFAs showed a general trend for increasing apoptosis with increasing degree of fatty acid unsaturation. However, arachidonic acid (AA; 20:4, n-6) stood out above the trend (in contrast to its behaviour in cancer cell lines, see below) as it induced apoptosis more strongly than both the more highly unsaturated (and more peroxidisable) EPA and DHA [Muralidhar et al. 2004], suggesting that other mechanisms for apoptosis-induction by PUFAs were at work. In vivo, PUFAs are also substrates of enzyme complexes, such as cyclooxygenase (COX) and lipoxygenase (LOX). For example, AA is metabolised to prostaglandins, leukotrienes etc. In our study [Muralidhar et al. 2004], AA-induced apoptosis was diminished by the COX inhibitor indomethacin and by the LOX inhibitor nordihydroguaiaretic acid, suggesting roles for these enzymes in the induction of apoptosis by AA. Moreover 15(S)-hydroperoxy-5,8,11,13-eicosatetraenoic acid (15-HPETE) was a very strong inducer of apoptosis in HMM, whereas 15(S)-hydroxy-5,8,11,13-eicosatetraenoic acid (15-HETE) was innocuous. The failure of sulindac (another COX inhibitor) to diminish AA-induced apoptosis might be due to lack of metabolism in vitro to its sulphide form, which is a more active COX inhibitor [Roberts and Morrow 2001].

Indomethacin can inhibit both COX-1 and COX-2, though is reportedly more active against the former [Mitchell et al. 1993]. Interestingly indomethacin was more strongly apoptosis-inducing (for HMM) when added without AA than when AA and indomethacin were added together. Also AA (no indomethacin) was less strongly apoptosis-inducing than indomethacin (no AA). Indomethacin is reported to be an agonist for PPARγ and PPARα [Lehmann et al. 1997] and the COX-2 gene possesses a PPAR response element so is under PPAR control [Pontsler et al. 2002]. Cross-talk between AA, indomethacin, COX-2 and PPAR might thus occur. Since we found that AA was a PPARγ activator in HMM (discussed in the section on PPARγ below), it is thus conceivable that competition between AA and indomethacin might explain the lower apoptosis induction for AA plus indomethacin than for indomethacin alone.

Another possible explanation for indomethacin's inhibitory effect on AA-induced apoptosis could be as follows. COX enzymes (strictly termed prostaglandin endoperoxide H synthases) possess 2 active sites per protein molecule, the cyclooxygenase site (that oxidises AA to PGG_2) and the peroxidase site (that reduces PGG_2 to PGH_2), and NSAIDs such as indomethacin inhibit the cyclooxygenase site but not the peroxidase site [Smith et al. 2000]. The latter site would thus remain capable of reducing, for example, toxic 15-HPETE to innocuous 15-HETE.

Recently, 4-hydroxynonenal (HNE) has been shown to induce COX-2 in a murine macrophage cell line (RAW264.7) [Kumagai et al. 2004]. HNE is a peroxidation product of n-6 PUFAs. Major n-6 PUFAs are linoleic (18:2) and arachidonic (20:4) acids; the latter is the more susceptible to peroxidation. Several other lipid oxidation products, including hydroxy- and hydroperoxy- octadecadienoic acids (peroxidation products of linoleic acid) and 7-ketocholesterol were ineffective at COX-2 induction [Kumagai et al. 2004]. The same study found COX-2 colocalised with HNE in human atherosclerotic lesions. The study thus suggests that lipid peroxidation can promote an inflammatory response, and that in this context HNE may be a significant pro-inflammatory molecule in atherosclerosis.

Various anti-inflammatory agents including indomethacin, and also a selective 15-lipoxygenase inhibitor, were anti-atherogenic in animal models of atherosclerosis [Bailey and Butler 1973; Pratico et al. 2001; Sendobry et al. 1997]. Recently, indomethacin phenethylamide, a highly selective inhibitor for COX-2 in vitro and which also partially inhibited COX-1 in vivo, significantly reduced early and intermediate-stage atherosclerotic lesions in apoE-deficient mice [Burleigh et al. 2005]. COX-1 is found in most tissues and mediates normal function requiring prostaglandin synthesis. COX-2 is induced in inflammation and is expressed in atherosclerotic lesions in humans [Baker et al. 1999; Schonbeck et al. 1999] and mice [Burleigh et al. 2002], in macrophages, smooth muscle cells and endothelial cells. However COX-2 inhibitors to date do not appear to have any clear beneficial effect on atherosclerosis in the advanced stages. Moreover, in patients taking the COX-2 inhibitor Vioxx (rofecoxib), there were increased cardiovascular events, in the Adenomatous Polyp Prevention on Vioxx (APPROVe) trial [Bresalier et al. 2005]. As a consequence, Vioxx was removed from the market. The relationships of COX-1 and COX-2 to atherosclerosis appear complex and incompletely understood.

DNA Oxidative Damage and Atherosclerosis

DNA oxidative damage is an aspect of oxidative stress emerging as of potential importance in atherosclerosis. It can be measured in terms of the well-established marker 8-hydroxy-2′-deoxyguanosine (8OHdG, also termed 8-oxo-dG, and the corresponding base 8-oxoG), one of the most abundant DNA "lesions" generated by oxidative stress [Helbock et al. 1998, Helbock et al. 1999]. Elevated DNA oxidative damage (8OHdG) was reported in human carotid plaques (relative to non-atherosclerotic mammary arteries) (Martinet et al., 2002), in tunica media of severely atherosclerotic human aortas [De Flora et al. 1997], and in cholesterol diet-induced atherosclerotic lesions in rabbits [Martinet et al. 2001]. Associated with 8OHdG elevation were increased DNA strand breaks, and elevations in p53 and phospho-p53 and DNA repair enzymes [Martinet et al. 2002, Martinet et al. 2001]; in rabbits these changes were reversed by normal diet [Martinet et al. 2001]. In human plaques, 8OHdG was found in smooth muscle cells (SMC), macrophages and endothelial cells [Martinet et al., 2002].

"The guardian of the genome", p53 (wild-type) can be triggered by DNA oxidative damage, and can either cause growth arrest (to allow DNA repair) or stimulate apoptosis. p53 kills mostly by transcriptional activation/repression of specific target proteins, most of which work through mitochondria, bringing about cytochrome c release into the cytosol leading to caspase cleavage, and thence to cell death [Ferri and Kroemer 2001]. Human SMC isolated from plaques are more sensitive to p53-mediated apoptosis than those from normal artery [Bennett et al. 1997].

A characteristic repeat motif TTAGGG found in telomeres is susceptible to oxidative damage, compared with a non-telomeric control TGTGAG [Oikawa and Kawanishi, 1999, Oikawa et al., 2001]. Telomere shortening, a characteristic of senescence and aging, is associated with DNA oxidative damage [von Zglinicki, 1998]. Recently, Matthews et al. [2006] found that SMC in fibrous caps of plaques expressed markers of senescence, and that plaque SMC had shorter telomeres than SMC from normal vessels. Moreover, plaque SMC exhibited DNA oxidative damage in vivo, whilst in vitro oxidants induced telomere shortening in SMC and reduced telomerase activity.

We found evidence linking lipid peroxidation-induced DNA oxidative damage with apoptosis, using 4 established, well-characterised [Abdel-Rahman et al. 2000] human colorectal cancer (CRC) cell lines as test models, with measurement of 8OHdG in DNA by HPLC with electrochemical detection and apoptosis by flow cytometric measurement of DNA fragmentation [K.L.H. Carpenter, K. Müller, M.T. O'Connell. and M.J. Arends, unpublished data]. CRC cells were cultured in the presence or absence of individual fatty acids and/or the natural lipophilic antioxidant alpha-tocopherol, and enabled exploration of the effects of p53 status (wild-type (wt) in CRC cell lines LoVo and C70, or mutant (mut) in HCT116 and HT29) and also status one of the major DNA repair pathways, mismatch repair (MMR; proficient in C70 and HT29, or deficient in LoVo and HCT116). The MMR system, which can respond to oxidative DNA damage [DeWeese et al. 1998] is a complex, multi-enzyme pathway for proof-reading newly synthesised DNA. MMR mutations can be germ-line or somatic [Toft and Arends 1998]. The MMR is capable of acting, at least in part, via p53 to induce apoptosis after DNA damage [Toft et al. 1998 and 1999].

The CRC cell lines treated with PUFAs in vitro demonstrated that apoptosis increased with degree of fatty acid unsaturation. Notably, DHA was more potent than the less highly unsaturated PUFAs at inducing DNA fragmentation, indicative of apoptosis, in these CRC cells, whilst oleic acid, a monounsaturate, was innocuous. This structure-activity relationship suggests a peroxidative mechanism of apoptosis induction, as there is a well-known rise in the susceptibility of lipids to peroxidation with increasing degree of unsaturation (i.e. with greater numbers of carbon-carbon double bonds per molecule). Our data for CRC cells follow the same pattern of increasing induction of apoptosis in pancreatic cancer and leukaemic cells with increasing degree of unsaturation of PUFAs shown in previous work [Hawkins et al. 1998]. The results for the CRC cell lines were consistent with the idea that lipid peroxidation can promote DNA oxidative damage leading to apoptosis, especially in the presence of p53-wt. The combination of MMR deficiency with p53-wt (in LoVo) permitted accumulation of high levels of 8OHdG in response to PUFAs. MMR deficiency conferred a partial sensitisation to apoptosis, though the influence on apoptosis of MMR status appeared subordinate to p53 status. Alpha-tocopherol (100 μM) inhibited DHA-induced 8OHdG accumulation, tested in HCT116 and HT29 cells. The effect of alpha-tocopherol on PUFA-induced death of CRC cells was not tested.

Although cell death was not measured directly in parallel to 8OHdG accumulation, these studies suggested that DNA oxidation precedes cell death. These CRC cell lines are habitually adherent; dead or dying cells tend to detach. The 8OHdG measurements were for adherent cells at 24 or 48 h, times chosen to minimise loss of cells, whereas the cell death measurements were for combined adherent and non-adherent cells after 72 h. Fatty acid concentrations were 200 μM for the apoptosis experiments and 100 or 200 μM for the 8OHdG experiments. Alpha-tocopherol was 100 μM.

We also measured 8OHdG in DNA from 17 human colorectal tumours, which had been characterised for MMR status. For the 9 tumours with 8OHdG levels greater than or equal to the median level, incidence of MMR deficiency (evidenced by microsatellite instability in 7 out of 9 tumours) was greater than for the 8 tumours with 8OHdG levels below the median (microsatellite instability in 3 out of 8 tumours).

Some human plaques (20% of cases) have shown microsatellite instability (MSI) indicating deficiency in MMR [Spandidos et al. 1996], and loss of heterozygosity (28% of cases) in MMR genes [Flouris et al. 2000]. MMR deficiency at the gene level (mutation or silencing) can result in high-degree MSI. More insidiously, sub-toxic oxidative stress can functionally inactivate MMR at the protein level in vitro, and may cause low-degree MSI seen in various chronically inflamed tissues without genetic inactivation of MMR [Chang et al. 2002]. Other DNA repair pathways, e.g. base excision repair, can also become compromised by oxidative stress, as shown in a cell line [Chen et al. 2000].

DNA oxidative damage may play a pivotal role in promoting death of SMC and macrophages. Lipid peroxidation (including LDL oxidation) may promote DNA oxidation, leading to p53 activation and apoptosis. An exacerbating factor may be the maiming of DNA repair mechanisms by oxidative damage. Appropriate antioxidants that protect DNA may spare macrophages and SMC from death, potentially combating atherosclerosis by stabilising plaques against rupture.

Vitamin E and Inhibition of Lipid Peroxidation in Atherosclerosis

The majority of epidemiological studies suggest a protective role for dietary vitamin E against cardiovascular events [Pryor, 2000]. Vitamin E comprises a family of molecules, the tocopherols and tocotrienols, which are lipophilic radical scavengers biosynthesised by plants and algae. Vitamin E is not biosynthesised by mammals, which therefore acquire vitamin E via the food chain. Alpha-tocopherol is the vitamin E species with the highest plasma concentration in humans, and is also the species that has been the subject of most study. Natural alpha-tocopherol is the RRR-form, whereas synthetic alpha-tocopherol is usually the all-racemic (all-rac) form.

Vitamin E's apparent protective role is supported by a great many experimental studies on vitamin E, including experiments involving plasma low-density lipoprotein (LDL) oxidation and cells in vitro, and oral vitamin E supplementation studies in animals. For example, alpha-tocopherol inhibited both LDL oxidation (mediated by Cu^{2+} or by HMM) and the ensuing toxicity to HMM in vitro [Marchant et al. 1995 and 1996; Müller et al. 1999]. Vitamin E reduced atherosclerosis progression in Apo-E-deficient mice [Practico et al. 1998] and in LDL-receptor-deficient mice [Cyrus et al. 2003]. In contrast, several large clinical trials of oral vitamin E in high-risk human subjects/patients found no protective effect for vitamin E, e.g. GISSI [1999], HOPE [Yusuf et al. 2000] and the Heart Protection Study [2002], whilst only a minority of trials demonstrated benefit of vitamin E, e.g. CHAOS [Stephens et al. 1996].

Various explanations have been proposed to attempt to rationalise this paradox, which at the same time reveal significant gaps in knowledge. One such gap is the issue of whether oral vitamin E exerts a biochemical effect, not only within plasma, but also more importantly within atherosclerotic lesions, the location where the majority of lipid peroxidation appears to take place. Particularly important is the question of whether oral vitamin E is able to exert an antioxidant effect within established, advanced atherosclerotic lesions (plaques). In an attempt to address this issue, an analytical study of oral alpha-tocopherol supplementation (all-rac, 500 IU/day), which was placebo-controlled and double-blind, was performed in 104 patients (53 treated; 51 placebo) undergoing endarterectomy for symptomatic carotid disease [Carpenter et al. 2003b]. Results for plasma and plaques were evaluated statistically, with alpha-tocopherol levels (concentrations) expressed standardised for cholesterol and also expressed independently of cholesterol.

In the above study, oral alpha-tocopherol supplementation significantly increased plasma alpha-tocopherol levels. Plasma LDL-associated alpha-tocopherol levels were significantly increased (by ca. 40%), thereby rendering LDL less susceptible to ex vivo oxidation. However, there was no significant increase in alpha-tocopherol mean concentration within plaques. Even so, alpha-tocopherol concentrations (expressed independently of cholesterol) in plaques correlated significantly with those in plasma, suggesting that plasma alpha-tocopherol levels can influence those in plaques. Also, there was a significant inverse correlation between cholesterol-standardised levels of alpha-tocopherol in plaques and cholesterol-standardised levels of 7beta-hydroxycholesterol, a free radical oxidation product of cholesterol, in plaques, suggesting an antioxidant effect of alpha-tocopherol.

The results of the above study suggest that within plasma and plaques, alpha-tocopherol can act as an antioxidant. However, the fact that in plaques the antioxidant effect took the form of a trend, but not a clear-cut difference, may partly explain the predominantly disappointing results for vitamin E in other clinical trials. The findings of the above studies, together with other studies, have highlighted the issues of individual variations and the need for better understanding of the pharmacodynamics of oral vitamin E and its interactions with other dietary antioxidants and therapeutic agents, to guide future trials in human subjects and patients.

PUFAs and Activation of Peroxisome Proliferator Activated Receptors

Various PUFAs and their oxidation products are able to activate peroxisome proliferator activated receptors (PPARs) [Forman et al. 1997; Kliewer et al. 1997; Nagy et al. 1998]. Three isoforms are known: PPARα, PPARγ and PPARδ (also termed PPARβ). PPARs are ligand-dependent transcription factors belonging to the nuclear hormone gene superfamily, and have many regulatory activities, especially those involving lipid handling. Activation of PPARγ plays an important role in differentiation of adipocytes and of other cell types as well as in glucose utilisation, whilst PPARα target genes are involved in fatty acid catabolism and utilisation. PPARγ activation can also be involved in apoptosis induction, at least partly by negatively interfering with the anti-apoptotic NFκB signalling pathway. NFκB activation appears to play a role in oncogenesis [Baldwin 2001]. The inhibitory effect of PPARγ on NFκB appears to be due to direct interaction between PPARγ and NFκB forming a transcriptionally inactive complex [Chung et al. 2000]. PPARγ may be able to exert an anticancer effect by promoting differentiation and apoptosis. Recently the PPARγ ligand troglitazone was shown to induce apoptosis in liver cancer cells [Toyoda et al. 2002]. Treatment of HT-29 colon cancer cells with ciglitazone, a PPARγ-activator, down-regulated COX-2 expression [Yang and Frucht 2001], which could constitute an anti-cancer mechanism. Although incompletely understood, PPARγ is considered to be a tumour suppressor and anti-inflammatory [Patel et al. 2001], although some exceptions exist in certain animal models [Saez et al. 1998]. PPARδ appears to function mainly as a tumour promotor [Park et al. 2001]. PPARγ is expressed in human colon tumours and appears predominantly non-mutated (51/55 sporadic cases) [Sarraf et al. 1999]. PPARγ has been suggested to be a potential therapeutic target for colon cancer [Yang and Frucht 2001].

In our study of PUFA-induced HMM apoptosis, we tested the effect of the 2 most potent apoptosis inducers (AA and DHA) and the 2 least potent apoptosis inducers (LIN and OA) on PPARγ expression [Muralidhar et al. 2004]. We measured PPARγ at 24 h (an early time point in apoptosis induction preceding execution phase), whereas our apoptosis measurements were at 48 h. We found that AA and DHA significantly increased PPARγ expression in both cytoplasm and nuclei, suggestive of activation, whereas LIN and OA did not increase PPARγ expression, relative to control HMM. We used a well-known PPARγ activator 15-deoxy-delta^{12,14}-prostaglandin J_2 (15d-PGJ_2) as a positive control, giving increased PPARγ expression in HMM. 15d-PGJ_2 is a COX product of AA, and is formed naturally in the resolution phase of inflammation. Whether significant amounts of 15d-PGJ_2 arise from AA incubated with HMM in vitro is unknown. We found that 15d-PGJ_2 at 1-10 μM for 24 h induced death of HMM [Muralidhar et al. 2004]; our PPARγ measurements were therefore done with 1 μM 15d-PGJ_2 at 8 h to minimise loss of cells. Our findings for 15d-PGJ_2 were consistent with those of other researchers, who reported that 15d-PGJ_2 activated PPARγ and induced apoptosis in HMM at 1 μM for 24 h [Chinetti et al. 1998] and in an endothelial cell line at 10 μM for 20 h [Bishop-Bailey and Hla 1999]. Apoptosis induction by 15d-PGJ_2 might not necessarily involve PPARγ. For example, 15d-PGJ_2 was reported to induce apoptosis by intracellular ROS production and activation of caspase 3 cascade in HL-60 human leukaemic cells [Chen et al. 2005].

PPARγ activation is, as discussed above, widely regarded as apoptosis-promoting. However, it may in some cases protect against cell death. Ciglitazone and rosiglitazone, both PPARγ activators, had biphasic effects on T-cell death [Wang et al. 2002]. In HMM, ciglitazone was innocuous when tested at 3 μM [Carpenter et al. 2003a], its reported EC_{50} for PPARγ activation in CV-1 cells [Willson et al. 1996]. As mentioned earlier, (in the section on Lp-PLA_2 and apoptosis) evidence from experiments with appropriate inhibitors of PPARγ and of Lp-PLA_2, and activator of PPARγ, suggested that non-hydrolysed oxidised phospholipids in oxLDL appeared to activate PPARγ in a defence mechanism against cell death [Carpenter et al. 2003a]. Oxidised alkyl phosphatidylcholine (the *O*-alkyl linkage in the *sn*-1 position, and the oxidised chain ester-linked in the *sn*-2 position), a sub-class of oxidised phosphatidylcholine in oxLDL, can specifically bind to and activate PPARγ [Davies et al. 2001]. The binding appeared a characteristic of the intact (non-hydrolysed) form since oxNEFAs were inefficient competitors. Oxidised phosphatidylcholine can activate PPARα [Lee et al. 2000], but this requires phospholipase A_2 activity [Delerive et al. 2000], suggesting that the oxNEFA thereby liberated were the actual PPARα ligands. In our own study [Carpenter et al. 2003a] PPARγ thus appears likely to be more important than PPARα in the putative defence mechanism triggered by non-hydrolysed oxidised phosphatidylcholine in HMM.

Atherosclerosis is a chronic inflammatory disease. PPARγ activation in macrophages in vitro has mixed consequences which if true in vivo could be pro- or anti-inflammatory and pro- or anti-atherogenic. These include reduction of inflammatory cytokines [Jiang et al. 1998], inhibition of MMP-9 gelatinolytic activity [Marx et al. 1998], and stimulation of cholesterol efflux via the ABCA1 pathway [Chinetti et al. 2001]. Activation of PPARγ by oxLDL upregulates CD36 (scavenger receptor B), of which oxLDL is a ligand, leading to enhanced uptake [Tontonoz et al. 1998]. This might promote foam cell formation, but appears to be offset by enhanced cholesterol efflux (see above).

PPARγ occurs in macrophages in atherosclerotic lesions, in a pattern highly correlated with oxidation-specific epitopes [Ricote et al. 1998; Marx et al. 1998]. PPARγ activation leading to macrophage apoptosis might be anti-inflammatory and hence anti-atherogenic, particularly as macrophages are able to kill SMC [Boyle et al. 2001] and thereby erode the fibrous cap. However, if apoptotic macrophages are inefficiently scavenged and contribute to the lipid core debris, together with necrotic macrophages, then death induction by peroxidised PUFAs, especially AA, could exert a pro-atherogenic influence. Evidence for the lack of phagocytosis of a proportion of apoptotic bodies is provided by the presence of free, intact, apoptotic bodies within the acellular lipid core of human advanced atherosclerotic lesions [Hegyi et al. 2001]. If, on the other hand, PPARγ activation promotes macrophage survival, then this might result in smaller lipid cores within lesions, and perhaps also less plaque rupture, particularly as macrophage apoptosis at the vulnerable shoulders of plaques was found associated with rupture of "culprit" plaques in sudden coronary death [Kolodgie et al. 2000].

Cardiolipin and Apoptosis

An important component of mitochondria is the phospholipid cardiolipin, which in mammals is virtually unique to mitochondria. It is most abundant in the inner mitochondrial membrane. The fatty acid chains of cardiolipin have a naturally high PUFA content, e.g. bovine heart cardiolipin contains > 80 % linoleic acid. Moreover cardiolipin composition is more responsive than other phospholipids to dietary PUFA in vivo, or supplementation of culture medium with PUFA in vitro. Cardiolipin was enriched to 48 % DHA by dietary fatty acid manipulation in mammals [Berger et al. 1992], and to 50 % DHA in HT-29 colon cancer cells by culturing with 50 μM DHA for 36 h [Watkins et al. 1998]. Cardiolipin fatty acid composition affects electron transport complex activity [Daum 1985], which will affect electron leakage and hence mitochondrial ROS production. HT-29 colorectal cancer cells produced elevated intracellular ROS as a result of DHA enrichment [Watkins et al. 1998]. Raising the degree of unsaturation of the cardiolipin will also increase its susceptibility to peroxidation.

Cytochrome c in the inter-membrane space of mitochondria is bound to native cardiolipin on that face of the inner membrane [Ott et al. 2002]. Peroxidation of cardiolipin releases cytochrome c from the bound state to the free state within the intermembrane space [Ott et al. 2002]. Cardiolipin is a major constituent of contact sites where the inner and outer mitochondrial membranes meet [Lutter et al. 2000 and 2001]. Increasing the PUFA content of cardiolipin appears to favour the formation of contact sites [Gasnier et al. 1998]. Truncated Bid or tBid (a Bcl family member that links the death receptor pathways to the mitochondrial effector mechanisms of apoptosis) appears targeted to cardiolipin at the contact sites, where pores form [Lutter et al. 2000]. It is plausible that cardiolipin might also play a role in permeabilisation of mitochondria by Bax in a similar fashion, since Bax appears to act at contact sites [Doran and Halestrap 2000]. Recently, caspase 2 has been shown to permeabilise the outer mitochondrial membrane and disrupt the binding of cytochrome c to anionic phospholipids, notably cardiolipin [Enoksson et al. 2004].

An interesting paper that supports the pro-apoptotic role of cardiolipin peroxidation is Nomura et al. [2000], entitled: "Mitochondrial phospholipid hydroperoxide glutathione peroxidase inhibits the release of cytochrome c from mitochondria by suppressing the peroxidation of cardiolipin in hypoglycaemia-induced apoptosis". Mitochondria-targeted antioxidants MitoQ and MitoVit E added in vitro were more effective than their untargeted counterparts at protecting Friedreich Ataxia fibroblasts against death induced by intracellular oxidative stress [Jauslin et al. 2003].

Interestingly, palmitic (16:0) and stearic (18:0) fatty acids induced apoptosis in myocytes in vitro, whereas the effect was counteracted by oleic acid (18:1) [de Vries et al. 1997]. These effects could be attributed to alteration of phospholipid membranes, including in mitochondria, though analysis of fatty acid chains was done for total cellular phospholipid, rather than a specific mitochondrial fraction. A complex dynamic mechanism seems to exist linking dietary fatty acid species with mitochondrial structure-function changes and energy metabolism, illustrated by studies in animals by Innis and Clandinin in the 70's and 80's [Renner et al. 1979; Innis and Clandinin 1981a,b,c; Clandinin and Innis 1983]. Interestingly, dietary fatty acid composition seems to influence not only the fatty acid composition of the cardiolipin (the most diet-responsive lipid) and other phospholipids in mitochondria, but also the phospholipid class distribution, e.g. the ratio of cardiolipin to phosphatidylcholine in mitochondria, without affecting the total phospholipid level in mitochondria (micrograms/mg protein).

The issue of variation in cardiolipin relative to phosphatidylcholine is interesting bearing in mind Barth Syndrome, an X-linked cardiomyopathy with abnormal mitochondria. In Barth Syndrome there is a four-fold reduction, compared to normal, in cardiolipin pool size (% of total cellular phospholipids), shown in fibroblasts. This reduction in cardiolipin is due to defective remodelling, i.e. diminished ability to incorporate linoleic acid into phosphatidyl glycerol and cardiolipin after de novo cardiolipin biosynthesis, followed by degradation of the abnormally acetylated cardiolipin [Vreken et al. 2000]. Apart from cardiolipin, there were no other differences between Barth Syndrome and normal, for pool size of any of the other classes of phospholipids (% of total cellular phospholipids).

The defects of Barth Syndrome highlight the requirement for incorporation into cardiolipin of PUFA, principally linoleic acid (18:2, n-6), for normal function of mitochondria. Linoleic acid cannot be biosynthesised by mammals so has to come from diet.

We have already mentioned that cardiolipin is susceptible to auto-oxidation. Notably, the preparation (coating) of plates for testing serum for "anti-phospholipid" and "anti-cardiolipin" antibodies, which are inflammatory markers, involves the drying (overnight at 4°C) of an ethanol solution of cardiolipin, during which time auto-oxidation of the cardiolipin occurs [Horkko et al. 1996]. Monoclonal antibodies to oxLDL also bound to oxidised cardiolipin. Probably this is because anti-phospholipid/anti-cardiolipin and anti-oxLDL antibodies all recognise epitopes of oxidised phospholipid. Possibly, oxidised cardiolipin might constitute an epitope on apoptotic bodies, if leftovers of mitochondria are exposed, which might be pro-inflammatory. Although the vast majority of the literature regards cardiolipin as an exclusively mitochondrial lipid, it has been reported as a minor phospholipid in plasma, where it is carried mostly in LDL [Deguchi et al. 2000]. These authors established that plasma cardiolipin was not due to cell remnants in their samples, and suggested that circulating anti-cardiolipin antibodies might arise as a response to oxidised cardiolipin within LDL. Cardiolipin is susceptible to hydrolysis, at least under some conditions. For example, in kidney homogenates, deacylation of endogenous cardiolipin, by endogenous phospholipases, was described as "the most prevalent lipolytic event" [Helmy et al. 2004]. However, hydrolysis of cardiolipin by endogenous mitochondrial phospholipase A_2 was quoted as being relatively slow compared to hydrolysis of phosphatidylethanolamine [de Winter et al. 1987]. Storage of cardiolipin in solution in chloroform (a solvent that usually contains traces of HCl due to decomposition) resulted in auto-oxidation and hydrolysis [Parinandi et al. 1988]. Whether oxidised cardiolipin is less or more susceptible to hydrolysis than non-oxidised cardiolipin is not known. It cannot be ruled out that oxidised cardiolipin might be susceptible to some kind of phospholipase that hydrolyses oxidised chains but not non-oxidised, like Lp-PLA_2, also known as. platelet-activating factor acetylhydrolase (PAF-AH). As mentioned earlier, this enzyme is secreted by monocytes and macrophages, and is carried predominantly on LDL. Moreover, intracellular isoforms of PAF-AH have been reported in the literature, but the area is not well explored, discussed in Carpenter et al. [2001].

Toxicity of Saturated Fatty Acids

So far we have focussed on the toxicity of polyunsaturated fatty acids, as a consequence of their susceptibility to peroxidation, as contrasted with the innocuousness of the monounsaturate oleic acid, which is relatively insusceptible to peroxidation. Saturated fatty acids might thus be expected to be innocuous also, as they are not prone to peroxidation. However, perhaps surprisingly, saturated fatty acids are not necessarily innocuous but appear to be involved in the phenomenon of lipoapoptosis as a consequence of inappropriate over-accumulation of saturated fatty acids in non-adipose tissues. In some cases, it appears that over-accumulation of saturates gives rise to increased cellular production of ROS and reactive nitrogen species, as described below. So, paradoxically, abnormal accumulation of non-peroxidisable saturated fatty acids can give rise to increased oxidative stress, which might conceivably in turn damage cellular polyunsaturated fatty acids.

Elevated plasma levels of free fatty acids (FFA; also termed non-esterified fatty acids, NEFA) have been implicated in obesity-associated health risks, such as hyperlipidemia, cardiomyopathy, kidney failure, reproductive disorders, insulin resistance and diabetes. All of these may be caused by the failure of leptin-mediated liporegulation and ensuing lipotoxicity/lipoapoptosis [Unger 2002; Unger and Orici 2002].

Leptin, a hormone produced by adipocytes, is now thought to act by promoting lipid-storage in adipocytes in order to prevent ectopic fat deposition in non-adipose tissues. Genetic disorders can lead to leptin deficiency or tissue non-responsiveness to leptin resulting in intracellular lipid accumulation (steatosis) and ultimately lipotoxicity in non-adipose tissues, associated with dysfunction of pancreatic β-cells, myocardium, kidney and skeletal muscle. In diet-induced obesity, leptin levels initially increase, allowing fat storage in adipose tissues without ectopic fat deposition or adverse effects. However, resistance to leptin activity develops eventually, resulting in ectopic fat storage in non-adipose tissues, lipotoxicity/lipoapoptosis and ultimately organ failure. Several studies suggest that lipoapoptosis results mainly from the accumulation of long-chain fatty acids, particularly saturated fatty acids [Eitel et al. 2002; Maestre et al. 2003; Listenberger et al. 2003; Okuyama et al. 2003; El-Assaad et al. 2003; Welters et al. 2004; Mishra and Simonson 2005].

The loss of pancreatic β-cells is a characteristic of both type 1- and type 2-diabetes. In type 1-diabetes, an autoimmune reaction leads to infiltration of pancreatic islets by macrophages and T-cells, which secrete cytokines, such as IFN-β, IL-1β and TNF-α. This leads to increased nitric oxide production (NO) in pancreatic islets cells and apoptosis. In type 2-diabetes, β-cell death is thought to be mainly due to lipoapoptosis, possibly aggravated by increased plasma glucose levels [Welters et al. 2004]. Saturated fatty acids, mainly palmitate or stearate, have been shown to induce apoptosis in rat INS 832/13 cells and human islet β-cells [Eitel et al. 2002; El-Assaad et al. 2003; Maestre et al. 2003], in the β-cell line HIT-T15 [Okuyama et al. 2003], but also in human mesangial cells [Mishra and Simonson 2005], in human ovarian granuloma cells [Mu et al. 2001], rat testicular Leydig cells [Lu et al. 2003], human breast cancer cells [Hardy et al. 2003] and in CHO cells [Listenberger et al. 2003].

The mechanisms by which saturated fatty acids induce apoptosis are still debated. In β-cells inhibition of FA β-oxidation was shown to aggravate palmitate-induced apoptosis [El-Assaad et al. 2003]. NO synthase inhibitors prevented palmitate-induced toxicity, indicating that nitric oxide production is involved in apoptosis induction [Okuyama et al. 2003]. In INS-1 cells incubation with palmitate led to increased superoxide production, cytochrome c and AIF release into the cytosol and increased bax expression [Maestre et al. 2003]. FFAs induced apoptosis in β-cells also by the induction of an ER-stress response independent of NFκB and nitric oxide formation [Kharroubi et al. 2004]. In CHO cells, palmitate-induced apoptosis was associated with an increase in the generation of ROS and ceramide [Listenberger et al. 2003]. In cardiomyocytes and breast cancer cells palmitate is thought to induce apoptosis by reducing cardiolipin synthesis, [El-Assaad et al. 2003 and refs therein; Hardy et al. 2003]. In human mesangial cells, palmitate and stearate induced apoptosis via caspase-9/3-dependent and -independent pathways. The caspase-9/3-independent pathway was probably mediated by the release of endonuclease G from mitochondria. [Mishra and Simonson 2005]. Palmitate-induced apoptosis *in vitro* can be aggravated by the simultaneous presence of high glucose concentrations [El-Assaad et al. 2003; Okuyama et al. 2003]. Okuyama et al. suggested that palmitate toxicity via increased NO production was aggravated by glucose-induced superoxide production through enhanced cellular formation of toxic peroxynitrite [Okuyama et al. 2003].

In contrast to the toxicity of saturated fatty acids, monounsaturated fatty acids, such as oleate or linoleate, were mostly found to be innocuous or even protected against saturated FA toxicity [Eitel et al. 2002; El-Assaad et al. 2003; Listenberger et al. 2003; Hardy et al. 2003; Welters et al. 2004; Mishra and Simonson 2005].

One possible mechanism for the protective effect of monounsaturated FFA is their stabilizing effect on mitochondria. In the rat β-cell line BRIN-BD11 inhibitor studies showed that the protective effect of palmitoleate could be due to attenuation of cytochrome c release from mitochondria via increases in cardiolipin synthesis [Welters et al. 2004]. In CHO cells, oleate protection was associated with an increased ability of the cells to store FA in the form of neutral lipid, i.e. oleate channels palmitate away from apoptosis-inducing pathways to non-toxic lipid storage pathways. Studies on genetically manipulated cells suggest that endogenous unsaturated FA promote neutral lipid storage. Furthermore, cells with increased neutral lipid storage are resistant to palmitate-induced apoptosis. Alternatively, cells with decreased capacity for triglyceride synthesis are more sensitive to palmitate-induced cell death [Listenberger et al. 2003]. In MDA-MB-231 breast cancer cells treated with palmitate, cardiolipin levels decreased significantly after 4 h, but remained unchanged in oleate-treated cells. Cardiolipin decrease was responsible for the release of cytochrome c and induction of apoptosis. The data indicate that cell survival depends on an adequate pool of unsaturated phospholipids necessary for cardiolipin synthesis. Oleate inhibits palmitate-induced apoptosis, probably by channelling palmitate to inert triglyceride stores and by sustaining CL synthesis [Hardy et al. 2003].

Diabetes therapy aiming at maintaining or restoring the existing β-cell mass could be achieved by β-cell transplantation, β-cell neogenesis, or prevention of β-cell apoptosis. GLP-1 (glucagon-like peptide) and liraglutide (a GLP-1 analogue) blocked the pro-apoptotic activities of both cytokines and fatty acids in rat islet cells. This anti-apoptotic activity of liraglutide was mediated via the GLP-1 receptor. Liraglutide inhibition of apoptosis was not mediated by inhibition of ceramide synthase or by inhibition NO production. Rather, the anti-apoptotic effect of liraglutide was mediated by intracellular cAMP and PI3 kinase activity [Bregenholt et al. 2005]. In the β-cell line RIN m5F, palmitate-induced apoptosis was also inhibited by elevating intracellular cAMP-levels. However, anti-apoptotic activity of cAMP was mediated via protein kinase A at low concentrations and through the cAMP-GEF pathway (cAMP – guanine nucleotide exchange factor) at high concentrations [Kwon et al. 2004]. These results indicate that GLP-1 agonist treatment may be a rational regimen for retaining/restoring pancreatic β-cell mass critical for both type 1 and type 2 diabetes.

Long-term treatment with TZDs (thiazolidinediones) has been shown to result in lowering of FFA levels in plasma, prevention of lipid deposition in β-cells, skeletal muscle, cardiac muscle and liver and in a redistribution of intracellular lipid from insulin-responsive organs to peripheral adipocytes. This also has a positive effect on cardiovascular risk factors, such as endothelial dysfunction, VSMC proliferation, and lipoprotein profile [Wyne 2003].

Conclusion

Epidemiological evidence suggests that diets rich in PUFAs, especially EPA and DHA, are beneficial against atherosclerosis. In vitro work has shown that PUFAs can induce apoptosis by many mechanisms: peroxidation with production of reactive oxygen species and toxic degradation products, formation of pro-apoptotic metabolites via COX and LOX, activation of PPARgamma, or effects on cardiolipin synthesis and oxidisability. Similarly, high levels of saturated fatty acids have been shown to be detrimental to pancreatic beta-cells and can lead to diabetes etc., and in turn to cardiovascular complications. This article highlights the need to tie together in vitro research and in vivo effects, with the view to the development of improved dietary or drug-based strategies for preventing and combating these diseases.

Acknowledgements

We thank the British Heart Foundation (KLHC, MJA, KM, IRC), Cancer Research UK (MJA), the Research Advisory Group and Charities Committee of Addenbrooke's Hospital (KLHC, MJA) and the Wellcome Trust (JNS) for financial support.

References

[1] Abdel-Rahman WM, Katsura K, Rens W, Gorman PA, Sheer D, Bicknell D, Bodmer WF, Arends MJ, Wyllie AH, Edwards PA. (2001) Spectral karyotyping suggests additional subsets of colorectal cancers characterized by pattern of chromosome rearrangement. *Proc Natl Acad Sci USA* 98:2538-2543.

[2] Bailey JM, Butler J. (1973) Anti-inflammatory drugs in experimental atherosclerosis. I. Relative potencies for inhibiting plaque formation. *Atherosclerosis* 17:515-522.

[3] Baker CS, Hall RJ, Evans TJ, Pomerance A, Maclouf J, Creminon C, Yacoub MH, Polak JM. (1999) Cyclooxygenase-2 is widely expressed in atherosclerotic lesions affecting native and transplanted human coronary arteries and colocalizes with inducible nitric oxide synthase and nitrotyrosine particularly in macrophages. *Arterioscler Thromb Vasc Biol.* 19:646-55.

[4] Baldwin AS. (2001) Control of oncogenesis and cancer therapy resistance by the transcription factor NF-kappaB. *J Clin Invest* 10:241-246.

[5] Bartsch H, Nair J, Owen RW. (1999) Dietary polyunsaturated fatty acids and cancers of the breast and colorectum: emerging evidence for their role as risk modifiers. *Carcinogenesis* 20:2209-18.

[6] Bennett MR LT, Schwartz SM, Weissberg PL. (1997) Increased sensitivity of human vascular smooth muscle cells from atherosclerotic plaques to p53-mediated apoptosis. *Circ Res* 81:591-9.

[7] Berger A, Gershwin ME, German JB. (1992) Effects of various dietary fats on cardiolipin acyl composition during ontogeny of mice. *Lipids* 27:605-612.

[8] Bishop-Bailey D and Hla T. (1999) Endothelial cell apoptosis induced by the peroxisome proliferator- activated receptor (PPAR) ligand 15-deoxy-delta12, 14-prostaglandin J2. *J Biol Chem* 274: 17042-17048.

[9] Boyle JJ, Bowyer DE, Weissberg PL and Bennett MR. (2001) Human blood-derived macrophages induce apoptosis in human plaque- derived vascular smooth muscle cells by Fas-ligand/Fas interactions. *Arterioscler Thromb Vasc Biol* 21: 1402-1407.

[10] Bregenholt S, Moldrup A, Blume N, Karlsen AE, Friedrichsen BN, Tornhave D, Knudsen LB, Petersen JS. (2005) The long-acting glucagons-like peptide-1 analogue, liraglutide, inhibits β-cell apoptosis in vitro. *Biochem Biophys Res Commun* 330: 577-584.

[11] Bresalier RS, Sandler RS, Quan H, Bolognese JA, Oxenius B, Horgan K, Lines C, Riddell R, Morton D, Lanas A, Konstam MA, Baron JA; Adenomatous Polyp Prevention on Vioxx (APPROVe) Trial Investigators. (2005) Cardiovascular events associated with rofecoxib in a colorectal adenoma chemoprevention trial. *N Engl J Med* 352:1092-102.

[12] Burleigh ME, Babaev VR, Oates JA, Harris RC, Gautam S, Riendeau D, Marnett LJ, Morrow JD, Fazio S, Linton MF. (2002) Cyclooxygenase-2 promotes early atherosclerotic lesion formation in LDL receptor-deficient mice. *Circulation* 105:1816-1823.

[13] Burleigh ME, Babaev VR, Patel MB, Crews BC, Remmel RP, Morrow JD, Oates JA, Marnett LJ, Fazio S, Linton MF. (2005) Inhibition of cyclooxygenase with indomethacin phenethylamide reduces atherosclerosis in apoE-null mice. *Biochem Pharmacol* 70:334-342.

[14] Carpenter KL, Challis IR, Arends MJ. (2003a) Mildly oxidised LDL induces more macrophage death than moderately oxidised LDL: roles of peroxidation, lipoprotein-associated phospholipase A_2 and PPARgamma. *FEBS Lett* 553:145-150.

[15] Carpenter KL, Dennis IF, Challis IR, Osborn DP, Macphee CH, Leake DS, Arends MJ, Mitchinson MJ. (2001) Inhibition of lipoprotein-associated phospholipase A_2 diminishes the death-inducing effects of oxidised LDL on human monocyte macrophages. *FEBS Lett* 505:357-363.

[16] Carpenter KL, Kirkpatrick PJ, Weissberg PL, Challis IR, Dennis IF, Freeman MA, Mitchinson MJ. (2003b) Oral alpha-tocopherol supplementation inhibits lipid oxidation in established human atherosclerostic lesions. *Free Rad Res* 37: 1235-1244.

[17] Carpenter KL, Taylor SE, van der Veen C, Williamson BK, Ballantine JA, Mitchinson MJ. (1995) Lipids and oxidised lipids in human atherosclerotic lesions at different stages of development. *Biochim Biophys Acta* 1256:141-150.

[18] Chang CL, Marra G, Chauhan DP, Ha HT, Chang DK, Ricciardiello L, et al. (2002) Oxidative stress inactivates the human DNA mismatch repair system. *Am J Physiol Cell Physiol* 283:C148-54.

[19] Chen KH, Srivastava DK, Singhal RK, Jacob S, Ahmed AE, Wilson SH. (2000) Modulation of base excision repair by low density lipoprotein, oxidized low density lipoprotein and antioxidants in mouse monocytes. *Carcinogenesis* 21:1017-22.

[20] Chen YC, Shen SC, Tsai SH. (2005) Prostaglandin D(2) and J(2) induce apoptosis in human leukemia cells via activation of the caspase 3 cascade and production of reactive oxygen species. *Biochim Biophys Acta* 1743:291-304.

[21] Chinetti G, Griglio S, Antonucci M, Torra IP, Delerive P, Majd Z, Fruchart JC, Chapman J, Najib J, Staels B. (1998) Activation of proliferator-activated receptors alpha and gamma induces apoptosis of human monocyte-derived macrophages. *J Biol Chem* 273:25573-25580.

[22] Chinetti G, Lestavel S, Bocher V, Remaley AT, Neve B, Torra IP, Teissier E, Minnich A, Jaye M, Duverger N, Brewer HB, Fruchart JC, Clavey V and Staels B. (2001) PPAR-alpha and PPAR-gamma activators induce cholesterol removal from human macrophage foam cells through stimulation of the ABCA1 pathway. *Nat Med* 7: 53-58.

[23] Chung SW, Kang BY, Kim SH, Pak YK, Cho D, Trinchieri G and Kim TS. (2000) Oxidized low density lipoprotein inhibits interleukin-12 production in lipopolysaccharide-activated mouse macrophages via direct interactions between peroxisome proliferator-activated receptor-gamma and nuclear factor-kappa B. *J Biol Chem* 275: 32681-32687.

[24] Clandinin MT, Innis SM. (1983) Does mitochondrial ATP synthesis decline as a function of change in the membrane environment with ageing. *Mech Ageing Dev.* 22:205-8.

[25] Clare K, Hardwick SJ, Carpenter KL, Weeratunge N, Mitchinson MJ. (1995) Toxicity of oxysterols to human monocyte-macrophages. *Atherosclerosis* 118:67-75.

[26] Connor WE. (2000) Importance of n-3 fatty acids in health and disease. *Am J Clin Nutr* 71(suppl) 171S-175S.

[27] Cyrus T, Yao Y, Rokach J, Tang LX, Pratico D (2003) Vitamin E reduces progression of atherosclerosis in low-density lipoprotein receptor-deficient mice with established vascular lesions. *Circulation* 107: 521-3.

[28] Daum G. (1985) Lipids of mitochondria. *Biochim Biophys Acta* 822:1-42.

[29] Davies SS, Pontsler AV, Marathe GK, Harrison KA, Murphy RC, Hinshaw JC, Prestwich GD, Hilaire AS, Prescott SM, Zimmerman GA, McIntyre TM. (2001) Oxidized alkyl phospholipids are specific, high affinity peroxisome proliferator-activated receptor gamma ligands and agonists. *J Biol Chem* 276:16015-23.

[30] de Lorgeril M, Renaud S, Mamelle N, Salen P, Martin JL, Monjaud I, Guidollet J, Touboul P, Delaye J. (1994) Mediterranean alpha-linolenic acid-rich diet in secondary prevention of coronary heart disease. *Lancet* 343:1454-9.

[31] de Vries JE, Vork MM, Roemen TH, de Jong YF, Cleutjens JP, van der Vusse GJ, van Bilsen M. (1997) Saturated but not mono-unsaturated fatty acids induce apoptotic cell death in neonatal rat ventricular myocytes. *J Lipid Res.* 38:1384-94.

[32] de Winter JM, Lenting HB, Neys FW, van den Bosch H. (1987) Hydrolysis of membrane-associated phosphoglycerides by mitochondrial phospholipase A_2. *Biochim Biophys Acta.* 917:169 -77.

[33] De Flora S, Izzotti A, Walsh D, Degan P, Petrilli GL, Lewtas J. (1997) Molecular epidemiology of atherosclerosis. *FASEB J* 11:1020-31.

[34] Deguchi H, Fernandez JA, Hackeng TM, Banka CL, Griffin JH. (2000) Cardiolipin is a normal component of human plasma lipoproteins. *Proc Natl Acad Sci USA.* 97:1743-8.

[35] Delerive P, Furman C, Teissier E, Fruchart J, Duriez P, Staels B. (2000) Oxidized phospholipids activate PPARalpha in a phospholipase A_2-dependent manner. *FEBS Lett.* 471:34-8.

[36] DeWeese TL, Shipman JM, Larrier NA, Buckley NM, Kidd LR, Groopman JD, Cutler RG, te Riele H, Nelson WG. (1998) Mouse embryonic stem cells carrying one or two

defective Msh2 alleles respond abnormally to oxidative stress inflicted by low-level radiation. *Proc Natl Acad Sci USA* 95:11915-20.

[37] Doran E, Halestrap AP. (2000) Cytochrome c release from isolated rat liver mitochondria can occur independently of outer-membrane rupture: possible role of contact sites. *Biochem J* 348 Pt 2:343-50.

[38] Eitel K, Staiger H, Brendel MD, Brandhorst D, Bretzel RG, Häring H-U, Kellerer M. (2002) Different role of saturated and unsaturated fatty acids in β-cell apoptosis. *Biochem Biophys Res Comm* 299: 853-856.

[39] El-Assaad W, Buteau J, Peyot M-L, Nolan C, Roduit R, Hardy S, Joly E, Dbaibo G, Rosenberg L, Prentki M. (2003) Saturated fatty acids synergize with elevated glucose to cause pancreatic β-cell death. *Endocrinology* 144: 4154-4163.

[40] Enoksson M, Robertson JD, Gogvadze V, Bu P, Kropotov A, Zhivotovsky B, Orrenius S. (2004) Caspase-2 permeabilizes the outer mitochondrial membrane and disrupts the binding of cytochrome c to anionic phospholipids. *J Biol Chem.* 279:49575-8.

[41] Ferri KF, Kroemer G. (2001) Organelle-specific initiation of cell death pathways. *Nature Cell Biology* 3: E255-E263.

[42] Flouris GA, Arvanitis DA, Parissis JT, Arvanitis DL, Spandidos DA. (2000) Loss of heterozygosity in DNA mismatch repair genes in human atherosclerotic plaques. *Mol Cell Biol Res Commun* 4:62-5.

[43] Forman BM, Chen J, Evans RM. (1997) Hypolipidemic drugs, polyunsaturated fatty acids, and eicosanoids are ligands for peroxisome proliferator-activated receptors alpha and delta. *Proc Natl Acad Sci USA* 94: 4312-4317.

[44] Gasnier F, Rey C, Hellio Le Graverand MP, Benahmed M, Louisot P. (1998) Hormone-induced changes in cardiolipin from Leydig cells: possible involvement in intramitochondrial cholesterol translocation. *Biochem Mol Biol Int* 45:93-100.

[45] GISSI-Prevenzione Investigators. (1999) Dietary supplementation with n-3 polyunsaturated fatty acids and vitamin E after myocardial infarction: results of the GISSI-Prevenzione trial. *Lancet* 354: 447-455.

[46] Guyton JR, Lenz ML, Mathews B, Hughes H, Karsan D, Selinger E, Smith CV. (1995) Toxicity of oxidized low density lipoproteins for vascular smooth muscle cells and partial protection by antioxidants. *Atherosclerosis* 118:237-249.

[47] Hakkinen T, Luoma JS, Hiltunen MO, Macphee CH, Milliner KJ, Patel L, Rice SQ, Tew DG, Karkola K, Yla-Herttuala S. (1999) Lipoprotein-associated phospholipase A_2, platelet-activating factor acetylhydrolase, is expressed by macrophages in human and rabbit atherosclerotic lesions. *Arterioscler Thromb Vasc Biol* 19: 2909-17.

[48] Hardwick SJ, Hegyi L, Clare K, Law NS, Carpenter KL, Mitchinson MJ, Skepper JN. (1996) Apoptosis in human monocyte-macrophages exposed to oxidized low density lipoprotein. *J Pathol* 179:294-302.

[49] Hardy S, El-Assaad W, Przybytkowski E, Joly E, Prentki M, Langelier Y. (2003) Saturated fatty acid-induced apoptosis in MDA-MB-231 breast cancer cells. A role for cardiolipin. *J. Biol. Chem* 278: 31861-31870.

[50] Hawkins RA, Sangster K, Arends MJ. (1998) Apoptotic death of pancreatic cancer cells induced by polyunsaturated fatty acids varies with double bond number and involves an oxidative mechanism. *J Pathol* 185:61-70.

[51] Heart Protection Study Collaborative Group (2002) MRC/BHF Heart Protection Study of antioxidant vitamin supplementation in 20,536 high-risk individuals: a randomised placebo-controlled trial. *Lancet* 360: 23-33.

[52] Helbock HJ, Beckman KB, Shigenaga MK, Walter PB, Woodall AA, Yeo HC, et al. (1998) DNA oxidation matters: the HPLC-electrochemical detection assay of 8-oxo-deoxyguanosine and 8-oxo-guanine. *Proc Natl Acad Sci U S A* 95:288-93.

[53] Helbock HJ, Beckman KB, Ames BN. (1999) 8-Hydroxydeoxyguanosine and 8-hydroxyguanine as biomarkers of oxidative DNA damage. *Methods Enzymol* 300:156-66.

[54] Hegyi L, Hardwick SJ, Siow RC and Skepper JN. (2001) Macrophage death and the role of apoptosis in human atherosclerosis. *J Hematother Stem Cell Res* 10: 27-42.

[55] Helmy FM, Hassanein M, Juracka A. (2004) Studies on the endogenous phospholipids of mammalian kidney and their in vitro hydrolysis by endogenous phospholipases: a thin layer chromatographic and densitometric study. *Cell Biochem Funct* 22:379-87.

[56] Horkko S, Miller E, Dudl E, Reaven P, Curtiss LK, Zvaifler NJ, Terkeltaub R, Pierangeli SS, Branch DW, Palinski W, Witztum JL. (1996) Antiphospholipid antibodies are directed against epitopes of oxidized phospholipids. Recognition of cardiolipin by monoclonal antibodies to epitopes of oxidized low density lipoprotein. *J Clin Invest* 98:815-25.

[57] Innis SM, Clandinin MT. (1981a) Dynamic modulation of mitochondrial inner-membrane lipids in rat heart by dietary fat. *Biochem J* 193:155-67.

[58] Innis SM, Clandinin MT. (1981b) Dynamic modulation of mitochondrial membrane physical properties and ATPase activity by diet lipid. *Biochem J* 198:167-75.

[59] Innis SM, Clandinin MT. (1981c) Mitochondrial-membrane polar-head-group composition is influenced by diet fat. *Biochem J* 198:231-4.

[60] Jauslin ML, Meier T, Smith RA, Murphy MP. (2003) Mitochondria-targeted antioxidants protect Friedreich Ataxia fibroblasts from endogenous oxidative stress more effectively than untargeted antioxidants. *FASEB J* 17:1972-4.

[61] Jiang C, Ting AT and Seed B. (1998) PPAR-gamma agonists inhibit production of monocyte inflammatory cytokines. *Nature* 391: 82-86.

[62] Kharroubi I, Ladriere L, Cardozo AK, Dogusan Z, Cnop M, Eizirik DL. (2004) Free fatty acids and cytokines induce pancreatic β-cell apoptosis by different mechanisms: role of nuclear factor-κB and endoplasmic reticulum stress. *Endocrinology* 145: 5087-5096.

[63] Kliewer SA, Sundseth SS, Jones SA, Brown PJ, Wisely GB, Koble CS, Devchand P, Wahli W, Willson TM, Lenhard JM and Lehmann JM. (1997) Fatty acids and eicosanoids regulate gene expression through direct interactions with peroxisome proliferator-activated receptors alpha and gamma. *Proc Natl Acad Sci USA* 94: 4318-4323.

[64] Kolodgie FD, Narula J, Burke AP, Haider N, Farb A, Hui-Liang Y, Smialek J, Virmani R. (2000) Localization of apoptotic macrophages at the site of plaque rupture in sudden coronary death. *Am J Pathol* 157:1259-1268.

[65] Kumagai T, Matsukawa N, Kaneko Y, Kusumi Y, Mitsumata M, Uchida K. (2004) A lipid peroxidation derived inflammatory mediator: identification of 4-hydroxy-2-nonenal as a potential inducer of cyclooxygenase-2 in macrophages. *J Biol Chem* 279:48389-96.

[66] Kwon G, Pappan KL, Marshall CA, Schaffer JE, McDaniel ML. (2004) cAMP dose-dependently prevents palmitate-induced apoptosis by both protein kinase A- and cAMP-guanine nucleotide exchange factor-dependent pathways in β-cells. *J Biol Chem* 279: 8938-8945.

[67] Lee H, Shi W, Tontonoz P, Wang S, Subbanagounder G, Hedrick CC, Hama S, Borromeo C, Evans RM, Berliner JA, Nagy L. (2000) Role for peroxisome proliferator-activated receptor alpha in oxidized phospholipid induced synthesis of monocyte chemotactic protein-1 and interleukin-8 by endothelial cells. *Circ Res* 87:516-21.

[68] Lehmann JM, Lenhard JM, Oliver BB, Ringold GM, Kliewer SA (1997) Peroxisome proliferator-activated receptors alpha and gamma are activated by indomethacin and other non-steroidal anti-inflammatory drugs. *J Biol Chem* 272:3406-3410.

[69] Leigh-Firbank EC, Minihane AM, Leake DS, Wright JW, Murphy MC, Griffin BA and Williams CM (2002) Eicosapentaenoic acid and docosahexaenoic acid from fish oils: differential associations with lipid responses. *Br J Nutr* 87: 435-45.

[70] Listenberger L., Han X, Lewis SE, Cases S, Farese RV, Ory DS, Schaffer JE. (2003) Triglyceride accumulation protects against fatty acid-induced lipotoxicity. Proc Natl *Acad Sci* USA 100: 3077-3082.

[71] Lu Z-H, Mu Y-M, Wang B-A, Li X-L, Lu J-M, Li J-Y, Pan C-Y, Yanase T, Nawata H. (2003) Saturated free fatty acids, palmitic acid and stearic acid, induce apoptosis by stimulation of ceramide generation in rat testicular Leydig cell. *Biochem Biophys Res Commun* 303: 1002-1007.

[72] Lutter M, Fang M, Luo X, Nishijima M, Xie X, Wang X. (2000) Cardiolipin provides specificity for targeting of tBid to mitochondria. *Nat Cell Biol* 2:754-61.

[73] Lutter M, Perkins GA, Wang X. (2001) The pro-apoptotic Bcl-2 family member tBid localizes to mitochondrial contact sites. *BMC Cell Biol* 2:22.

[74] Macphee C, Benson GM, Shi Y, Zalewski A. (2005) Lipoprotein-associated phospholipase A_2: a novel marker of cardiovascular risk and potential therapeutic target. *Expert Opin Investig Drugs* 14: 671-679.

[75] MacPhee CH, Moores KE, Boyd HF, Dhanak D, Ife RJ, Leach CA, Leake DS, Milliner KJ, Patterson RA, Suckling KE, Tew DG, Hickey DM. (1999) Lipoprotein-associated phospholipase A_2, platelet-activating factor acetylhydrolase, generates two bioactive products during the oxidation of low-density lipoprotein: use of a novel inhibitor. *Biochem J* 338:479-87.

[76] Macphee CH, Nelson J, Zalewski A. (2006) Role of lipoprotein-associated phospholipase A2 in atherosclerosis and its potential as a therapeutic target. *Curr Opin Pharmacol* 6:154-61.

[77] Maestre I, Jordan J, Calvo S, Reig JA, Cena V, Soria B, Prentki M, Roche E. (2003) Mitochondrial dysfunction is involved in apoptosis induced by serum withdrawal and fatty acids in the beta-cell line Ins-1. *Endocrinology* 144: 335-345.

[78] Marchant CE, Law NS, van der Veen C, Hardwick SJ, Carpenter KL, Mitchinson MJ. (1995) Oxidized low-density lipoprotein is cytotoxic to human monocyte macrophages: protection with lipophilic antioxidants. *FEBS Lett* 358:175-178.

[79] Marchant CE, van der Veen C, Law NS, Hardwick SJ, Carpenter KL, Mitchinson MJ. (1996) Oxidation of low-sensity lipoprotein by human monocyte-macrophages results in toxicity to the oxidising culture. *Free Rad Res* 24: 333-342.

[80] Martinet W, Knaapen MW, De Meyer GR, Herman AG, Kockx MM. (2001) Oxidative DNA damage and repair in experimental atherosclerosis are reversed by dietary lipid lowering. *Circ Res* 88:733-9.

[81] Martinet W, Knaapen MW, De Meyer GR, Herman AG, Kockx MM. (2002) Elevated levels of oxidative DNA damage and DNA repair enzymes in human atherosclerotic plaques. *Circulation* 106:927-32.

[82] Matthews C, Gorenne I, Scott S, Figg N, Kirkpatrick P, Ritchie A, Goddard M, Bennett M. (2006) Vascular smooth muscle cells undergo telomere-based senescence in human atherosclerosis: effects of telomerase and oxidative stress.*Circ Res* 99:156-64.

[83] Marx N, Sukhova G, Murphy C, Libby P and Plutzky J. (1998) Macrophages in human atheroma contain PPARgamma: differentiation- dependent peroxisomal proliferator-activated receptor gamma(PPARgamma) expression and reduction of MMP-9 activity through PPARgamma activation in mononuclear phagocytes in vitro. *Am J Pathol* 153: 17-23.

[84] Min JH, Jain M., Wilder C, Paul L, Apitz-Castro R, Aspleaf DC, Gelb MH. (1999) Membrane-bound plasma platelet activating factor acetylhydrolase acts on substrate in the aqueous phase. *Biochemistry* 38: 12935-42.

[85] Min JH, Wilder C, Aoki J, Arai H, Inoue K, Paul L, Gelb MH. (2001) Platelet-activating factor acetylhydrolases: broad substrate specificity and lipoprotein binding does not modulate the catalytic properties of the plasma enzyme. *Biochemistry* 40: 4539-49.

[86] Mishra R, Simonson MS. (2005) Saturated free fatty acids and apoptosis in microvascular mesangial cells: palmitate activates pro-apoptotic signalling involving caspase 9 and mitochondrial release of endonuclease *G. Cardiovascular Diabetology* 4: 2.

[87] Mitchell JA, Akarasereenont P, Thiemermann C, Flower RJ, Vane JR. (1993) Selectivity of nonsteroidal antiinflammatory drugs as inhibitors of constitutive and inducible cyclooxygenase. *Proc Natl Acad Sci U S A* 90:11693-11697.

[88] Mu Y-M, Yanase T, Nishi Y, Tanaka A, Saito M, Jin CH, Mukasa C, Okabe T, Nomura M, Goto K, Nawata H. (2001) Saturated FFAs, palmitic acid and stearic acid, induce apoptosis in human granulosa cells. *Endocrinology* 142:3590-3597.

[89] Müller K, Carpenter KL, Mitchinson MJ. (1998) Cell-mediated oxidation of LDL: comparison of different cell types of the atherosclerotic lesion. *Free Radic Res* 29:207-220.

[90] Müller K, Carpenter KL, Freeman MA, Mitchinson MJ. (1999) Antioxidant BO-653 and human macrophage-mediated LDL oxidation. *Free Radic Res* 30:59-71.

[91] Müller K, Hardwick SJ, Marchant CE, Law NS, Waeg G, Esterbauer H, Carpenter KL, Mitchinson MJ. (1996) Cytotoxic and chemotactic potencies of several aldehydic components of oxidised low density lipoprotein for human monocyte-macrophages. *FEBS Lett* 388:165-168

[92] Muralidhar B, Carpenter KL, Müller K, Skepper JN, Arends MJ. (2004) Potency of arachidonic acid in polyunsaturated fatty acid-induced death of human monocyte-macrophages: implications for atherosclerosis. *Prostaglandins Leukot Essent Fatty Acids* 71:251-262.

[93] Nagy L, Tontonoz P, Alvarez JG, Chen H, Evans RM. (1998) Oxidized LDL regulates macrophage gene expression through ligand activation of PPARgamma. *Cell* 93: 229-240.

[94] Nomura K, Imai H, Koumura T, Kobayashi T, Nakagawa Y. (2000) Mitochondrial phospholipid hydroperoxide glutathione peroxidase inhibits the release of cytochrome c from mitochondria by suppressing the peroxidation of cardiolipin in hypoglycaemia-induced apoptosis. *Biochem J* 351:183-93.

[95] Oikawa S, Kawanishi S. (1999) Site-specific DNA damage at GGG sequence by oxidative stress may accelerate telomere shortening. *FEBS Lett* 453:365-8.

[96] Oikawa S, Tada-Oikawa S, Kawanishi S. (2001) Site-specific DNA damage at the GGG sequence by UVA involves acceleration of telomere shortening. *Biochemistry* 40:4763-8.

[97] Okuyama R, Fujiwara T, Ohsumi J. (2003) High glucose potentiates palmitate-induced NO-mediated cytotoxicity through generation of superoxide in clonal β-cell HIT-T15. *FEBS Lett* 545: 219-223.

[98] Ott M, Robertson JD, Gogvadze V, Zhivotovsky B, Orrenius S. (2002) Cytochrome c release from mitochondria proceeds by a two-step process. *Proc Natl Acad Sci U S A* 99:1259-1263.

[99] Parinandi NL, Weis BK, Schmid HH. (1988) Assay of cardiolipin peroxidation by high-performance liquid chromatography. *Chem Phys Lipids* 49:215-20.

[100] Park BH, Vogelstein B, Kinzler KW. (2001) Genetic disruption of PPARdelta decreases the tumorigenicity of human colon cancer cells. *Proc Natl Acad Sci U S A* 98:2598-2603.

[101] Patel L, Pass I, Coxon P, Downes CP, Smith SA, Macphee CH. (2001) Tumor suppressor and anti-inflammatory actions of PPARgamma agonists are mediated via upregulation of PTEN. *Curr Biol* 11:764-768.

[102] Pontsler AV, St Hilaire A, Marathe GK, Zimmerman GA, McIntyre TM. (2002) Cyclooxygenase-2 is induced in monocytes by peroxisome proliferator activated receptor gamma and oxidized alkyl phospholipids from oxidized low density lipoprotein. *J Biol Chem* 277:13029-13036.

[103] Pratico D, Tangirala RK, Rader DJ, Rokach J, FitzGerald GA (1998) Vitamin E suppresses isoprostane generation in vivo and reduces atherosclerosis in ApoE-deficient mice. *Nat Med 4*:1189-92.

[104] Pratico D, Tillmann C, Zhang ZB, Li H, FitzGerald GA. (2001) Acceleration of atherogenesis by COX-1-dependent prostanoid formation in low density lipoprotein receptor knockout mice. *Proc Natl Acad Sci U S A* 98:3358-3363.

[105] Pryor WA (2000) Vitamin E and heart disease: basic science to clinical intervention trials. *Free Radic Biol Med* 28: 141-64.

[106] Renner R, Innis SM, Clandinin MT. (1979) Effects of high and low erucic acid rapeseed oils on energy metabolism and mitochondrial function of the chick. *J Nutr* 109:378-87.

[107] Ricote M, Huang J, Fajas L, Li A, Welch J, Najib J, Witztum JL, Auwerx J, Palinski W and Glass CK. (1998) Expression of the peroxisome proliferator-activated receptor gamma (PPARgamma) in human atherosclerosis and regulation in macrophages by colony stimulating factors and oxidized low density lipoprotein. *Proc Natl Acad Sci U S A* 95: 7614-7619.

[108] Roberts LJ and Morrow JD. (2001) Analgesic-antipyretic and antiinflammatory agents and drugs used in the treatment of gout. In: *Goodman and Gilman's The Pharmacological Basis of Therapeutics*, pp. 687-731 [JG Hardman, LE Limbird and AG Gilman, editors]: 10th Edn., McGraw-Hill, New York.

[109] Saez E, Tontonoz P, Nelson MC, Alvarez JG, Ming UT, Baird SM, Thomazy VA, Evans RM. (1998) Activators of the nuclear receptor PPARgamma enhance colon polyp formation. *Nat Med* 4:1058-1061.

[110] Sarraf P, Mueller E, Smith WM, Wright HM, Kum JB, Aaltonen LA, de la Chapelle A, Spiegelman BM, Eng C. (1999) Loss-of-function mutations in PPARgamma associated with human colon cancer. *Mol Cell* 3: 799-804.

[111] Schonbeck U, Sukhova GK, Graber P, Coulter S, Libby P. (1999) Augmented expression of cyclooxygenase-2 in human atherosclerotic lesions. *Am J Pathol* 155:1281-91.

[112] Sendobry SM, Cornicelli JA, Welch K, Bocan T, Tait B, Trivedi BK, Colbry N, Dyer RD, Feinmark SJ, Daugherty A. (1997) Attenuation of diet-induced atherosclerosis in rabbits with a highly selective 15-lipoxygenase inhibitor lacking significant antioxidant properties. *Br J Pharmacol* 120:1199-1206.

[113] Siow RC, Richards JP, Pedley KC, Leake DS, Mann GE. (1999) Vitamin C protects human vascular smooth muscle cells against apoptosis induced by moderately oxidized LDL containing high levels of lipid hydroperoxides. *Arterioscler Thromb Vasc Biol* 19:2387-2394.

[114] Smith WL, DeWitt DL, Garavito RM. (2000) Cyclooxygenases: structural, cellular, and molecular biology. *Annu Rev Biochem* 69:145-182.

[115] Spandidos DA, Ergazaki M, Arvanitis D, Kiaris H. (1996) Microsatellite instability in human atherosclerotic plaques. *Biochem Biophys Res Commun* 220:137-40.

[116] Stafforini DM, Elstad MR, McIntyre TM, Zimmerman GA, Prescott SM. (1990) Human macrophages secret platelet-activating factor acetylhydrolase. *J Biol Chem* 265: 9682-7.

[117] Stephens NG, Parsons A, Schofield PM, Kelly F, Cheeseman K, Mitchinson MJ, Brown MJ (1996) Randomised controlled trial of vitamin E in patients with coronary disease: Cambridge Heart Antioxidant Study (CHAOS). *Lancet* 347: 781-6.

[118] Thies F, Garry JM, Yaqoob P, Rerkasem K, Williams J, Shearman CP, Gallagher PJ, Calder PC and Grimble RF (2003) Association of n-3 polyunsaturated fatty acids with stability of atherosclerotic plaques: a randomised controlled trial. *Lancet* 361: 477-85.

[119] Tjoelker LW, Wilder C, Eberhardt C, Stafforini DM, Dietsch G, Schimpf B, Hooper S, Le Trong H, Cousens LS, Zimmerman GA, et al. (1995) Anti-inflammatory properties of a platelet-activating factor acetylhydrolase. *Nature* 374: 549-53.

[120] Toft NJ, Arends MJ. (1998) DNA mismatch repair and colorectal cancer. *J Pathol* 185: 123-129.

[121] Toft NJ, Arends MJ, Wyllie AH, te Riele H, Clarke AR. (1998) No evidence of female embryonic lethality in mice nullizygous for both *Msh2* and *p53*. *Nature Genetics* 18:17-18.

[122] Toft NJ, Winton DJ, Kelly J, Howard LA, Dekker M, te Riele H, Arends MJ, Wyllie AH, Margison GP, Clarke AR. (1999) *Msh2* status modulates both apoptosis and mutation frequency in the murine small intestine. *Proc Natl Acad Sci USA* 96:3911-3915.

[123] Tontonoz P, Nagy L, Alvarez JG, Thomazy VA, Evans RM. (1998) PPARgamma promotes monocyte/macrophage differentiation and uptake of oxidized LDL. *Cell* 93: 241-252.

[124] Toyoda M, Takagi H, Horiguchi N, Kakizaki S, Sato K, Takayama H, Mori M. (2002) A ligand for peroxisome proliferator activated receptor gamma inhibits cell growth and induces apoptosis in human liver cancer cells. *Gut* 50: 563-567.

[125] Unger RH. (2002) Lipotoxic diseases. *Annu Rev Med* 53: 319-336.

[126] Unger RH, Orci L. (2002) Lipoapoptosis: its mechanism and its diseases. *Biochim Biophys Acta* 1585: 202-212.

[127] von Zglinicki T. (1998) Telomeres: influencing the rate of aging. Ann N Y Acad Sci 854:318-27.

[128] Vreken P, Valianpour F, Nijtmans LG, Grivell LA, Plecko B, Wanders RJ, Barth PG. (2000) Defective remodeling of cardiolipin and phosphatidylglycerol in Barth syndrome. *Biochem Biophys Res Commun* 279:378-82.

[129] Waddington E, Sienuarine K, Puddey I, Croft K. (2001) Identification and quantitation of unique fatty acid oxidation products in human atherosclerotic plaque using high performance liquid chromatography. *Analytical Biochemistry* 292:234-244.

[130] Wander RC and Du S-H. (2000) Oxidation of plasma proteins is not increased after supplementation with eicosapentaenoic and docosahexaenoic acids. *Am J Clin Nutr* 72: 731-737.

[131] Wang YL, Frauwirth KA, Rangwala SM, Lazar MA and Thompson CB. (2002) Thiazolidinedione activation of peroxisome proliferator-activated receptor gamma can enhance mitochondrial potential and promote cell survival. *J Biol Chem* 277: 31781-31788.

[132] Watkins SM, Carter LC, German JB. (1998) Docosahexaenoic acid accumulates in cardiolipin and enhances HT-29 cell oxidant production. *J Lipid Res* 39:1583-1588.

[133] Welters HJ, Tadayyon M, Scarpello JHB, Smith SA, Morgan NG. (2004) Mono-unsaturated fatty acids protect against β-cell apoptosis induced by saturated fatty acids, serum withdrawal or cytokine exposure. *FEBS Lett* 560: 103-108.

[134] Willson TM, Cobb JE, Cowan DJ, Wiethe RW, Correa ID, Prakash SR, Beck KD, Moore LB, Kliewer SA, Lehmann JM. (1996) The structure-activity relationship between peroxisome proliferator- activated receptor gamma agonism and the antihyperglycemic activity of thiazolidinediones. *J Med Chem* 39: 665-668.

[135] Wyne KL. (2003) Free fatty acids and type 2 diabetes mellitus. *Am J Med* 115:29S-36S.

[136] Yang WL and Frucht H. (2001) Activation of the PPAR pathway induces apoptosis and COX-2 inhibition in HT-29 human colon cancer cells. *Carcinogenesis* 22: 1379-1383.

[137] Yla-Herttuala S, Palinski W, Rosenfeld ME, Parthasarathy S, Carew TE, Butler S, Witztum JL, Steinberg D. (1989) Evidence for the presence of oxidatively modified low density lipoprotein in atherosclerotic lesions of rabbit and man. *J Clin Invest* 84:1086-1095.

[138] Yla-Herttuala S, Rosenfeld ME, Parthasarathy S, Glass CK, Sigal E, Witztum JL, Steinberg D. (1990) Colocalization of 15-lipoxygenase mRNA and protein with epitopes of oxidized low density lipoprotein in macrophage-rich areas of atherosclerotic lesions. *Proc Natl Acad Sci U S A* 87:6959-6963.

[139] Yusuf S, Dagenais G, Pogue J, Bosch J, Sleight P (2000) Vitamin E supplementation and cardiovascular events in high-risk patients. The Heart Outcomes Prevention Evaluation Study Investigators. *N Engl J Med* 342: 154-60.

In: Frontiers in Atherosclerosis Research
Editor: Karin F. Kepper, pp. 29-48
ISBN 1-60021-371-5

Chapter 2

PROGRESS IN ATHEROSCLEROSIS RESEARCH – ACAT ENZYME AND INHIBITION

T. Heinonen
Tampere University of Technology, Finland

ABSTRACT

The mortality rate resulting from atherosclerosis is a large enough incentive to continue research efforts toward disease prevention and treatment. But the stakes are raised when one considers the enormous burden placed on society as a result of lost productivity and health care expenditure. The complexities of atherosclerosis pathophysiology are numerous and new facets continue to unfold at a rapid pace. Following the completion of several landmark trials over the past decades, the importance of altering lipid metabolism through the inhibition of HMG-CoA reductase has been demonstrated. The role of cholesterol absorption, has also led to the development of cholesterol absorption inhibitors which add to the portfolio of effective medications in the fight against coronary artery disease. Other metabolic pathways and factors are currently being explored which include cholesterol ester transfer protein (CETP), microsomal transfer protein (MTP), peroxisome proliferator-activated receptor (PPAR), and Acyl coenzymeA: cholesterol acyltransferase (ACAT). Excess cholesterol is stored as cholesteryl ester (CE) through an esterification process regulated in part by ACAT. The ACAT enzyme is found in many tissues types which require the storage of cholesterol. Since cholesterol is both an essential building block, but also a risk factor for cardiovascular a clear understanding of the role of ACAT in human metabolism is important. While cholesterol is an essential component of steroid, hormones, bile acids, and cellular membranes, high levels of serum cholesterol increases the deposition in the arterial wall. Most notably for cardiovascular disease ACAT activity is significant in intestinal and hepatic tissue and arterial macrophages. ACAT has been evaluated in cell cultures, experimental animal models and clinical trials for several decades. Much information has been gained regarding the contribution of this enzyme and it continues to be evaluated as a potential target for therapeutic intervention. Several ACAT inhibitors have been investigated for their potential to favorably alter serum lipoprotein levels by blocking intestinal absorption, hepatic inhibition and/or slow the progression of atherosclerosis through a non-lipid arterial inhibition. However, no ACAT inhibitor to date has proven to be a safe and effective therapy for the management of patients with atherosclerotic disease or at risk for cardiovascular events. Recent evaluations of ACAT and ACAT inhibitors have provided some insight into the therapeutic potential and risks of ACAT inhibition as a means of treating atherosclerosis.

INTRODUCTION

Atherosclerosis is a major contributor to coronary artery disease and stroke, which are currently the first and third highest causes of death in the United States. While the mortality rate resulting from atherosclerosis is a large enough incentive continue research efforts toward disease prevention and treatment, the stakes are raised when one considers the enormous burden placed on society as a result of lost productivity and health care expenditure. Atherosclerosis is often thought of as a disease of the "older" population, but evidence of atherosclerotic plaque formation is evident in the first decades of life. Atherosclerotic does not discriminate by race or gender, and is prevalent in all populations, particularly in developed and developing countries. As a result of the ubiquitous and chronic nature of atherosclerosis, as well as the persistently high incidence of cardiovascular morbidity and mortality, research efforts in this area remain vital. In recent years these efforts have changed our understanding of atherosclerosis significantly. A process which was once though of a static accumulation of fat in the arteries is now realized to be a very dynamic process in which numerous environmental, genetic, and individual factors contribute. Research which at one time focused almost exclusively on cholesterol metabolism has now branched out to provide further insight into the role other processes such as inflammatory contributors. A number of chemokines and cytokines involved in the inflammatory process have now been identified, and potential markers of disease progression and regression are under evaluation. Additionally, our ability to understand the process of atherosclerosis and the causative factors has gained sophistication with the experimental and clinical employment of various high-technology tools. These tools include the use of genomics, proteomics, the identification of soluble plasma markers, as well as imaging technologies such as quantitative coronary angiography, intravascular coronary and peripheral ultrasound, B-mode carotid ultrasound, positron emission tomography, computed tomography, and magnetic resonance imaging, to name a few.

The complexities of atherosclerosis pathophysiology are numerous and new facets continue to unfold at a rapid pace. In adolescence, atherosclerosis begins with the accumulation of lipids. This accumulation appears to be regulated by several different factors including plasma lipoprotein concentrations, blood pressure, vascular tone, and anatomical location. Injury to the endothelium, may then accelerate the rate of lipid deposition in the wall of the artery and contribute to the subsequent risk of cardiovascular disease. The artery wall is made of three main structural layers: the intima, media, and adventitia. The intima consists of a single layer of endothelial cells, connective tissue, and some smooth muscle cells. The endothelial layer maintains vascular tone, helps metabolize plasma lipids, and regulates the thrombotic and inflammatory processes. The media is the middle layer and contains mainly smooth muscle cells which are responsible for vasoconstriction and vasodilation. The outer layer, the adventitia, consists of fibroelastic tissue, vessels, and nerves and acts as the protective covering. Disruption of the structure and/or function of the vascular wall can predispose to major cardiovascular events such as myocardial infarction, stroke or sudden cardiac death.

Atherosclerotic lesions are categorized as Types I-VI, depending on the development stage and complexity. Type I lesions are those in which lipids have just started to accumulate. Lipid accumulation within the arterial wall primarily results from the transportation of cholesterol by low-density lipoprotein (LDL). Accumulating cholesterol may also be removed from the arterial wall by high-density lipoprotein (HDL) through a process known as reverse cholesterol transport. Lipid accumulation triggers an inflammatory response which then furthers the accumulation of lipids and initiates a set of reactions which may lead to luminal obstruction or plaque rupture. Type II lesions are also known as fatty streaks. These lesions are visible to the naked eye and are located on the intimal surface. Type II lesions consist of lipid-laden macrophages or "foam cells". Type III lesions are those which have further progressed to the point of extracellular lipid accumulation and cause a disruption of the normal intimal structure. Type IV and V lesions have advanced to the stage of significant lipid accumulation, and more extensive disruption of the intimal architecture. Complicated, or Type VI lesions are those which have developed fissures, ulcerations, hematomas, hemorrhages and thrombi. Atherosclerotic lesions which are Type III-VI can lead to an array of clinical symptoms depending on location, severity, and other factors. These symptoms include chest pain, or angina due to myocardial ischemia, leg pain, or claudication due to ischemia of peripheral skeletal muscle, transient ischemic attacks, stroke, myocardial infarction, or cardiac death.

Research findings continue to build additional layers in the scaffolding of our understand ding as the role of lipids, lipoproteins and inflammatory processes in atherosclerotic disease become more evident. With the continuous refinement of research tools such as genetic engineered experimental animal models, diagnostic sciences, and imaging technologies, we are better able to unravel some of the remaining mystery. One avenue of research that has benefited from advancements in technology is in the area of cholesterol metabolism and foam cell formation. A variety of enzymes are now known to be involved in cholesterol metabolism. One enzyme, 3-hydroxy-3-methylglutaryl coenzyme A (HMG-CoA) has been identified as a key enzyme in intracellular cholesterol synthesis. Inhibition of HMG-CoA with the class of drugs known as the statins has been extensively studied. Inhibiton of intracellular HMG-CoA reductase results in the expression of more LDL receptors. Since hepatic LDL receptors function to promote the clearance of LDL from plasma, statins are effective agents used primarily for the reduction of LDL cholesterol. The statins are now very broadly used to reduce LDL-cholesterol in people at risk for coronary artery disease and their evaluation in clinical trials continues.

Acyl coenzymeA: cholesterol acyltransferase (ACAT) is another enzyme involved in cholesterol metabolism. ACAT catalyzes the conversion of free cholesterol and fatty acyl CoA to the storage form of cholesterol, cholesteryl ester (CE). ACAT is believed to be a key enzyme involved in the production and secretion of cholesterol as well as in the storage of cholesterol in lipid-laden macrophages or "foam cells". ACAT has been evaluated in cell cultures, experimental animal models and clinical trials for several decades. Much information has been gained regarding the contribution of this enzyme and it continues to be evaluated as a potential target for therapeutic intervention. However, no ACAT inhibitor to date has proven to be a safe and effective therapy for the management of patients with atherosclerotic disease or at risk for cardiovascular events. This review aims to outline the role of ACAT in lipid metabolism and atherosclerosis pathogenesis and to review results of studies designed to assess the effects of ACAT inhibition on slowing atherosclerosis progression.

ACAT OVERVIEW

Mouse tissue expression studies and the disruption of the mouse ACAT gene have demonstrated that two forms of ACAT exist in humans and other mammals [1]. The first ACAT gene, which was cloned in 1993 [2] is now designated ACAT-1. The ACAT-1 protein has been shown to be highly expressed in human atherosclerotic lesions and is predominantly expressed in macrophages. Involvement of ACAT-1 in the development of human atheroma are supported by studies which have shown that when monocytes spontaneously differentiate into macrophages, ACAT-1 protein content increases by up to 10-fold. This result demonstrating an increase in ACAT-1 protein coinciding with the monocyte differentiation process [3] suggests an important role for this enzyme isoform. ACAT-1 appears to contain two types of sterol binding sites [4]. One of the sterol binding sites is an ACAT-1 activator site. This site appears to be relatively selective for cholesterol. The second sterol binding site is the ACAT-1 substrate site. This substrate site has been shown to utilize a variety of sterols as substates. The second characterized mammalian ACAT enzyme, designated ACAT -2, is 44% identical to the ACAT-1 in the mouse [5]. ACAT-2 is expressed primarily in mouse liver and small intestine, as well as the liver and intestines of primates [6] supporting the hypothesis that ACAT-2 contributes at least in part to the esterification of cholesterol in these tissues. ACAT-2 has a configuration that most likely places the active site in the lumen of the endoplasmic reticulum [6]. This orientation of ACAT-2 in the endoplasmic reticular membrane, in addition to its selective expression in liver and intestine, suggests that this enzyme may primarily function to promote the formation of cholesteryl esters into apolipoprotein (apo) B-containing lipoproteins. This hypothesis has been supported by evaluations of ACAT and ACAT inhibitors in cell cultures, animal models and clinical trials.

ACAT – A POTENTIAL DUAL ROLE IN ATHEROSCLEROSIS

Lipids and lipoproteins have been known to have an important role in the development and progression of atherosclerotic disease. Lipids are essential for normal cell structure and function, and can be classified as cholesterol and triglycerides. Most of the body's cholesterol is produced in the liver, but some is absorbed from the diet by the small intestines. While cholesterol is an essential component of steroid, hormones, bile acids, and cellular membranes, high levels of serum cholesterol increases the deposition in the arterial wall. Cholesterol is deposited in the arterial wall in the form of cholesteryl ester and contributes to the formation of atherosclerotic plaques. Triglyceride, on the other hand, does not accumulate in the arterial wall. However high levels of triglyceride and triglyceride containing lipoprotein particles have been associated with increased development of atherosclerotic plaque. Lipids, which are not water soluble, are transported throughout the body by attaching to proteins called apolipoproteins. The resulting lipoproteins are a heterogeneous mix of particles composed of a core of triglycerides and/or cholesterol esters and surrounded by a layer of phospholipids and apolipoproteins. Lipoproteins are commonly classified according to density and size as chylomicrons, very low-density lipoproteins (VLDL), intermediate-density lipoproteins (IDL), low-density lipoproteins (LDL) and high-density lipoprotoens (HDL).

Chylomicrons, which are the largest of the lipoproteins, consist primarily of triglycerides. Chylomicrons function to transport dietary cholesterol and triglycerides from the small intestine to the liver. VLDL is the second largest lipoprotein and also consists primarily of triglycerides. VLDL and chylomicron remnants can contribute to foam cell formation and atherosclerotic plaque progression. However, most of human cholesterol is contained within LDL particles. LDL transports cholesterol from the liver to other tissues and has also been identified as a strong risk factor in the development of atherosclerotic disease. HDL particles which are the smallest lipoprotein particles function in part to transport cholesterol from the body tissues back to the liver for processing, and therefore may be protective against atherosclerotic disease.

With the completion of several landmark trials over the past decades, the importance of altering lipid metabolism through the inhibition of HMG-CoA reductase has been demonstrated. The role of cholesterol absorption, has also led to the development of cholesterol absorption inhibitors which add to the portfolio of effective medications in the fight against coronary artery disease. Other metabolic pathways and factors are currently being explored which include cholesterol ester transfer protein (CETP), microsomal transfer protein (MTP), and peroxisome proliferators-activated receptor (PPAR). These proteins and receptors are being evaluated to better understand factors important in the pathophysiology of atherosclerotic disease and also as potential targets for drug therapy. Due to its role in the absorption, storage, and production of lipids, ACAT has been explored as a potential target for pharmacologic intervention. Additionally, since the role of the macrophage as a promoter, and instigator of plaque formation, has rightfully gained much attention over the last few years the direct role of ACAT in plaque progression and stabilization is being persistently examined.

Lipid Metabolism

ACAT-2 is the enzyme responsible for converting free cholesterol to cholesteryl ester in the intestine and liver. Conversion of free cholesterol to cholesteryl ester is believed to be essential for the intestinal absorption of cholesterol. Similarly, the conversion of free cholesterol to cholesterol ester through the actions of ACAT-2 is believed to be essential for the production and secretion hepatic VLDL particles. Since VLDL particles are metabolized to LDL particles, ACAT-2 is believed to play a role in plasma concentrations of both of these apoB containing lipoproteins. Much has been learned about the role of ACAT in lipid metabolism through the evaluation of compounds known to inhibit ACAT in the intestine and liver. Not all ACAT inhibitors have demonstrated equivalent effects on intestinal and hepatic ACAT, but rather appear to be selective based on a variety of factors. The relative contribution of ACAT inhibitors on these two tissues may be a function of bioavailability, tissue selectivity, or the interrelationship between these areas of plasma lipid regulation. The pharmacological effect of the ACAT inhibitor, YM17E (Yamanouchi Pharmaceutical Co. Ltd., Japan) could be explained by differences in plasma concentrations after oral or intravenous administration with increased plasma concentrations resulting in a shift from the small intestinal to hepatic ACAT inhibition [7]. In contrast, when the effects of a selective intestinal ACAT inhibitor, EAB309 (Mitsubishi Chemical, Japan), were studied in cholesterol-fed rats, results demonstrated that EAB309 significantly suppressed both intestinal and hepatic CE output and stimulated chylomicron removal. These findings suggest that the inhibition of intestinal ACAT can subsequently suppress hepatic ACAT by decreasing the delivery of cholesteryl ester to the liver [8]. Furthermore, studies with the ACAT inhibitor YIC-708-424 in rats suggest that the metabolic stability of ACAT inhibitors in the liver and intestine has a strong influence on their pharmacological activities in vivo [9]. Differences in metabolic stability, bioavailability, the relative contribution of these pathways, and the interrelationship between these pathways may explain some of the seemingly disparate clinical results currently reported.

Cholesterol Absorption

One function of the ACAT enzyme is to facilitate intestinal cholesterol absorption. Chylomicron formation requires the esterification of dietary cholesterol within the mucosal cells [10] and the role of ACAT in regulating this process has been firmly established [11-14]. Studies of ACAT-2 have demonstrated that this enzyme has a strong preference for cholesterol over the plant sterol sitosterol in cholesterol loaded and sitosterol loaded microsomes containing ACAT. This preference may reflect a role in sorting dietary sterols during intestinal absorption [15]. ACAT inhibitors have demonstrated significant cholesterol-absorption characteristics in animal studies, but their subsequent inability to significantly modify lipids in clinical trials has been disappointing. The effects of ACAT inhibition on the esterification of cholesterol has been studied using CaCo-2 cells derived from a human colonic adenocarcinoma cell line which is useful for studying hormonal control of lipid metabolism in enterocytes. CaCo2 cells were used to evaluate the effects of the ACAT inhibitor CL277082 on apoB48 secretion. Results from experiments suggest that apoB48 secretion may regulated by ACAT since ACAT inhibition significantly attenuated apoB48 secretion under basal and stimulatory conditions by a mechanism which enhanced apoB48 degradation [16]. Another supportive piece of information comes from the evaluation of the areca nut, which is grown in Southeast Asia. Areca nut extract has been found to lower the absorption of dietary cholesterol ester. When areca nut extract was administered to an experimental rat model, it was found to also decrease intestinal ACAT activity. The effect of this extract on dietary absorption of cholesterol and on intestinal ACAT activity further suggests a link ACAT and cholesterol absorption [17].

Studies evaluating the ACAT inhibitors CL277082 (American Cyanamid Co, USA) and CP113818 (CV Therapeutics, USA) determined that the uptake of cholesterol from bile salt mixed-micelles was not regulated by cellular ACAT, but that the subsequent esterification of exogenous sterol was completely dependent on ACAT activity [18]. This dissociation of cholesterol uptake from ACAT activity suggests that the factors controlling the transfer of sterol from extracelular media to the cell are different from the factors regulating the cellular level of cholesterol esterification. Additionally, the effect of the ACAT inhibitor, avasimibe (CI-1011, Pfizer Inc., USA) on clearance of postprandial triglyceride-rich lipoproteins was examined using miniature pigs [19]. Following an oral fat load, avasimibe significantly increased triglyceride-rich lipoprotein clearance which appeared to have decreased hepatic VLDL by decreasing the competition for its removal.

The importance of ACAT regulation within the intestinal cells in humans has been dfficult to determine. In a separate study designed to clarify the relationship between ACAT-2 gene mutations and hyperlipidemia in humans, a single nucleotide polymorphism (SNP) in the ACAT-2 gene was identified. The presence of this ACAT-2 SNP in subjects did not affect plasma concentration of lipids or apolipoproteins in either hypercholesterolemic or normaolipidemic subjects suggesting that the ACAT-2 gene may not substantially affect lipid levels in humans [20]. Overall, mechanistic studies in this area have demonstrated that ACAT does play a role in cholesterol absorption, but the importance of this role in humans has yet remains uncertain.

Hepatic Cholesterol Production

ACAT is an important enzyme in the production of hepatic cholesterol. One recent piece of evidence supporting the role of ACAT in hepatic cholesterol production comes from an evaluation of a rat model of chronic renal failure. Chronic renal failure is associated with profound abnormalities of lipid metabolism and accelerated atherosclerosis. A study of rats with chronic renal failure and exhibiting marked hyertriglyceridemia and modest hypercholesterolemia had significant up-regulation of hepatic tissue ACAT-2 protein and mRNA abundance. This up-regulation of ACAT expression and activity may contribute to the associated lipid disorders in this model, and may also explain the lipid disorder in humans with chronic renal failure. Given this association between chronic renal failure and ACAT, further research in this area is warranted [21]. Also of interest is the hypothesis that increased ACAT activity may contribute to the disregulation of cholesterol metabolism and increased risk of atherosclerosis associated with diabetes. O'Rourke et al. demonstrated in cultured macrophages that in the presence of glucose, both insulin and leptin caused a significant increase in ACAT activity [22], again outlining the possible role of ACAT in the metabolic abnormalities associated with a disease which carries high risk for atherosclerotic cardiovascular disease.

ACAT appears to be necessary for the full development and secretion of apoB containing lipoproteins in the liver. In cultured human HepG2 cells, the ACAT inhibitor, avasimibe was evaluated for its effects on apoB secretion. Results demonstated that the additiona of avasimibe resulted in a decreased secretion of apo B and its associated lipoproteins and a concomitant accumulation of secretion incompetent apoB in HepG2 cells [23]. When apoB kinetic studies were carried out in cholesterol-fed miniature pigs treated with avasimibe, treatment significantly decreased the VLDL apoB pool size and the hepatic secretion rate of VLDL apoB, but did not alter its fractional catabolism [24]. Results suggest inhibition of hepatic ACAT reduces both plasma VLDL and LDL apoB concentrations, primarily by decreasing apoB secretion. Further evaluations indicate that the mechanism for decreased apoB secretion involved enhanced intracellular degradation of apoB [25].

The hepatic effects of ACAT inhibition have also been evaluated through evaluations of bile acid and bile acid synthesis. In one experiment, the effect of ACAT inhibition with avasimibe on bile acid synthesis and cholesterol 7alpha-hydroxylase was evaluated using cultured rat hepatocytes and rats fed different diets [26]. Hepatocytes treated with avasimibe showed a shift from storage and secretion of cholesteryl esters to conversion of cholesterol into bile acids. A potential concern has been that ACAT inhibition would result in increased lithogenicity of bile. However in this trial of avasimibe, no increase in the ratio of biliary excreted cholesterol to bile acids was found, indicating that ACAT inhibition does not result increased lithogenicity. Further evaluations demonstrate that avasimibe increases bile acid synthesis in cultured hepatocytes by enhancing the supply of free cholesterol both as substrate and inducer of cholesterol 7alpha-hydroxylase. These results demonstrate the complex role of ACAT in lipid regulation and may partially explain the cholesterol-lowering effects of ACAT inhibitors.

While some agents which have been developed for their ACAT inhibitory properties, have demonstrated an ability to alter plasma cholesterol levels, other agents which have first demonstrated an ability to lower plasma cholesterol levels have subsequently demonstrated ACAT inhibitory activity. For these agents, it has been proposed that the ACAT effects has been partially responsible for the lipid-lowering effects. For example, SMP-500 (Sumitomo, Japan) reduces total serum cholesterol, hepatic free cholesterol, and hepatic esterified cholesterol content in animal models through the inhibition of ACAT and potentially another mechanism [27, 28]. Several flavenoids and soya-derived phytoestrogens which have demonstrated hypocholesterolemic properties also inhibit ACAT expression and activity [29-32]. While these agents have demonstrated an effect on other enzymes involved in lipid metabolism such as MTP and HMG-CoA, the effect on ACAT is an interesting one. Fish oil has also demonstrated ACAT inhibitory properties and this has been proposed as a possible mechanism for its effect on decreasing in VLDL production and secretion [33].

Foam Cell Formation and Atherosclerotic Lesions

The high levels of ACAT-1 present in cultured macrophages may account for the high level of ACAT-1 measured in atherosclerotic lesions. Data now supports the hypothesis that ACAT-1 plays an important role in differentiating monocytes and in forming foam cells during the development of human atherosclerosis [34]. Additionally, ACAT appears to have a pivotal role in the storage and release of cholesterol within foam cells and ACAT inhibitors have recently demonstrated an ability to limit lipid storage in human macrophages [35]. Studies evaluating the ACAT inhibitor HL-004 (TS-962, Taisho, Japan) in macrophages and foam cells from aortic intima of high cholesterol fed rabbits demonstrate that HL-004 suppresses the synthesis of cholesterol and decreases cholesterol ester content in foam cells [36]. These data suggested that ACAT inhibition can decreases cholesterol ester in foam cells by increasing the release of cholesterol. The exact mechanism by which ACAT inhibitors promote the removal of cholesterol from the macrophages located in the atherosclerotic plaque is yet unknown, but one hypothesis is that free cholesterol becomes more available for removal by HDL [37].

Since ACAT inhibitors have historically demonstrated remarkably good lipid-regulating abilities in animal models, it has been challenging at times to separate lipid effects from direct anti-atherosclerotic effects. A few carefully designed studies have now demonstrated ACAT inhibitors ability to reduce atherogenesis independent of their cholesterol-lowering effects. Evaluations of at least four ACAT inhibitors, avasimibe, F1394 (Fujirebio, Japan), R-755 (Nihon Nohyaku, Japan), and KV-2920 have demonstrated direct antiatherosclerotic activity.

Treatment of ApoE3-Leiden mice with avasimibe resulted in reduced monocyte adherence to the endothelium and lesion severity which were independent of lipid changes [38]. Avasimibe has also demonstrated independent anti-atherosclerotic effects in the fat fed hamsters, [39] and hyperlipidemic rabbit models [40]. Apolipoprotein E-deficient mice treated with the ACAT inhibitor, F-1394 showed a decreased lesional area and reduced lesional immunostaining for macrophages as compared with controls with no obvious signs of systemic or vessel wall toxicity [41, 42]. F-1394 also reduced the extent of atherosclerotic lesions as well as the total and esterified cholesterol in lesions without effecting serum total cholesterol levels in cholesterol fed rabbits [43]. In a separate study, F-1394 reduced neointimal thickening and macrophage involvement without having an effect on serum cholesterol. This affect indicates a possible utility of ACAT inhibition in the treatment of restenosis following percutaneous transluminal coronary angioplasty (PTCA) [44]. In rabbits with pre-established aortic atherosclerosis, administration of the ACAT inhibitor R-755 resulted in a tendency for a dose-dependent reduction in the surface area of atherosclerotic involvement and cholesterol content in the thoracic aorta and abdominal aorta, in the absence of a significant effect on plasma total cholesterol [45]. KV-2920-human LDL complex was injected into atherogenic mice resulting in significant decreases in CE content of aorta despite no change in serum cholesterol levels [46]. Finally, taurine, which has hypocholesterolemic effects and anti-atherosclerotic properties has been evaluated in Watanabe heritable hyperlipidemic rabbits (WHHL). Treatment with taurine in this model resulted in a significant decrease in ACAT activity as well as an anti-atherosclerotic effect as demonstrated by decreases in CE content of vessel walls and decreased intimal thickening, in the absence of any apparent effect on blood pressure and serum cholesterol levels [47].

These histologically measured improvements in the plaque burden may result in physiologic improvements. ACAT inhibition has demonstrated beneficial effects on vascular function in rabbits with dietary hypercholesterolemia, with results supporting a decrease in the vascular oxygen free-radical generation and improvements in endothelium-dependent vascular relaxation [48]. This finding suggests that noninvasive measures of endothelial function may be applied to clinical trials designed to assess the efficacy of various ACAT inhibitors.

Inflammation and Plaque Stability

The ACAT enzyme has been measured in several cellular sites including a cytoplasmic reticular/nuclear membrane site, a perinuclear cytoplasmic site, and a cell-surface site in non-attached macrophages.[49]. Therefore it is possible that there are some physiological differences between ACAT in these locations and that they may have different roles in cholesterol regulation and macrophage foam cell formation. There is also new evidence that ACAT inhibition promotes lesion stability by limiting macrophage enrichment and thereby a source of matrix metalloproteinases (MMP) in addition to promoting atherosclerotic lesion regression. Since sudden cardiac death in asymptomatic patients accounts for nearly a third of all cardiac deaths, the prevention of plaque rupture is an important consideration for therapeutic targeting and a clarified understanding of ACAT's role in this process is important.

In male New Zealand white rabbits fed a cholesterol/fat diet and treated with avasimibe, an examination of the iliac-femoral artery revealed a decreased monocyte-macrophage content and reduced macrophage/lesion ratio [40]. Within the aortic arch, catalytic activity of latent and active MMP-1,-3 and-9 were significantly reduced. Therefore ACAT inhibition appears to directly limit macrophage accumulation and potentially stabilize pre-established atherosclerotic lesions by reducing MMP expression within the lesion. The anti-atherosclerotic properties of F 12511 were studies in rabbits with endogenous hypercholesterolemia and an induced endothelial injury. Administration of F 12511 produced a 50% reduction in total plasma cholesterol, a 50% reduction in incidence of lesions, decreased macrophage accumulation, and increase in smooth muscle cells suggesting that ACAT inhibition may result in lesion stability [50]. In an experiment designed to ascertain the role of cholesteryl ester pathways in human vascular smooth muscle cell cycle progression, Batetta et al. demonstrated that serum induced vascular smooth muscle cell proliferation was preceded by an increased ability of cells to esterify cholesterol and an increased expression of ACAT [51].

Combination ACAT Inhibition and HMG Co-A Reductase Inhibition

Since HMG-CoA reductase inhibitors have clearly demonstrated significant efficacy while maintaining a high safety profile, the evaluation of ACAT inhibition with HMG-CoA reducatase inhibition is important for possible combination therapy. Combination therapy has now been evaluated in cell cultures, in animal models of atherosclerotic disease progression and regression, and using histopathological an non-invasive imaging techniques – all with encouraging results.

One of the earliest evaluations of this combination in animal models was a study of the effects of the ACAT inhibitor, CI-976 (Pfizer, Inc, USA) and Lipitor (atorvastatin, Pfizer Inc., USA) in cholesterol-fed rabbits [52]. With co-administration, plasma total cholesterol levels as well as liver cholesterol ester content were reduced more significantly than with either treatment alone. Indices of atherosclerotic progression (lesion CE content, lesion area, macrophage content) were also more significantly reduced with coadministration than with either alone suggesting that inhibition of HMG-CoA reductase and ACAT acts synergistically to lower plasma total cholesterol and to limit the development of atherosclerotic lesions. Using another ACAT inhibitor, eflucimibe (F 12511, Lilly, USA and bioMerieux-Pierre Fabre, France), Junquero et al. subsequently demonstrated in rabbits with pre-established endogenous hypercholesterolemia, that co-administration of eflucimibe and atorvastatin lowered plasma total cholesterol and apo B-100 containing lipoproteins to a greater extent and more rapidly than either agent alone. [53].

Combination ACAT and HMG-CoA reductase inhibitors were evaluated in a rabbit model of atherosclerosis progression. Despite similar changes in plasma total and lipoprotein cholesterol exposure and lipoprotein composition, co-administration of avasimibe and Zocor (simvastatin, Merck, USA) had a more significant effect on decreasing lesion progression, and also promoted the regression of pre-established atherosclerotic lesions [54]. A recent study by Worthley et al. has provided further evidence of the utility of this combination therapy while also providing some additional support for non-invasive methods of lesion evaluation [55]. In this trial, the effects atorvastatin in combination with avasimibe in Watanabe Heritable Hyperlipidaemic (WHHL) rabbits were examined. The effects of the different treatments on atherosclerotic lesion progression were assessed by magnetic resonance imaging (MRI) and histopathology using vessel wall area as a surrogate of atherosclerotic burden. The combination of atorvastatin and avasimibe induced a significant regression of the previously established lesions with excellent agreement between MRI and histopathology assessments. These important findings not only confirm that ACAT inhibition is a potent addition to statin therapy for the regression of atherosclerotic but demonstrates that the changes can be measured serially and noninvasively with MRI. These studies lend credence to the hypothesis that ACAT inhibiton and HMG-CoA reductase inhibition are complementary and may represent a better approach to prevent atherosclerotic disease progression (Figure 2).

POTENTIAL RISKS

Adrenal Toxicity

The alteration of any enzume system always raises concern about adverse affects of such alteration. Early studies of ACAT unveiled concerns about adrenal toxicity. It was hypothesized that by inhibiting ACAT, intracellular free-cholesterol levels would increase to levels no longer supporting cell viability [56]. In early studies, cholesterol-enriched mouse peritoneal macrophages incubated with ACAT inhibitors resulted in an increase in cell toxicity that paralled an increase in the cellular free-cholesterol content. Subsequent studies in 1998, by Kellner-Weibel et al. supported this finding [57] while later studies by Rodriguez have not [58, 59].

Interestingly, the adrenal toxicity of an ACAT inhibitor, FR 145237 (Fujisawa, Japan), was investigated using Japanese White (normal) and low density lipoprotein (LDL) receptor deficient Watanabe heritable hyperlipidemic (WHHL) rabbits. In the normal rabbits, severe necrosis of the cells in the zona fasciculate and reticularis was observed 24 hr after intravenous injection whereas no morphological changes could be found in the adrenal cells of the WHHL rabbits in spite of a higher plasma concentration of the drug [60]. These results suggest that the susceptibility of the adrenal cells differ between models and possibly species. Using a human cell line which has functional properties comparable to those of normal human adrenal cells, incubation with eflucimibe at concentrations well exceeding the IC 50 did not impair steroid production nor transcription of genes involved in steroidogenesis and lipoprotein uptake [61]. Results from other studies have suggested that adrenal toxicity observed with ACAT inhibitors may not be mechanism related [62] and that liver ACAT may be distinct from the adrenal counterpart [63].

The preclinical safety and toxicokinetics of avasimibe have been reported. Avasimibe was assessed in beagle dogs in an escalating-dose study of up to 52-weeks duration. Adrenal effects were noted only in the 52-week study and consisted of minimal to mild cortical cytoplasmic vacuolization and fibrosis [64]. While the question of adrenal toxicity certainly has not been fully addressed, evidence suggests that it is not a class effect. The safety and tolerability of individual ACAT inhibitors should best be determined by the careful evaluation of properly conducted toxicological evaluations and clinical trials.

Drug Interactions

Since any new developing therapy for atherosclerosis would be administeredto a population already treated with numerous other medications, interactions between new and existing agents must be carefully evaluated. Only avasimibe has reported drug-interation clinical trial data. In normal volunteers, administration of avasimibe resulted in a 3 and 8 fold reduction in levels of midazolam, suggesting a dose-dependent induction of cytochrome P450 3A4 activity [65]. Typically cytochrome P450 induction is less worrisome that inhibition since induction results in decreased exposure to agents metabolized by this pathway while inhibition results in increased exposure and possible toxicity. Since this enzyme system is responsible for the metabolism of many currently available drugs, including those frequently used in patients with coronary artery disease, an investigational drug which results in significant alterations in either direction may be problematic. However a drug that is administered chronically, may pose less of a burden. Reported data from a Phase II clinical trial in which patients have received avasimibe and other agents concomitantly have demonstrated an acceptable safety profile [66]. Data from additional clinical trials are expected to provide further insight into whether or not drug interactions will be a barrier for this and/or other ACAT inhibitors.

Accumulation of Unesterified Cholesterol

Results from a recently published evaluation of the effects of selective ACAT-1 deficiency in two mouse models of atherosclerosis have raised concern about a possible detrimental effect of ACAT inhibition. In the setting of severe hypercholesterolemia caused by deficiency in apoE or the LDL receptor, total ACAT-1 deficiency led to marked alterations in cholesterol homeostasis and extensive deposition of unesterified cholesterol in the skin and brain of the evaluated mice, without a beneficial effect on atherosclerotic lesions [67]. These results were evident despite lower serum cholesterol levels. Additionally, Perrey et al. reported in April 2001 that when selective macrophage ACAT inhibitors were tested in models of atherosclerosis (Fat-fed C57BL/6 mice, chow fed apo E-/- mice and KHC rabbits) the ACAT inhibitors either had no effect or increased indices of athoerosclerotic foam cell formation, possibly due to augmented free cholesterol [68]. These results suggest that inhibition of macrophage ACAT may actually aggravate atherosclerotic disease progression. Again, potential benefits and risks of individual ACAT inhibitors need to be carefully measured in long-term clinical trials.

CLINICAL TRIALS

As with all potential new therapies, clinical trial results will provide the essential information needed to determine whether or not ACAT inhibition should be included in future treatment strategies. The only ACAT inhibitor currently approved for use (Japan) is melinamide (Artes, Sumitomo Pharmaceuticals Co., Japan) and indicated for hyperchlesterolemia as a cholesterol absorption inhibitor. Melinamide inhibits cholesterol esterase and ACAT and it is thought that the gastrointestinal absorption of dietary cholesterol and reabsorption of cholesterol in the enterohepatic circulation are inhibited by these mechanisms [69]. The most frequent adverse events in clinical trials and in studies of post-approval use were gastrointestinal in nature (diarrhea, abdominal pain, and anorexia). Other adverse events occurring with an incidence of <5% include elevated liver enzymes, headache, dizziness, rash, pruritus, constipation and hot flashes. In clinical trials including over 700 subjects with hypercholesterolemia approximately 40% showed decreases in total serum cholesterol of 15% or more.

Few other ACAT inhibitors have been fully evaluated in clinical trials. Most of the ACAT inhibitors that have been evaluated in clinical trials have been discontinued due to disappointing lipid results. A few agents are currently reported to be in Phase II or III clinical development including KY-505 (Sankyo, Tokyo, Japan), F1394 (Fujirebio, Japan), eflucimibe (Lilly, USA and bioMerieux-Pierre-Fabre, France) and avasimibe (Pfizer, Inc., USA). Available clinical data from these trials is limited. In an 8-week multicenter trial involving 130 patients with combined hyperlipidemia and hypoalphalipoproteinemia, avasimibe treatment (50 – 500 mg/day capsules) significantly decreased plasma total TG and VLDL-C by 16-23% and 20-30% respectively, but a clear dose-response was not seen [66]. Plasma levels of TC, LDL-C, HDL-C, and apoB were unaffected. Another avasimibe clinical trial conducted in 27 patients with homozygous familial hypercholesterolemia demonstrated that avasimibe, when administered with atorvastatin, enhances the lipid-lowering properties of atorvastatin (22% vs. 18% LDL-C reduction, $p < .05$) [70]. Additionally, the co-administration of 750 mg avasimibe and 80 mg atorvastatin was well-tolerated over a 6-week treatment period. No clinical results have been reported for KY-505, F1394, or eflucimibe.

ALZHEIMER'S DISEASE

Although the primary focus of ACAT inhibitor development has been atherosclerosis, there is some new evidence that these agents may have utility in the treatment of Alzheimer's disease. A recently completed evaluation demonstrated that cholesteryl ester levels are correlated with the production of amyloid beta-peptide [71]. The researchers also demonstrate that ACAT inhibition modified the generation of amyloid beta-peptide, suggesting that these agents may have potential use in the treatment of Alzheimer's disease.

Conclusion

ACAT is the enzyme which catalyzes the conversion of free cholesterol and fatty acyl CoA to the storage form of cholesterol, cholesteryl ester. Excess cholesterol is stored as cholesteryl ester through an esterification process regulated in part by ACAT. Several ACAT inhibitors have been investigated for their potential to favorably alter serum lipoprotein levels by blocking intestinal absorption, hepatic inhibition and/or slow the progression of atherosclerosis through a non-lipid arterial inhibition. Evaluations of individual ACAT inhibitors have generally supported the hypothesis ACAT plays a significant role in cholesterol production, storage and subsequent atheroma formation and progression. Concerns about detrimental effects of ACAT inhibition including adrenal toxicity have persisted, and new concerns including drug-drug interactions and the promotion of atherosclerosis through the accumulation of free cholesterol have recently surfaced. Despite the number of ACAT inhibitors synthesized over the past several decades, with several ACAT inhibitors reported to be in Phase II – III development, clinical trial data remains sparse. Results from the ongoing clinical trials will need to be carefully evaluated in order to further understand the role of ACAT in human disease and to determine whether or not this line of investigation should continue to be pursued.

Few people would dispute that statins have made a major impact on our ability to treat and prevent coronary artery disease and that the primary mechanism by which statins are effective is lipid and lipoprotein lowering. However, regardless of its widespread use in risk assessment, plasma LDL-cholesterol is not the only factor that accounts for coronary disease progression and regression. The expectation that the next generation of anti-atherosclerotic drugs will be developed using a single, readily measured surrogate marker such as LDL-cholesterol may be a bit optimistic. Herein lies the challenge. ACAT inhibitors have not consistently demonstrated a significant lipid- or lipoprotein-lowering effect. Other possible soluble markers of inflammation and atherosclerosis progression have been identified which may be modified by new anti-atherosclerotic agents. However, despite remarkable progress in this area, clear and independent links between such markers and coronary artery disease still need to be strengthened to facilitate development of such direct anti-atherosclerotic agents. Other research efforts, directed at identifying clinically meaningful endpoints, using technologies such as intravascular and B-mode ultrasound, magnetic resonance imaging, positron emission tomography, computed tomographic imaging, and methods to assess total atherosclerotic burden and plaque vulnerability have increased the likelihood that such evaluations may facilitate the development of ACAT inhibitors. While the development of potentially anti-atherosclerotic agents such as ACAT inhibitors has and will continue to present challenges, coronary artery disease remains consistently prominent among the conditions responsible for morbidity and mortality worldwide. Therefore despite the magnitude of the developmental challenge, the reward of success should be even greater.

REFERENCES

[1] Oelkers P, Behari A, Cromley D, Billheimer Jt, Sturley Sl: Characterization of two human genes encoding acyl coenzyme A: Cholesterol acyltransferase-related enzymes. *J. Biol. Chem.* (1998) 273(41): 26765-26771.

[2] Chang CCY, Huh HY, Cadigan KM, Chang TY: Molecular cloning and functional expression of human acyl-coenzyme A-cholesterol acyltransferase cDNA in mutant Chinese hamster ovary cells. *J. Biol. Chem.* (1993) 268:20747-20755.

[3] Miyazaki A, Sakashita N, Lee O *et al.*: Expression of ACAT-1 protein in human atherosclerotic lesions and cultured human monocytes-macrophages. *Arterioscler. Thromb. Vasc. Biol.* (1998) 18(10): 1568-1574.

[4] Zhang Y, Yu C, Liu J, et al.: Cholesterol is superior to 7-ketocholesterol or 7 alpha-hydroxycholesterol as an allosteric activator for acyl-coenzyme A: cholesterol acyltransferase 1. J Biol Chem. 2003 Mar 28;278(13):11642-7.

[5] Cases S, Novak S, Zheng YW *et al.*: ACAT-2, a second mammalian acyl-CoA:cholesterol acyltransferase – Its cloning, expression, and characterization. *J. Biol. Chem.* (1998) 273(41):26755-26764.

[6] Anderson RA, Joyce C, Davis M *et al.*: Identification of a form of acyl-CoA:cholesterol acyltransferase specific to liver and intestine in nonhuman primates. *J. Biol. Chem.* (1998) 273(41): 26747-26754.

[7] Uchida T, Aoyama K, Watanabe T, Higuchi S: Relationship between bioavailability and hypocholesterolemic activity of YM17E, an inhibitor of ACAT, in cholesterol-fed rats. *Atherosclerosis* (1998) 137(1): 97-106.

[8] Umeda Y, Hirano T, Kako Y, Kamagata K, Okuyama K, Suzuki K: A selective inhibitor of intestinal ACAT, EAB309 suppresses both intestinal and hepatic cholesterol output and stimulates chylomicron removal. *Life Sci.* (1998) 63(13): 187-95.

[9] Ohishi K, Sawada H, Yoshida Y, et al. The Metabolic stability of acyl-coA:cholesterol 0-acyltransferase(ACAT) inhibitors, N-(4-Benzyloxy-3,5-dimethoxycinnamoyl)-N'-(2,4-dimethylphenyl)piperazine (YIC-708-424) and its derivatives in rat liver and intestinal epithelium. Biol Pharm Bull. 2003 May;26(5):600-7.

[10] Vahouny GV, Fawal I, Treadwell CR: Factors facilitating cholesterol absorption from the intestine via lymphatic pathways. *Am. J. Physiol.* (1957) 188: 742-746.

[11] Suckling KE, Stange EF: Role of acyl-CoA-cholesterol acyl-transferase in cellular cholesterol metabolism. *J. Lipid Res.* (1985) 26:647-671.

[12] Heider JG, Pickens CE, Kelly LA: Role of acyl CoA:cholesterol acyltransferase in cholesterol absorption and its inhibition of 57-118 in the rabbit. *J. Lipid Res.* (1983) 24:1127-1277.

[13] Bennett CS, Tercyak AM: Reduced cholesterol transmucosal transport in rats with inhibited mucosal acyl CoA:cholesterol acyltransferase and normal pancreatic function. (1984) *J Lipid Res.* 25:148-159.

[14] Largis EE, Wang CH, Devries VG, Schaffer SA: CL277082, a novel inhibitor of ACAT-catalyzed cholesterol esterification and cholesterol absorption. *J. Lipid Res.* (1989) 30:681-690.

[15] Temel RE, Gebre AK, Parks JS, Rudel LL. Compared to ACAT1 and LCAT, ACAT2 displays the greatest capacity to differentiate cholesterol from sitosterol. J Biol Chem. 2003 Sep 15.

[16] Pal S, Allister E, Thomson A, Mamo JC. Cholesterol esters regulate apoB48 secretion in CaCo2 cells. Atherosclerosis. 2002 Mar;161(1):55-63

[17] Park YB, Jeon SM, Byun SJ, Kim HS, Choi MS. Absorption of intestinalfree cholesterol is lowered by supplementation of Areca catechu L. extract in rats. Life Sci. 2002 Mar 8;70(16):1849-59.

[18] Ellsworth JL, Starr JR: Inhibition of acyl coenzyme A: cholesterol acyltransferase blocks esterification but not uptake of cholesterol in Caco-2 cells. *Metabolism* (1998) 47(3): 325-32.

[19] Burnett JR, Barrett PHR, Telford DE, Huff MW: The ACAT inhibitor avasimibe increases the fractional clearance rate of postprandial triglyceride-rich lipoproteins. *Atherosclerosis* (2000) 151:134 W16.

[20] Katsuren K, Fukuyama S, Takata K, Ohta T. Effects of a new single-nucleotide polymorphism in the Acyl-CoA:cholesterol acyltransferase-2 gene on plasma lipids and apolipoproteins in patients with hyperlipidemia. J Atheroscler Thromb. 2003;10(1):32-6.

[21] Liang K, Vaziri ND. Upregulation of acyl-CoA: cholesterol acyltransferase in chronic renal failure. Am J Physiol Endocrinol Metab. 2002 Oct;283(4):E676-81.

[22] O'Rourke L, Gronning LM, Yeaman SJ, Shepherd PR. Glucose-dependent regulation of cholesterol ester metabolism in macrophages by insulin and leptin. J Biol Chem. 2002 Nov 8;277(45):42557-62.

[23] Taghibiglou C, Van Iderstine S, Kulinski A, Rudy D, Adeli K: Intracellular Mechanisms Mediating the Inhibition of ApoB-Containing Lipoprotein Synthesis and Secretion in HepG2 Cells by avasimibe (CI-1011), a novel acyl-coenzyme A:cholesterol acyltransferase (ACAT) inhibitor. *Biochem. Pharmacol.* (2002) 63(3):349-360.

[24] Burnett JR, Wilcox LJ, Telford DE *et al.*: Inhibition of ACAT by avasimibe decreases both VLDL and LDL apolipoprotein B production in miniature pigs. *J. Lipid Res.* (1999) 40:1317-27.

[25] Wilcox LJ, Barrett PHR, Newton RS, Huff MW: ApoB 100 secretion from HepG2 cells is decreased by the ACAT inhibitor CI-1011: an effect associated with enhanced intracellular degradation of apoB. *Arterioscler. Thromb. Vasc. Biol.* (1999) 19:939-949.

[26] Post SM, Zoeteweij JP, Bos MHA *et al.*: Acyl-coenzyme A:cholesterol acyltransferase inhibitor, avasimibe, stimulates bile acid synthesis and cholesterol 7alpha-hydroxylase in cultured rat hepatocytes and in vivo in the rat. *Hepatology* (1999) 30(2):491-500.

[27] Ioriya K, Kino K, Sato YF, Ohashi N. Effect of SMP-500, a novel acyl-CoA:cholesterol acyltransferase inhibitor, on serum cholesterol level andLDL cholesterol clearance in hamsters with induced hyperlipidemia. Pharmacology. 2002 Oct;66(2):107-14.

[28] Ioriya K, Nishimura T, Ohashi N. Effect of SMP-500, a novel ACAT inhibitor, on hepatic cholesterol disposition in rats. Lipids. 2002 Apr;37(4):395-400.

[29] Borradaile NM, de Dreu LE, Barrett PH, Huff MW. Inhibition of hepatocyte apoB secretion by naringenin : enhanced rapid inracellular degradation independent of reduced microsomal cholesteryl esters. J Lipid Res. 2002 Sep;43(9):1544-54.

[30] Lee MK, Moon SS, Lee SE, et al. Naringenin 7-O-cetyl ether as inhibitor of HMG-CoA reductase and modulator of plasma and hepatic lipids in high cholesterol-fed rats. Bioorg Med Chem. 2003 Feb 6;11(3):393-8.

[31] Kim HK, Jeong TS, Lee MK, Park YB, Choi MS. Lipid-lowering efficacy of hesperetin metabolites in high-cholesterol fed rats. Clin Chim Acta. 2003 Jan;327(1-2):129-37.

[32] Borradaile NM, de Dreu LE, Wilcox LJ, Edwards JY, Huff MW. Soya phytoestrogens, genistein and daidzein, decrease apolipoprotein B secretion from HepG2 cells through multiple mechanisms. Biochem J. 2002 Sep 1;366(Pt 2):531-9.

[33] Botham KM, Zheng X, Napolitano M, et al. The effects of dietary n-3 polyunsaturated fatty acids delivered in chylomicron remnants on transcription of genes regulating the synthesis and secretion of very-low-density lipoprotein by the liver: modulation by cellular oxidative state. Exp Biol Med (Maywood). 2003 Feb;228(2):143-51.

[34] Miyazaki A, Sakashita N, Lee O *et al.*: Expression of ACAT-1 protein in human atherosclerotic lesions and cultured human monocytes-macrophages. *Arterioscler. Thromb. Vasc. Biol.* (1998) 18(10): 1568-1574.

[35] Rodriguez A, Wee SB, Usher DC: The acyl-CoA:Cholesterol acyltransferase inhibitor, avasimibe, effectively limits lipid storage in human macrophages. *Circulation* (1999)100(18):I613.

[36] Ishii I, Yokoyama N, Yanagimachi M *et al.*: Stimulation of cholesterol release from rabbit foam cells by the action of a new inhibitor for acyl CoA:cholesterol acyltransferase (ACAT), HL-004. *J. Pharmacol. Exp. Therap.* (1998) 287(1):115-121.

[37] Li L, Pownall HJ: Effects of high-density lipoprotein(2) on cholesterol transport and acyl-coenzyme A:cholesterol acyltransferase activity in P388D1 macrophages. *Biochem. Biophys. Acta* (2001) 1530 (1):111-122.

[38] Delsing DJM, Offerman EH, Van Duyvenvoorde W *et al.*: Acyl-CoA: Cholesterol acyltransferase inhibitor avasimibe reduces atherosclerosis in addition to its cholesterol-lowering effect in ApoE*3-Leiden mice. *Circulation.* (2001) 103:1778-1786.

[39] Nicolosi RJ, Wilson TA, Krause BR.: The ACAT inhibitor, CI-1011, is effective in the prevention and regression of aortic fatty streak area in hamsters. *Atherosclerosis* (1998) 137:77-85.

[40] Bocan TMA, Krause BR, Rosebury WS *et al.*: The ACAT inhibitor avasimibe reduces macrophages and matrix metalloproteinase expression in atherosclerotic lesions of hypercholesterolemic rabbits. *Arterioscler. Thromb. Vasc. Biol.* (2000) 20:70-79.

[41] Chiwata T, Aragane K, Fujinami K et al.: Direct effect of an acyl-CoA:cholesterol acyltransferase inhibitor, F-1394, on atherosclerosis in apolipoprotein E and low density lipoprotein receptor double knockout mice. *Br. J. Pharmacol.* (2001) 133(7):1005-1012.

[42] Kusunoki J, Hansoty DK, Aragane K, Falon JT, Badimon JJ, Fisher EA: Acyl-CoA:cholesterol acyltransferase inhibition reduces atherosclerosis in apolipoprotein E-deficient mice. *Circulation* (2001) 103(21):2604-2609.

[43] Aragane K, Kojima K, Fujinami K, Kamei J, Kusunoki J: Effect of F-1394, an acyl-CoA: cholesterol acyltransferase inhibitor, on atherosclerosis induced by high cholesterol diet in rabbits. *Atherosclerosis* (2001) 158(1) 139-145.

[44] Aragane K, Fujinami K, Kojima K, Kusunoki J: ACAT inhibitor F-1394 prevents intimal hyperplasia induced by balloon injury in rabbits. *J. Lipid Res.* (2001) 42(2) 480-488. This article describes a newly described effect of ACAT inhibition on preventing

intimal hyperplasia following balloon injury in an animal model of atherosclerotic disease.

[45] Matsui Y, Horiuchi K, Yamamoto K, Kanai K: Pharmacological properties of R-755, a novel acyl-CoA:cholesterol acyltransferase inhibitor, in cholesterol-fed rats, hamsters and rabbits. *Jpn. J. Pharmacol.* (2001) 5(4):423-433.

[46] Tauchi Y, Yoshimi A, Shirahase H, et al. Inhibitory effect of acyl-CoA:cholesterol acyltransferase inhibitor-low density lipoprotein complex on experimental atherosclerosis. Biol Pharm Bull. 2003 Jan;26(1):73-8.

[47] Murakami S, Kondo Y, Sakurai T, Kitajima H, Nagate T. Taurine suppresses development of atherosclerosis in Watanabe heritable hyperlipidemic (WHHL) rabbits. Atherosclerosis. 2002 Jul;163(1):79-87.

[48] Kurz S, Borthayre AB, Harrison DG: The effect of ACAT inhibition with avasimibe on vascular function in hypercholesterolemia. *Circulation* (1998) I109-I110 This study demonstrated a functional rather than histopathological improvement following exposure to an ACAT inhibitor.

[49] Khelef N, Buton X, Beatini N *et al.*: Immunolocalization of acyl-coenzyme A: Cholesterol O-acyltransferase in macrophages. *J. Biol.Chem.* (1998) 273(18): 11218-11224.

[50] Rival Y, Junquero D, Bruniquel F *et al.*: Anti-atherosclerotic properties of the acyl-coenzyme A:cholesterol acyltransferase inhibitor F 12511 in casein-fed New Zealand rabbits. *J. Cardiovasc. Pharmacol.* (2002) 39(2):181-191.

[51] Batetta B, Mulas MF, Sanna F, et al. Role of cholesterol ester pathway in the control of cell cycle in human aortic smooth muscle cells. FASEB J. 2003 Apr;17(6):746-8. Epub 2003 Feb 19.

[52] Bocan TMA, Mueller SB, Brown EQ *et al*: HMG-CoA reductase and ACAT inhibitors act synergistically to lower plasma cholesterol and limit atherosclerotic lesion development in the cholesterol-fed rabbit. *Atherosclerosis* (1998) 139(1):21-30.

[53] Junquero D, Bruniquel F, N'guyen X *et al.*: F 12511, a novel ACAT inhibitor, and atorvastatin regulate endogenous hypercholesterolemia in a synergistic manner in New Zealand rabbits fed a casein-enriched diet. *Atherosclerosis* (2001) 155(1):131-142.

[54] **Bocan TMA, Krause BR, Rosebury WS *et al.*: Inhibition of Both ACAT and HMG-CoA Reductase May Directly Induce Atherosclerotic Lesion Regression. *Atherosclerosis* (2001) 157(1):97-105. These study results demonstrate the benefit of coadministering an ACAT inhibitor and HMG-CoA reductase inhibitor in an animal model of atherosclerosis.

[55] **Worthley SG, Helft G, Osende JI et al.: Serial evaluation of atherosclerosis with in vivo MRI: Study of atorvastatin and avasimibe in WHHL rabbits. *Circulation* (2000)102:II809. This study provides evidence for non-invasive assessment of the anti-atherosclerotic effects of co-administration of atorvastatin and avasimibe.

[56] Warner GJ, Stoudt G, Bamberger M *et al.*: Cell toxicity induced by inhibition of acyl coenzyme A: cholesterol acyltransferase and accumulation of unesterified cholesterol. *J. Biol. Chem.* (1995) 270:5772-5778.

[57] Kellner-Weibel G, Jerone WG, Small DM *et al.*: Effects of intracellular free cholesterol accumulation on macrophage viability, a model for foam cell death. *Arterioscler. Thromb. Vasc. Biol.* (1998)18:423-431.

[58] Rodriguez A, Bachorik PS, Wee SB: Novel effects of the acyl-coenzyme A: cholesterol acyltransferase inhibitor 58-035 on foam cell development in primary human monocyte-derived macrophages. *Arterioscler. Thromb. Vasc. Biol.* (1999)19:2199-2206.

[59] Rodriguez A, Wee SK, Usher DC: The acyl-CoA: cholesterol acyltransferase inhibitor, avasimibe, effectively limits lipid storage in human macrophages. *Circulation* (1999) 100:613.

[60] Matsuo M, Hashimoto M, Suzuki J, Iwanami K, Tomoi M, Shimomura K: Difference between normal and WHHL rabbits in susceptibility to the adrenal toxicity of an acyl-CoA:cholesterol acyltransferase inhibitor, FR 145237. *Toxicol. Appl. Pharmacol.* (1996) 140 (2):387-392.

[61] Junquero D, Pilon A, Carilla-Durand E *et al.*: Lack of toxic effects of F 12511, a novel potent inhibitor of acyl-coenzyme A: cholesterol O-acyltransferase, on human adrenocortical cells in culture. *Biochem. Pharmacol.* (2001) 61(4):387-398.

[62] Sliskovic DR, Picard JA, O'brien PM *et al.*: Alpha-substituted malonester amides: tools to define the relationship between ACAT inhibition and adrenal toxicity. *J. Med. Chem.* (1998) 41(5): 682-90.

[63] Kawasaki T, Miyazaki A, Hakamata H, Matsuda H, Horiuchi S: Biochemical evidence for oligomerization of rat adrenal acyl-coenzyme A:cholesterol acyltransferase. *Biochem. Biophys. Res. Commun.* (1998) 244(2): 347-352.

[64] Robertson DG, Breider MA, Milad MA: Preclinical safety evaluation of avasimibe in beagle dogs: An ACAT inhibitor with minimal adrenal effects. *Toxicol. Sci.* (2001) 59:324-34.

[65] Milad MA, Stern R, Strenkoshki-Nix LC, Lathia CD. Dose dependent induction of oral midazolam metabolism by avasimibe. *Clin. Pharmacol. Ther.* (2000) 67(2):136.

[66] **Insull W, Koren M, Davignon J *et al.* Efficacy and short-term safety of a new ACAT inhibitor, avasimibe, on lipids, lipoproteins, and apolipoproteins, in patients with combined hyperlipidemia. *Atherosclerosis* (2001) 157: 137-144. This article describes the effects of the ACAT inhibitor, avasimibe, on lipid levels in pathients with combined hyperlipidemia. Signifidcant decdreases in VLDL-cholesterol and triglycerides were observed with no significant effect on other lipid fractions. A hepatic mechanism is proposed.

[67] *Accad M, Smith SJ, Newland DL *et al.:* Massive xanthomatosis and altered composition of atherosclerotic lesions in hyperlipidemic mice lacking acyl CoA:cholesterol acyltransferase. *J. Clin. Invest.* (2000) 105(6):711-719. This study demonstrates a pro-atherosclerotic effect in a genetically altered mouse model lacking ACAT.

[68] Perry S, Legendre C, Matsuura A et al.: Preferential pharmacological inhibition of macrophage ACAT increases plaque formation in mouse and rabbit models of atherogenesis. *Atherosclerosis* (2001) 155(2):359-370.

[69] Artes package insert.

[70] * *Klepack E, Raal FJ, Marais AD, Heinonen T: Effects of avasimibe in patients with severe hypercholesterolemia. Proceedings of the XIVth International Symposium on Drugs Affecting Lipid Metabolism (DALM), New York, USA (2001). Study results demonstrate a potential benefit of co-administering avasimibe and atorvastatin in patients with severe hypercholesterolemia.

[71] Puglielli L, Konopka G, Pack-Chung E, *et al.*: Acyl-coenzyme A: cholesterol acyltransferase modulates the generation of the anyloid beta-peptide. *Nat. Cell Biol.* (2001) 10:905-12.

In: Frontiers in Atherosclerosis Research
Editor: Karin F. Kepper, pp. 49-65
ISBN 1-60021-371-5

Chapter 3

PROTECTIVE EFFECT OF ALPHA-TOCOPHEROL (VITAMIN E) IN HEAD AND NECK CANCER RADIATION-INDUCED MUCOSITIS

Paulo Renato Ferreira and Marta Pereira-Lima
Department of Radiation Oncology, Hospital de Clinicas de Porto Alegre, Universidade Federal do Rio Grande do Sul (UFRGS), Porto Alegre, RS, Brazil

ABSTRACT

The fundamental principle of radiotherapy is to destroy malignant cells while minimizing damage to normal tissues. Almost all patients who receive radiotherapy to the head and neck area develop some grade of acute mucositis, which is not only painful, but may compromise tumor control by determining decrease in dose intensity and interruptions of the treatment. The term 'oral mucositis' describes the adverse effect of chemotherapy or radiation induced inflammation of the oral mucosa. Symptoms of mucositis vary from pain and discomfort to an inability to tolerate food or fluids. The degree and duration of mucositis in patients receiving radiotherapy are related to radiation source, cumulative dose, dose intensity, volume of irradiated mucosa, smoking/alcohol consumption and oral hygiene conditions. To our knowledge, there is no other controlled study which has evaluated vitamin E as a single radioprotective agent in patients with head and neck tumors treated with radiation therapy alone or post-operative. For this reason, we conducted a double-blind, randomized trial with the objective to investigate the potential mucosal protection of vitamin E in irradiated patients with head and neck cancer, motivated by its simplicity of administration, no severe toxicity in conventional doses, low cost and easy availability.

The fundamental principle of radiotherapy is to destroy malignant cells while minimizing damage to normal tissues. Almost all patients who receive radiotherapy to the head and neck area develop some grade of acute mucositis [1], which is not only painful, but may compromise tumor control by determining decrease in dose intensity and interruptions of the treatment [2]. The term 'oral mucositis' describes the adverse effect of chemotherapy or radiation induced inflammation of the oral mucosa [3]. Symptoms of mucositis vary from pain and discomfort to an inability to tolerate food or fluids. The degree and duration of mucositis in patients receiving radiotherapy are related to radiation source, cumulative dose, dose intensity, volume of irradiated mucosa, smoking/alcohol consumption and oral hygiene conditions [4, 5]. The pathogenesis of oral mucositis is thought to involve direct and indirect mechanisms. It is generally believed that oral mucositis is consequent to the direct inhibitory effects of therapy on DNA replication and mucosal cell proliferation [6]. Indirect effects result from release of inflammatory mediators, loss of protective salivary constituents, therapy-induced neutropenia, and the emergence of microorganisms on damaged mucosa [7]. Sonys et al [8] proposed a four phase hypothesis as to the mechanisms of the development of mucositis: 1) inflammatory or vascular phase, induced by toxic cytokines released from epithelial cells after chemotherapy or radiotherapy administration; 2) epithelial phase, characterized by atrophy and ulceration due to reduced renewal of the oral basal epithelium; 3) ulcerative or bacteriological phase, during which some areas of erosion become covered with a fibrinous pseudomembrane. Bacterial colonization occurs, producing endotoxins which contribute to further cytokines release; and 4) healing phase, with epithelial renewal and reestablishment of the local flora. Histopathologically, edema and vascular changes such as thickening of the tunica intima, reduction in the size of the lumen and destruction of the elastic and muscle fibers of the vessel walls are noted [9]. A number of agents with potentially mucosal protection capabilities and different mechanisms of action in radioinduced mucositis has been investigated in randomized trials. Most of them have reduced number of patients, and their efficacy and safety have not been clearly established [1,10,11]. Consequently, there is no standard intervention for oral radioinduced mucositis [7].

Prevention and Treatment of Radioinduced Mucositis

General Measures

Adequate mouth and dental hygiene during the radiotherapy period is one of the most effective measure to prevent mucositis [11,12]. Abrasive toothpastes, oral irritating solutions, smoking, alcohol, acid or excessively hot or cold foods should be avoided [13]. In a consensus conference, the National Institute of Health of the USA [14] recommended some previous measures for head and neck patients candidates to radiotherapy, such as patient and family counseling about side effects of therapy, treatment of preexisting dental cavities at least 14 days before treatment commencement, and intensive use of toothpaste, dental floss and frequent mouth washes with oral fluoride.

Oral Antiseptics, Antibiotics and Antiinflamatories

The oropharyngeal bacterial flora is composed mainly of anaerobics, streptococci and neisseria sp. Necrotic tumors are an adequate medium for many microorganisms, and radiotherapy may predispose to bacterial overgrowth by damaging dividing cells leading to colonization by abnormal bacteria and by reducing saliva. Oral antiseptics such as chlorhexidine, have been tested as mucosal protectants, but no significant effect has been observed [15,16,17]. By the other hand, iodine povidone was reported to decrease incidence, intensity and duration of oral mucositis when compared with placebo [18]. The antibiotic association of polimyxin E, tobramycin and anfotericin B was evaluated by three trials, which found different conclusions. Spijkervet *et al.* [15] conducted a three arm trial comparing polimixin E, tobramycin and anfotericin B versus chlorhexidine versus placebo in patients with head and neck tumors treated with radiotherapy alone. There was a significant reduction in mucositis intensity in the first arm. In a similar larger trial, Symonds *et al.* [19] confirmed these results. However, Okuno *et al.* [20] found no differences favouring these antibiotics association. In a trial conducted by Leborgne et al [21], prednisone reduced interruptions in radiotherapy necessary for recovering of oral toxicity, but it had no effect on intensity and duration of mucositis. Two additional pilot studies confirmed the efficacy of corticosteroids versus placebo [22,23].

Anti-Ulcer Agents

Because ulceration of the oral epithelium is part of the mucositis process, the preventive role of anti- peptic ulcer agents has been evaluated. Sucralfate has been the most investigated agent in randomized trials, but results are conflicting. Lievens *et al.* [24], Barker *et al.* [25], Epstein *et al.* [26], Makkonen *et al.* [27] and Ferreira [28] have found no significant differences between sucralfate and placebo, whereas Scherlacher *et al.* [29], Valls *et al.* [30] and Franzén *et al.* [31] found significant mucosal protection. In a literature review, Belka *et al.* [32] concluded that, except in pelvic tumors, sucralfate has limited benefit in radiation induced mucositis of the head and neck.

Prostaglandins and Antiprostaglandins

Prostaglandins are radioprotective drugs, especially of the gastrointestinal tract [11]. Some small trials found reduction in mucositis intensity with prostaglandin E (PGE_2) in irradiated patients with head and neck tumors [33,34,35]. The role of prostaglandins in the infammatory process envolved in mucositis was investigated by Pillsbury *et al.* [36]. Compared to placebo, indometacin, an anti-prostaglandin agent, reduced intensity and postponed the onset of mucositis in irradiated patients with head and neck tumors.

Colony Stimulating Factors

Granulocytes colony stimulating factor (G-CSF) and granulocytes and macrophages colony stimulating factor (GM-CSF) are glycoproteins related to neutrophille and monocytes/macrophages proliferation and differentiation [11]. GM-CSF may also stimulate proliferation and migration of oral mucosal cells [37,38]. Two phase II studies showed that GM-CSF reduced the incidence of mucositis in patiens undergoing total body irradiation (TBI) [39,40] and radiotherapy for head and neck cancer [41,42,43]. Keratinocyte growth factor-2 (KGF-2) is an new class of agent that has no in vitro or in vivo proliferative effects on human epithelial-like tumor, but it selectively induces epithelial cell proliferation, differentiation and migration. This failure to stimulate tumor cell growth characterizes the ability of this drug to speciffically target normal epithelial cells [44,45]

Amifostine

Amifostine, an aminothyol with radioprotective capabilities in normal tissues, was tested in some trials with patients with head and neck tumors. Büntzel *et al.* [46] evaluated 39 patients treated with radiotherapy and chemotherapy and found that amifostine reduced significantly the frequency of grade 3 and 4 mucositis, with apparently no interference on the therapeutic effect of therapy. Similar results were observed in a small trial conducted by Wagner *et al.* [47], where amifostine reduced both intensity and duration of oral mucositis. However, data for protection of mucositis are considered marginal and insufficient to recommend amifostine at this time [48].

Other Agents

Other agents with different mechanisms of action have been used as potential radioprotectants. Capsaicin, an agent which has been used in neuropathic syndroms, was topically employed in the oral mucosa of 11 patients with head and neck tumors undergoing chemoradiotherapy [49]. There was a significant reduction in pain intensity. Silver nitrate at 2% was investigated in 16 patients with head and neck tumors submitted to a split- course hiperfractionated radiotherapy. In the 5 days before and the 2 days after the onset of radiotherapy, left oral mucosa was topically treated with silver nitrate 3 times a day. The right size was kept as control without medication. Duration and intesity of mucositis were significantly reduced.

Vitamins

Several vitamins have shown radioprotective activity in animal and human models. Ascorbic acid (vitamin C) protected mouse spermatogonies against irradiation of ^{125}I [50]. In a randomized clinical trial, β-caroten, a vitamin A precursor, significantly reduced grades 3 and 4 oral mucositis in patients with head and neck tumors treated by radiotherapy and chemotherapy [51]. Although one study reported no radioprotective effect of vitamin E in rats by the criteria of chromosomal aberrations [52], many authors found significant evidence of intestinal [53,54,55,56] and oral mucosal protection [57] in irradiated rodents receiving systemic or topic vitamin E. Some phase III clinical trials also found significant oral mucosal protection when vitamin E was used alone in chemotherapy studies or combined to other protective agents in a chemoradiation study. In a randomized, double-blind trial with 18 evaluable patients treated with chemotherapy alone for several malignancies, Wadleigh et al [58] found that daily doses of 400 mg of vitamin E topically applied significantly speeded the healing of oral mucositis. The duration of mucositis (median of 3 days) was significantly shorter in the vitamin E group comparing to placebo group (only 1 among 9 patients had healing of mucosal lesions on the five days of observation). No toxicity was observed. The authors concluded that topical use of vitamin E is safe in preventing oral mucositis induced by chemotherapy.

One trial evaluated vitamin E and other similar drugs as radioprotective agents, in which vitamin E was not the experimental drug. Osaki et al. [59] randomized 63 patients with head and neck tumors treated with radiotherapy and concomitant chemotherapy. The experimental group received daily doses of azelastine, a histamin H1 antagonist with antioxidant activity, vitamin C, vitamin E and gluthation. The control group received identical treatment, but no azelastine. The study showed that 21 patients of the experimental group had grades 1 and 2 oral mucositis, and 16 had lesions grades 3 and 4. In the control group, only 5 patients had grades 1 and 2 oral mucositis, but 21 had lesions grades 3 and 4. The authors conclude that azelastine may be useful in the prevention of grades 3 and 4 oral mucositis induced by chemoradiotherapy.

In another randomized trial, Lopez et al [60] evaluated 19 patients with acute myelogenous leukemia treated with either induction or intensive chemotherapy followed by autologous bone marrow transplant. The duration of grades 3-4 of oral mucositis was significantly shorter in patients receiving 2 ml of topical vitamin E over the oral mucosa in the arm treated with induction chemotherapy. The plasmatic concentration of vitamin E was unexpectedly lower in patients receiving vitamin E than in patients receiving placebo. Their data suggested that the intestinal absorption of vitamin E does not seem significant, and that the mucosal protective action is mainly due to a local effect.

Rational for the Preventive Effect of Vitamin E in Radioinduced Mucositis

As experimentally demonstrated in the intestinal mucosa of rodents, there is substantial data to support that radiation induced oxygen free radicals act as mediators of cell injury following ionizing irradiation [53,54,61]. Free radicals induce DNA structural modifications which are incompatible with cell survival, if not repaired [62]. They also remove hydrogen atoms from cell membrane fatty acids, a reaction called lipidic peroxidation, which results in alterations of membrane permeability and, ultimately, in cell death [63].

Under physiological conditions, some protective mechanisms are important natural defensive agents against the oxidative action caused by free radicals, such as cytoprotective enzymes (superoxide dismutase, catalase, glutathione peroxidase) and antioxidants (tocopherols, carotenes, ascorbic acid, reduced glutathione) [64]. Providing ionizing radiation and many cytotoxic drugs are known to produce free radicals, and because they are implicated in the process of cell killing, mutagenesis, transformation and carcinogenesis, it is reasonable to assume that scavenging free radicals agents would play a significant role in modulating these processes [55].

Alpha-tocopherol, the main constituent of vitamin E, is the most important natural antioxidant present in the human blood [63]. Its main biological function is to scavenge peroxil free radicals (HO_2) in the cell membrane. Vitamin E has been reported as capable to stabilize cellular membranes and to improve herpetic gengivitis, possibly through its antioxidant activity [65,66,67]. According to Köstler et al [68], the rational for the topical use of vitamin E as a mucosal protective agent is based upon its antioxidant and membrane stabilizing action, which interferes with the inflammatory damage caused by reactive oxygen free radicals created in the course of chemotherapy or radiotherapy. Consequently, because vitamin E is inexpensive, readily available and well tolerated, confirmatory and prophylactic trials would be of great interest.

A Double-Blind, Randomized Trial on the Protective Effect of Vitamin E on Radioinduced Mucositis in Head and Neck Cancer

To our knowledge, there is no other controlled study which has evaluated vitamin E as a single radioprotective agent in patients with head and neck tumors treated with radiation therapy alone or post-operative. For this reason, we conducted a double-blind, randomized trial with the objective to investigate the potential mucosal protection of vitamin E in irradiated patients with head and neck cancer, motivated by its simplicity of administration, no severe toxicity in conventional doses, low cost and easy availability [69,70]. Our study admitted patients with confirmed histological diagnosis of cancer of the oral cavity and oropharynx referred to radiotherapy. They were evaluated at Hospital de Clinicas de Porto Alegre – Universidade Federal do Rio Grande do Sul (UFRGS) and received irradiation alone or post-operative at Hospital Sao Lucas da PUCRS - Pontificia Universidade Catolica do Rio Grande do Sul (HSL-PUCRS) in Porto Alegre, Southern Brazil. The trial was approved by the Scientific and Bioethics Committees of both institutions in accordance with the precepts established by the Helsinki Declaration. An informed consent was obtained from all patients. Admission requirements consisted of: 1) a minimal irradiated buccal mucosal area ≥ 12,2 cm^2. The limits of this area, measured on verification films, were the hard palate (superior), the floor of the mouth (inferior), the anterior border of the vertical portion of the mandible (posterior) and the distal border of the irradiation field (anterior); 2) age ≥ 21; 3) Zubrod [71] performance status grade 2 or lower, 4) tolerance of solid food at study entry, and 5) no trismus, concomitant use of oral anticoagulants, previous or current history of other cancers, previous history of radiotherapy in the head and neck area nor previous or concomitant chemotherapy. The initial evaluation consisted in history, physical/ otolaryngological/dental examination, computed tomography of the head and neck, chest x-ray study and complete blood count. Patients were staged according to the UICC (International Union Against Cancer) -TNM classification [72].

Randomization process was conducted by coworkers not directly involved in this study. Patient's names were picked out by lot and allocated in a grid with 5 blanks per line, according to the group of treatment: vitamin E or placebo. Intermittently, the line sequences were changed in order to improve the randomization. Neither the authors nor patients were aware of the identification of the prescribed drugs. Patients were given either 400 mg of vitamin E (Ephynal©, Produtos Roche Quimicos e Farmaceuticos, Sao Paulo, SP, Brazil) or 500 mg of placebo (Efamol Pure Evening Primrose Oil©, Kentville, NS, Canada). The drugs were available as an oil solution enclosed in capsules. Patients were taught to dissolve it in saliva, rinse it all over the oral cavity during 5 minutes, and then swallow it immediately before every session of irradiation, Monday through Friday, from the first to the last day of radiotherapy. A second capsule was similarly administered at patient's home after 8-12 hours. Both vitamin E and placebo capsules had the same size, shape, color and texture and were given to the patients in vials supplied weekly. The drug used as placebo is a combination of fatty acids (oleic, linoleic, gama-linoleic, palmitic, stearic and others), but also contains 2.5 % of vitamin E in its formula (13 I.U. per capsule of 500 mg). Prescribed analgesics were paracetamol/codeine or dipyrone whenever necessary.

Radiotherapy was provided by a Cobalt 60 unit (Theratron Phoenix) operating at 80 cm target-skin distance. Two parallel opposed fields were designed with customized alloy shielding blocks to include the tumor within a 2 cm safe margin and the upper cervical lymph nodes bilaterally. Anterior supraclavicular fields were added whether metastatic cervical lymph nodes were present or the primary tumor was located in tonsils or tongue. A daily dose of 2 Gy/section/5 days a week was calculated at the midline up to a cumulative dose of 44 Gy/4.5 weeks. A first field reduction was made for spinal cord sparing up to the dose of 60 Gy/6 weeks. A second reduction was made to encompass only the tumor within 1 cm margins up to the final dose of 70 Gy/7 weeks. Patients previously treated with complete or incomplete resections were planned to receive total doses of 50 or 60 Gy in 5 and 6 weeks, respectively, with a similar technique. Check films were obtained during patient set up and weekly for subsequent quality control, throughout radiotherapy. Protocol violations were established when patients: 1) did not receive the prescribed dose of irradiation, 2) interrupted radiotherapy more than 3 consecutive fractions, or 3) did not take the protocol medications adequately.

A comprehensive dentistry evaluation was made in order to assure adequate balancing of pre-treatment conditions related to secondary factors associated with mucositis severity. Patients had their weight recorded and oral mucositis evaluated and graded by the same investigator on the first day of radiotherapy, and then subsequently once a week until the last fraction. The RTOG/EORTC [73] (Radiation Therapy Oncology Group/European Organization for Research and Treatment of Cancer) objective grading system was used: grade 0- no changes over baseline; grade 1- Injection. May experience mild pain. No analgesics required; grade 2- patchy mucositis may produce inflammatory serosanguinous discharge. May experience moderate pain requiring analgesia; grade 3- confluent fibrinous mucositis. May experience severe pain requiring narcotic; grade 4-ulceration, hemorrhage or necrosis. For the purposes of this study, symptomatic mucositis was considered as grade ≥2. To evaluate the impact on quality of life, at the end of the treatment patients filled out a questionnaire based on the World Health Organization Grading of Mucositis/Stomatitis [7], where they informed the occurrence of pain and oral intake difficulty during radiotherapy. This subjective grading system consisted in the following scale: grade 0- no pain; grade 1- painful mucositis did not require modifications in oral intake; grade 2- painful mucositis, can eat but did require decrease in liquids intake any time during radiotherapy; grade 3- painful mucositis prevented oral intake; 4-painful mucositis required parenteral or enteral support any time during radiotherapy.

The main endpoint was the severity of oral mucositis. All randomized patients were counted for the analysis, according to the intention to treat principle. Not all the patients completed 7 weeks of radiotherapy because some had been submitted to previous surgery and required lower doses of irradiation. "Patients-week" were defined as the number of patients at risk who were in the study in every week of radiotherapy. For every patient-week, each record of symptomatic buccal mucositis was considered as a single event. The number of events of symptomatic mucositis was correlated with the number of patients-week, aiming to take into account the duration of time the patient suffered the toxicity. A density of incidences of symptomatic mucositis was calculated as a coefficient obtained by the number of symptomatic mucositis events divided by the number of patients-week in every week of radiotherapy. The study was designed to test a moderate to large effect. The expected sample size was estimated based on a 15% difference in the scores of symptomatic mucositis between vitamin E and placebo groups from a previous pilot study carried out with 28 patients reported elsewhere [74]. One hundred fifty-one patients-week were estimated as necessary in each arm. A significant level of 5% and a statistical power of 80% were adopted in order to test a minimal incidence difference of at least 15 events for every 100 patients-week. Secondary endpoints were duration of mucositis and weight loss. For the same significance level, statistical power and sample size, the estimated differences required for the duration of symptomatic mucositis and weight loss between both groups were at least 10 days and 11 kg, respectively.

Pre-treatment characteristics, as well as differences in the intensity of mucositis and complications, were analyzed by the Pearson's Chi-square test with a confidence interval of 95% (CI95%). Student's t test and Mann-Whitney test were utilized to compare differences between means and medians, respectively. Survival estimates were obtained by the Kaplan-Meier test [75], and the differences between survival curves by the Log Rank Test. All P values were two-tailed.

From December 1997 to December 1999, fifty-four patients were randomized. Twenty-eight were accrued to vitamin E group and 26 to the placebo group. Frequencies of gender, age, histological type, tumor location, stage, previous surgery, oral and dental evaluation, smoking and alcohol consumption were similar in both arms (table 1). Most of the patients were male. The mean age was 55.4 years (standard deviation [SD]=12.5). The most frequent histology and anatomical site were squamous cell carcinoma and oral cavity, respectively. Forty patients had stages III and IV disease: 24/28 (85.7%) belonged to the vitamin E group and 16/26 (61.5%) to the placebo group (RR [relative risk]=1.39; CI95%=0.99-1.96; P=0.086). Around 2/3 of the patients had been submitted to previous surgery. Most of them had some type of oral or dental alteration (23/28 and 16/26 patients in vitamin E and placebo groups, respectively), and history of cigarette and alcohol consumption. Three patients from the vitamin E group did not receive the prescribed doses: two due to intense mucositis and one due to death assigned to tumor progression. The median follow-up of the 54 patients was 12 months (range:2-24 months).

At twenty-four months, the estimated overall and median survivals for all patients were 44.8% and 9.5 months (range: 2-24) respectively. For patients of the vitamin E and placebo groups, these figures were 32.2% and 8.5 months (range: 2-24) and 62.9% and 12.5 months (range: 2-23) respectively (P=0.126).

Table 1. Patient characteristics

	Number of patients per treatment group (%)				
Characteristics	Vitamin E		Placebo		P
GENDER					0.999
Male	25	(89.3)	23	(88.5)	
Female	3	(10.7)	3	(11.5)	
AGE					0.268
Mean (standard deviation)	53.5 (9.1)		57.3 (15.3)		
HISTOLOGY					0.347
Squamous cell carcinoma	26	(92.8)	21	(80.8)	
Undifferentiated Carcinoma	1	(3.6)	4	(15.4)	
Adenoid cystic carcinoma	0	(0)	1	(3.8)	
Fibrossarcoma	1	(3.6)	0	(0)	
ANATOMICAL SITE					0.789
Tonsil	3	(10.7)	5	(19.2)	
Base of the tongue	4	(14.3)	2	(7.7)	
Retromolar trigone	3	(10.7)	2	(7.7)	
Soft palate	0	(0)	1	(3.8)	
Oral tongue	10	(35.7)	9	(34.6)	
Floor of the mouth	8	(28.6)	7	(26.9)	
STAGE					0.142
I	0	(0)	3	(11.5)	
II	4	(14.3)	7	(26.9)	
III	5	(17.8)	4	(15.4)	
IV	19	(67.9)	12	(46.2)	
PREVIOUS SURGERY					0.840
Yes	18	(64.3)	17	(65.4)	
No	10	(35.7)	9	(34.6)	
ORAL AND DENTAL EVALUATION					0.610
Normal teeth and oral mucosa	5	(17.8)	10	(38.5)	
Single alterations					
Periodontal disease	5	(17.8)	4	(15.4)	
Increased coating of the tongue	3	(10.7)	1	(3.8)	
Fibrous hyperplasia	2	(7.1)	1	(3.8)	
Gingivitis	1	(3.6)	1	(3.8)	
Multiple alterations					
Periodontal disease, cavities, pericoronitis, fibrous hyperplasia, increased coating of the tongue	8	(28.6)	4	(15.4)	
No evaluation	4	(14.3)	5	(19.2)	
CIGARRETTE SMOKING HISTORY	27	(96.4)	24	(92.3)	0.603
Yes					
No	1	(3.6)	2	(7.7)	
ALCOHOL HISTORY					0.878
Yes	21	(75.0)	20	(77.0)	
No	7	(25.0)	6	(23.0)	

All the patients developed varying degrees of mucositis during radiotherapy (table 2). Symptomatic mucositis was more frequent in the placebo group than in the vitamin E group: 36 events of symptomatic mucositis were observed in 167 patients-week (21.6%) of the vitamin E group, whereas 54 events of symptomatic mucositis were observed in 161 patients-week (33.5%) of the placebo group. These data were computed in the calculation of a density of incidences (RR= 0.643, 95CI%= 0.42-0.98, P= 0.038) (table 3). Accordingly, 8.3 patients-week were required for vitamin E avoiding one event of symptomatic mucositis. Maximum peaks of symptomatic mucositis occurred at the 6th week and 5th week for the vitamin E and placebo groups, respectively (figure 1). As shown in table 4, an analysis of the questionnaires answered by patients at the end of the treatment also revealed that vitamin E decreased pain and restriction in oral intake (grades 2-3) during radiotherapy (3/28 patients= 10.7% vs. 14/26 patients= 53.8%) (P=0.0001).

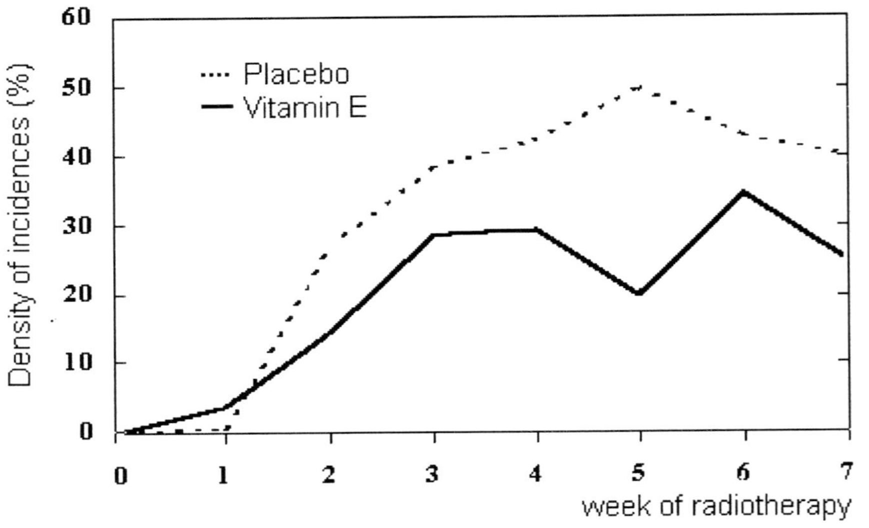

Figure 1. Density of incidences of symptomatic mucositis according to the week of radiotherapy.

Table 2. Events of symptomatic mucositis according to the radiotherapy week and the number of patients-week

	Vitamin E group (28 patients)			Placebo group (26 patients)		
Week	Patients-week	Number of events	(%)	Patients-week	Number of events	(%)
1	28	1	(3.6)	26	0	(0)
2	28	4	(14.3)	26	7	(27.0)
3	28	8	(28.6)	26	10	(38.5)
4	27	8	(29.6)	26	11	(42.3)
5	25	5	(20.0)	26	13	(50.0)
6	23	8	(34.8)	21	9	(42.9)
7	8	2	(25.0)	10	4	(40.0)
TOTAL	167 (100)	36	(21.6)	161 (100)	54	(33.5)

Table 3. Density of incidences of symptomatic mucositis

Group	Number of events		
	Symptomatic mucositis	Patients-week	Incidence per 100 patients-week
Vitamin E	36	167	21.6
Placebo	54	161	33.5

*RR= 0.643, 95CI%= 0.42-0.98, P= 0.038

Table 4. Pain and oral intake restriction based on subjective data provided by patients at the end of the treatment*

Grade	Vitamin E Number of patients (%)		Placebo Number of patients (%)	
0	13	(46.4)	3	(11.5)
1	12	(42.8)	9	(34.6)
2	3	(10.7)	9	(34.6)
3	0	(0)	5	(19.2)
4	0	(0)	0	(0)
Total	28	(100)	26	(100)

*P= 0.0001

Total doses of radiotherapy were similarly distributed in both arms (table 5). There was no dose-response relationship or mucosal area-dependence with the severity of mucositis. Mean doses at the primary site for the vitamin E and placebo groups were 61 Gy and 62 Gy (P=0.664) and mean durations of radiotherapy were 5.9 and 6.1 weeks, respectively (P=0.520). The median area of buccal mucosal irradiation for the vitamin E and placebo groups were 20.7 cm^2 (range:12.2-33.8) and 22.9 cm^2 (range:12.5-35.0), respectively (P=0.176).

The median duration of symptomatic mucositis in patients of the vitamin E and placebo groups was one week (range: 0-5) and two weeks (range: 0-5), respectively (P=0.102). The initial mean weight in patients of the vitamin E and placebo groups (60.4 kg [SD= 10.4] and 66.2 kg [SD= 14.0], respectively) was compared to the mean weight during radiotherapy (55.5 kg [SD=20.8] and 60.7 kg [SD=22.1], respectively). The observed differences in weight were 4.9 kg and 5.5 kg, respectively (P=0.249).

Two thirds of the patients presented acute complications during the treatment (table 6). Mild nausea was the most frequent, but the majority of them may be related to the disease's natural history or to irradiation itself. Their frequencies in both treatment arms were similar (P=0.216). No late reactions were observed.

Table 5. Frequency of the total doses of radiotherapy according to the treatment group*

	Vitamin E	Placebo
Total dose (Gy)	Number of patients (%)	Number of patients (%)
50	5 (17.8)	5 (19.2)
60	15 (53.5)	11 (42.3)
70	8 (28.6)	10 (38.4)
Total	28 (100)	26 (100)

* P=0.68

Table 6. Frequency of acute complications according to treatment group*

	Treatment group§			
Complication	Vitamin E 28 patients (%)		Placebo 26 patients (%)	
None	10	(35.7)	9	(34.6)
Mild nausea	12	(42.8)	10	(38.5)
Vomit	4	(14.3)	5	(19.2)
Fever	4	(14.3)	1	(3.8)
Candidiasis	2	(7.1)	4	(15.4)
Bleeding	2	(7.1)	9	(34.6)

*P=0.216.

§Some patients had more than one complication simultaneously.

In the vitamin E treated group, 6/9 patients had complete resolution of their mucositis within 4 days of initiating therapy, whereas in the placebo group only one patient had resolution of the lesions during the same time.

The proper assessment of the oral mucosa is of great importance before initiating therapy and throughout a treatment course. A variety of protocols and grading systems has been established and at least two of them incorporate both subjective and objective criteria: the RTOG/EORTC and the Wold Health Organization Grading of Mucositis/Stomatitis [7]. We used both scales based on their simplicity. Some studies define grade 3 and 4 as severe mucositis. No conventions for such reporting have been published. Many studies only report the incidence of severe reactions, whereas others combine "grade 2-3" reactions [76]. We considered RTOG grade 2 as symptomatic mucositis because it also expresses impairment in quality of life as consequence of inflammatory reaction, moderate to significant pain and necessity of analgesics. The frequency of symptomatic mucositis in the experimental arm was 64% of that observed in the placebo arm, which means that vitamin E reduced the risk of symptomatic mucositis development by 36%. By the other hand, since the differences in duration of mucositis and weight loss were lower than the minimal differences detectable by the sample size, our study had no sufficient statistical power to, conclusively, define whether vitamin E was capable or not to significantly influence these secondary endpoints.

The concentration of vitamin E in our placebo was considered acceptable for the purpose of this study because it corresponds to only 3.1% of drug concentration present in the active drug. The presence of vitamin E in placebo capsules has been reported in similar studies [58].

Although there was a trend of poorer survival in the experimental arm, it is unlikely that vitamin E has influenced short term survival, since the differences between both curves were non significant. We attribute this trend to the higher frequency of stages III and IV prevailing in the vitamin E arm, although these differences were also non significant. Mild nausea was more frequently reported by patients in the vitamin E group, whereas bleeding was more frequent in the placebo group. However, many of these symptoms may be attributable to radiotherapy and the tumor itself. Differences in complications between both groups were non significant, suggesting that vitamin E did not induce relevant toxicity.

We conclude that patients of the vitamin E group had lower frequencies of symptomatic mucositis than patients of the placebo group. On the other hand, our study had no sufficient statistical power to conclusively assess differences in the duration of symptomatic mucositis and weight loss. The administration of vitamin E was simple, side effects had low toxicity and no significant influence in survival was observed. We consider that vitamin E has a potential protective effect on the oral mucosa of irradiated patients with tumors of the oral cavity and oropharynx. The most effective dose, frequency of administration, and synergistic role of other natural antioxidants with vitamin E are issues still to be investigated. New studies are necessary to confirm our results and address further questions.

References

[1] Loprinzi CL, Gastineau DA, Foote RL: Oral complications. In: Abeloff M, Armitage JO, Lichter AS, Niederhuber JE, editors. *Clinical Oncology*. 2nd ed. New York: Churchill Livingstone; 2000. pp. 965-979.

[2] Parsons J: the effect of radiation on normal tissues of the head and neck. In: Million R, Cassisi N, editors. *Management of the head and neck cancer: A multidisciplinary approach*. 2nd ed. Philadelphia: JB Lippincott; 1994, pp. 245-289.

[3] Naidu MU, Ramana GV, Rani PU, Mohan IK et al: Chemotherapy-induced and/or radiation therapy-induced oral mucositis-complicating the treatment of cancer. *Neoplasia*. 2004;6:423-431.

[4] Franzen L, Funegard U, Ericson T, and Henriksson R (1992). Parotid gland function during and following radiotherapy of malignancies in the head and neck. *Eur J Cancer* 1992:28, 457– 462.

[5] Verdi CJ: Cancer therapy and oral mucositis—an approval of drug prophylaxis. *Drug Saf* 1993:9: 185 – 195.

[6] Lockhart PB, Sonis ST: Alterations in the oral mucosa caused by chemotherapeutic agents. *J Dermatol Surg* 1981;7:1019-1025.

[7] Wilkes JD: Prevention and treatment of oral mucositis following cancer chemotherapy. *Semin Oncol* 1998;5:538-551.

[8] Sonis ST: Mucositis as a biological process: a new hypothesis for the development of chemotherapy-induced stomatotoxicity. *Oral Oncol* 1998;34: 39-43.

[9] Berger A, Kilroy T: Oral complications. In: De Vita VT, Hellman S, Rosenberg SA, editors. *Cancer, Principles and Practice of Oncology*. 5th ed. Philadelphia: JB Lippincott; 2001. pp. 2714-2725.

[10] Berger A, Kilroy T: Oral complications. In: De Vita VT, Hellman S, Rosenberg SA, editors. *Cancer, Principles and Practice of Oncology*. 6th ed. Philadelphia: JB Lippincott; 2001. pp. 2881.

[11] Symonds RP: Treatment-induced mucositis: An old problem with new remedies. *Br J Cancer* 1998;77:1689-1695.

[12] Feber T. Management of mucositis in oral irradiation. *Clin. Oncol* (R. Coll. Radiol.) 1996;8: 106-111.

[13] Loprinzi CL.; Gastineau DA; Foote RL: Oral complications. In: Abeloff M., Armitage JO; Lichter AS; Niederhuber JE; (ed.) . *Clinical Oncology*. 2.ed. New York. Churchill Livingstone; 2000. p. 965-979.

[14] NIH Consens Statement Online - 1989 April 17-19. Oral complications of cancer therapy. *Diagnosis, prevention and treatment.* National Institutes of Health Consensus Development Conference Statement 1989;7: 1-11.

[15] Spijkervet FL; Van Saene HK; Panders AK et al:Effect of chlorhexidine rinsing on the oropharyngeal ecology in patients with head and neck cancer who have irradiation mucositis. *Oral Surg. Oral Med. Oral Path*1989;67: 154-158.

[16] Foote RL; Loprinzi CL; Frank R et al: Randomized trial of a chlorhexidine mouthwash for the alleviation of radiation induced mucositis. *J Clin. Oncol* 1994;12: 2630, 2633.

[17] Samaranayake LP; Robertson AG; Macfarlane TW et al: The effect of chlorhexidine and benzydamine on mucositis induced by therapeutic irradiation. *Clin. Radiat* 1988;39: 291-294.

[18] Adamietz I; Rahn R; Böttcher H et al: revention of radiochemotherapy-induced mucositis: Value of the prophylactic mouth rinsing with PVP-iodine solution. *Strahlenther Onkol* 1998; 174:149-155.

[19] Symonds RP, McIlroy P, Khorrami J et al: The reduction of radiation mucositis by selective decontamination antibiotic pastilles: a placebo-controlled double-blind trial. *Br J Cancer* 1996;74:312-317.

[20] Okuno S; Foote R; Loprinzi C et al: A randomized trial of nonabsorbable antibiotic lozenge given to alleviate radiation-induced mucositis. *Cancer* 1997;79: 2193-2199.

[21] Leborgne J; Leborgne F; Zubizarreta E et al:Corticosteroids and radiation mucositis in head and neck cancer. A double-bind placebo controlled randomized trial. Radiother. *Oncol* 1998; 47: 145-148.

[22] Rothwell BR; Speltor WS: Palliation of radiation-related mucositis. *Special Care Dentistry* 1990;10: 21-25.

[23] Abdelaal A; Barker D; Fergusson M. Treatment for irradiation-induced mucositis. *Lancet,* 1987;1:97-102.

[24] Lievens Y; Haustemans K; Van den Weyngaert D *et al:* Does sucralfate reduce the acute side effects in head and neck cancer treated with radiotherapy? A double-bind randomized trial. *Radiother Oncol* 1998;47: 149-153.

[25] Barker G; Loftus L; C et al: The effects of sucralfate suspension and diphenhydramine syrup plus kaolin-pectin on radiotherapy-induced mucositis. *Oral Surg. Oral Méd. Oral Pathol* 1991; 71:288-293.

[26] Epstein JB; Wong FL: The efficacy of sucralfate suspension in the prevention of oral mucositis due to radiation therapy. *Int J. Radiat Oncol Biol Phys* 1994;28: 693-698.

[27] Makkonen T; Böstrom P; Vilja P et al: Sucralfate mouth washing in the prevention of radiation-induced mucositis: a placebo-controlled double-bind randomized study. *Int J Radiat Oncol Biol. Phys* 1994;30:177-182,.

[28] Ferreira PR: Utilização de sucralfato para a prevenção de mucosite na radioterapia dos tumores da cabeça e pescoço: um estudo randomizado. *Radiol Bras* 1993; 26: 71-80.

[29] Scherlacher A; Beufort-Spontin E: Radiotherapy of head and neck neoplasms: prevention of the inflamation of the mucosa by sucralfate treatment. *HNO* 1990;38: 24-28.

[30] Valls A; Algara M; Domènech M et al: Efficacy of sucralfate in the prophylaxis of diarrhea secondary to acute radiation-induced enteritis. Preliminary results of a double-bind randomized trial. *Med Clin (Barc.)* 1991;96: 449-452.

[31] Franzén L; Henriksson R; Littbrand B et al: Effects of sucralfate on mucositis during and following radiotherapy of malignancies in the head and neck region. A double-blind placebo-controlled study. *Acta Oncol* 1995;34: 2, 219-223.

[32] Belka C; Hoffmann W; Paulsen F et al: The use of sucralfate in radiation oncology. *Strahlenter Onkol* 1997;173:247-2525 (abst).

[33] Matejka M; Nell A; Kment G et al: Local benefit of prostaglandin E2 in radiochemotherapy-induced oral mucositis. *Br J Oral Maxillofac Surg* 1990;28: 89-94.

[34] Sinzinger H; Porterder H; Matejka M et al: Prostaglandins in irradiation induced mucositis. *Lancet* 1989;1:556-558.

[35] Porteder H; Rausch E; Kment G et al: Local prostaglandin E_2 in patients with oral malignancies undergoing chemo and radiotherapy. *J . Craniomaxillo Surg* 1988;16: 371.

[36] Pillsbury H; Webster W; Rosenman J: Prostaglandin inhibitor and radiotherapy in advanced head and neck cancers. *Arch. Otolaryngol. Head Neck Surg* 1986;112:552-553.

[37] Dinarello C: Interleukin 1 and interleukin antagonism. *Blood* 1991;77:1627-1652.

[38] Zaghloul MS; DORIE M; KALLMAN RF: Interleukin 1 increases thymidine labeling index of normal tissues of mice but not the tumor. *Int J Radiat Oncol Biol Phys* 1994;29: 805-811.

[39] Troussard X; Macro M.; Vie B et al: Human recombinant granulocyte macrophage colony stimulating factor (hr GM-CSF) improves double hemibody irradiation (DHBI) tolerance in patients with stage III multiple myeloma. a pilot study. *Br J Hematol* 1995;89: 191-195.

[40] Taylor K; Jagannath S; Spitzer G et al: Recombinant human granulocyte colony stimulating factor hastens granulocyte recovery after high dose chemotherapy and autologous bone marrow transplantation in Hodgkin's disease. *J Clin Oncol* 1989;7: 791-1799.

[41] Kannan V; Bapsy P; Anantha N et al: Efficacy and safety of granulocyte macrophage colony stimulating factor (GM-CSF) on the frequency and severity of radiation mucositis in patients with head and neck carcinoma. *Int. J. Radiat. Biol. Phys* 1997;37:1005-1010.

[42] Rosso M; Blasi G; Gherlone E et al: Effect of of granulocyte macrophage colony stimulating factor (GM-CSF) on prevention of mucositis in head and neck cancer patients treated with chemo-radiotherapy. *J. Chemother* 1997;9:382-385.

[43] Throuvalas M; Antonadou D; Pulizzi M et al: Evaluation of the efficacy and safety of GM-CSF in the prophylaxis of patients with head and neck cancer treated by RT. *Apresentado na European Conference of Clinical Oncology* (ECCO), p. 593. Federation of European Cancer Societies, Paris, 1995 (abst 431).

[44] Meropol NJ, Somer RA, Gutheil J et al: Randomized phase I trial of recombinant keratinocyte growth factor plus chemotherapy: potential role as mucosal protectant. *J Clin Oncol* 2003;1452 – 1458.

[45] Alderson R, Gohari-Fritsch S, Olsen H et al: In vitro and in vivo effects of repifermin (keratinocyte growth factor-2, KGF-2) on human carcinoma cells. *Cancer Chemother Pharmacol* 2002;50,202 – 212.

[46] Büntzel J; Küttner K; Fröhlich D et al: Selective radioprotection with amifostine in concurrent radiochemotherapy for head and neck cancer. *Annals Onco* 1998;9: 505-509.

[47] Wagner W; Prott F; Schonekas K:. Amifostine: a radioprotector in locally advanced head and neck tumors. *Oncol. Rep* 1998;5:1255-1257.

[48] Wasserman T, Chapman J: Radiation response modulator. In: *Principles and practice of radiation oncology*. Perez C, Brady L, Halperin E, Schmidt-Ullrich R (eds.). Philadelphia: Lippincott Williams and Wilkins, 2004. P. 679.

[49] Berger A; Ederson M; Madoolman W et al: Oral capsaicin provides temporary relief for oral mucositis pain secondary to chemotherapy/radiation therapy. *J. Pain Symptom Manage* 1995;10: 243-248.

[50] Narra V Harpanhalli R; HOWELL R et al: Vitamins as radioprotectants in vivo. I. Protection by vitamin C against internal radionuclides in mouse testes: implications to the mechanisms of the Auger effect *Radiat Res* 1994137: 394-399.

[51] Mills E: The modifying effect of beta-carotene on radiation and chemotherapy induced oral mucositis. *Br J Cancer* 1988;57: 416-42.

[52] El-Nahas SM, Mattar FE, Mohamed AA: Radioprotective effect of vitamins C and E. *Mutat Res* 1993;301:143-147.

[53] Felemovicius I, Bonsak ME, Baptista ML: Intestinal radioprotection by vitamin E (alpha tocopherol). *Ann Surg* 1995;222: 4,504-508.

[54] Delaney JP, Bonsak M, Hall P: Intestinal radioprotection by two new agents applied topically. *Ann Surg* 1992;216: 417-421,

[55] Empey LR, Papp JD, Jewell LD, et al: Mucosal protective effects of vitamin E and misoprostol during acute radiation-induced enteritis in rats. *Dig Dis Sci* 1992;37:205-214.

[56] Blumenthal RD, Lew W, Reising A, et al: Anti-oxidant vitamins reduce normal tissue toxicity induced by radio-immunotherapy. *Int J Cancer* 2000;86:276-280.

[57] Shaheen AA, Hassan SM: Radioprotection of whole body gamma-irradiation-induced alteration in some haematological parameters by cysteine, vitamin E, and their combination in rats. *Strahlenther Onkol* 1991;167:498-501.

[58] Wadleigh RG, Redman RS, Graham ML, et al: Vitamin E in the treatment of chemotherapy-induced mucositis. *Am J Med* 1992;92: 481-484.

[59] Osaki T, Ueta E, Yoneda K, et al: Prophylaxis of oral mucositis associated with chemoradiotherapy for oral carcinoma by Azelastine hydrochloride (Azelastine) with other antioxidants. *Head Neck* 1994;16:331-339.

[60] Lopez I, Goudou C, Ribrag V, et al: Traitement des mucines par la vitamine E lors de l'administration d'anti-neoplastiques neutropéniants. *Ann Med Interne* 1994;145: 405-408.

[61] Schofield FF, Holden D, Carr HD: Bowel disease after radiotherapy. *J R Soc Med* 1983;76:463-466.

[62] Brock WA: Kinectis of micronucleus expression in synchronized irradiated Chinese hamster ovary cells. *Cell Tissue Kinet* 1985;18: 247-252.

[63] Van Acker SA, Hoyman L, Bast A: Molecular pharmacology of vitamin E: Structural aspects of antioxidant activity. *Free Radic Biol Med* 1993;15: 311-328.

[64] Ward R, Peters T: Free radicals. In: Marshal W, Bangert S, editors. *Clinical Biochemistry – Metabolic and Clinic Aspects*. London: Church Livingstone; 1995. pp. 765-777.

[65] Regan V.; Servinova E.; Packer L: Antioxidant effects of ubiquinones in microsomes and mitochondria are mediated by tocopherol recycling. *Biochem Biophys Res Commun* 1990;169: 851-856.

[66] Tampo Y, Yonaha M: Vitamin E and gluthatione are required for preservation of microsomal gluthatione S-transferase from oxidative stress in microsomes. *Pharmacology* 66:259, 1990.

[67] Starasoler S, Haber GS: Use of vitamin E oil in primary herpes gingivostomatitis in an adult. NY State Dentristy 1978;44:382.

[68] Köstler WJ, Hejna M, Wenzel C, et al: Oral Mucositis Complicating Chemotherapy and/or Radiotherapy: Options for Prevention and Treatment. *CA Cancer J Clin* 2001;51: 290-315.

[69] Ferreira PR, Fleck JF, Diehl A et al: Protective effect of vitamin E (VE) in head and neck cancer radiation induced mucositis: a double-blind randomized trial. *Presented in the annual meeting of American Society of clinical Oncology*, 2002 (abstr 909).

[70] Ferreira PR, Fleck JF, Diehl A et al: Protective effect of alpha-tocopherol in head and neck cancer radiation-induced mucositis: a double-blind randomized trial. *Head Neck* 2004;26:313-21.

[71] Zubrod CG, Scheiderman M: Appraisal of methods for the study of chemotherapy of cancer in man. *J Chronic Dis* 1960;11:7-33.

[72] UICC, *International Union Against Cancer. TNM Classification of Malignant Tumours*. 5th ed. Wiley-Liss Inc. 1997. p. 19.

[73] Cox JD, Stetz J, Pajak TF: Toxicity criteria of the Radiation Therapy Oncology Group (RTOG) and the European Organization for Research and Treatment of Cancer (EORTC). *Int J Radiat Oncol Biol Phys* 1995;31: 1341-1346.

[74] Ferreira PR, Fleck JF, Diehl AS, et al: Vitamin E preventing radiation-induced mucositis in head and neck cancer: Interim analysis of a randomized, double-blind clinical trial. Proceedings of the 29th Paulista Meeting of Radiology, Sao Paulo, Brazil. *Rev Imagem* 1999, p. 22 (suppl).

[75] Kaplan G, Meier P: Non-parametric estimation from incomplete observations. *J Am Stat* 1958;53: 457-481.

[76] Trotti A: Toxicity in head and neck cancer: A review of trends and issues. *Int J Radiat Oncol Biol Phys* 2000;47:1-12.

In: Frontiers in Atherosclerosis Research
Editor: Karin F. Kepper, pp. 67-92

ISBN 1-60021-371-5

Chapter 4

THE ROLE OF VITAMIN E ON INTRACELLULAR SIGNALING PATHWAYS IN BRAIN: MOLECULAR BASIS FOR THE TREATMENT OF NEURODEGENERATIVE PROCESSES

Selma A. Serra, Gerard Ill-Raga, Mireia Coma, Francesc X. Guix and Francisco J. Muñoz*

Grup de Canalopaties i Fisiologia Molecular, Unitat de Senyalització Cel·lular, Departament de Ciències Experimentals i de la Salut, Facultat de Ciències de la Salut i de la Vida, Universitat Pompeu Fabra, Barcelona, Spain

ABSTRACT

Recent research on Vitamin E (vit E) has pointed out novel mechanisms of action in addition to its well-known antioxidant activity. One of the main non-antioxidant actions of vit E is the modulation of intracellular signaling cascades. Vit E has been reported to directly or indirectly modulate different kinases such as protein kinase C (PKC), phosphatidylinositol-3-phosphate kinase (PI3K), glycogen syntase kinase-3β (GSK-3β), phosphatases such as protein phosphatase type 2A (PP2A), and key regulatory enzymes such as phospholipase A2 (PLA2) and cyclooxygenase-2 (COX-2). The neuroprotective effects attributed to vit E show complex mechanisms of action, in which its non-antioxidant activities are also playing a key role. In the present work, we have reviewed the effects of vit E in the intracellular signaling pathways in brain, focusing on its modulation of neuronal survival and growth, glial inflammatory response and vascular function. We will conclude with a note on the putative protective role of vit E in neurodegenerative processes.

Keywords: vitamin E, non-antioxidant, brain, neurodegeneration, Alzheimer's disease

---

* To whom correspondence should be addressed: Dr. Francisco J. Muñoz, Laboratori de Fisiologia Molecular; Universitat Pompeu Fabra, Carrer Dr. Aiguader, 80, Barcelona 08003, Spain, Phone: +34 93 542 28 84; Fax: + 34 93 542 28 02; e-mail: paco.munoz@upf.edu

ABBREVIATIONS

AA,	arachidonic acid;
Aß,	amyloid ß-peptide;
AD,	Alzheimer's disease;
AGEs,	advanced glycation end products;
Akt/PKB,	serine/threonine kinase Akt/protein kinase B;
AP-1,	activator protein-1;
AMPA,	α-amino-3-hydroxy-5-methyl-4-isoxasole-proprionic acid;
AVED,	ataxia with isolated vit E deficiency;
BBB,	blood brain barrier;
CNS,	central nervous system;
COX,	cyclooxygenase;
CRALBP,	cellular retinal binding protein;
CRAL_TRIO,	hydrophobic lipid binding pocket of cellular retinal binding protein;
DAG,	diacylglycerol;
E_2,	17β-estradiol;
ERK,	extracellular signal-regulated kinase;
GSK-3β,	glycogen synthase 3β;
GOLD,	Golgi dynamics;
HDLs,	high density lipoproteins;
H2O2,	hydrogen peroxide;
hTAP,	human tocopherol-associated protein;
JNK,	c-Jun N-terminal kinase;
KA,	kainic acid;
LDLs,	low density lipoproteins;
LOX,	lipooxygenase;
LPL,	Lipoprotein lipase;
NMDA,	n-methyl-D-aspartic acid;
NO,	nitric oxide;
NOX,	NADPH-oxidase;
NSAIDs,	non steroidal anti-inflammatory drugs;
OS,	oxidative stress;
PA,	phosphatidic acid;
PC,	phosphatidylcholine;
PG,	phosphatidylglycerol;
PGE_2,	prostaglandin E_2;
PI,	phosphoinositide;
PI3K,	phosphatidylinositol-3-phosphate kinase;
PKC,	protein kinase C;
PLA_2,	phospholipase A_2;
PP1,	protein phosphatase type 1;
PP2A,	protein phosphatase type 2A;
ROS,	reactive oxygen species;
SR-BI,	scavenger receptor class B type I;

TAPs,	tocopherol-associated proteins;
TRF,	tocotrienol-rich fraction;
α-TTP,	α-tocopherol transfer protein;
TRF,	tocotrienol-rich fraction;
vit C,	vitamin C;
vit E,	vitamin E;
VLDLs,	very low density lipoproteins;
VSMCs,	vascular smooth muscle cells.

INTRODUCTION

Oxidative stress (OS) is involved in pathological processes that affect human tissues. Particularly, the central nervous system (CNS) accumulates reactive oxygen species (ROS) throughout the life of the individual due to its high glucose metabolism and the lack of neuronal regeneration. OS is particularly relevant in the context of neurodegenerative disorders such as Alzheimer's disease (AD), Parkinson's disease and brain ischemia, all of them proposed to be related to high OS levels.

Increasing number of evidences suggest a protective role of antioxidants in neurodegeneration. Vitamin E (vit E) has been used as a therapeutic approach in many degenerative processes due to its bioavailability and antioxidant capacity. But in addition to its antioxidant properties, vit E interacts with different intracellular proteins usually anchored to the cell membrane, where vit E can be inserted easily. It turns out that vit E, through modulation of specific targets, can exert different roles in cell metabolism, thereby contributing to the beneficial effects previously attributed to its antioxidant property only. In the present work, we are reviewing the current knowledge of the non-antioxidant functions of vit E in neurons and its putative protective role on neurodegenerative processes.

PHYSIOLOGICAL BIOCHEMISTRY OF VIT E

Molecular Characteristics and Antioxidant Properties of Vit E

Vit E was originally described by Evans and Bishop in 1922 as a fat soluble factor necessary for normal reproduction in rats [1]. Natural occurring components of vit E include two groups of closely related compounds, tocopherols and tocotrienols (Fig.1). In 1966, the antioxidant properties of vit E were evidenced for the first time [2]. The heterocyclic chromanol ring of tocopherols and tocotrienols can act *in vitro* and *in vivo* as an antioxidant molecule *per se* (Fig.2).

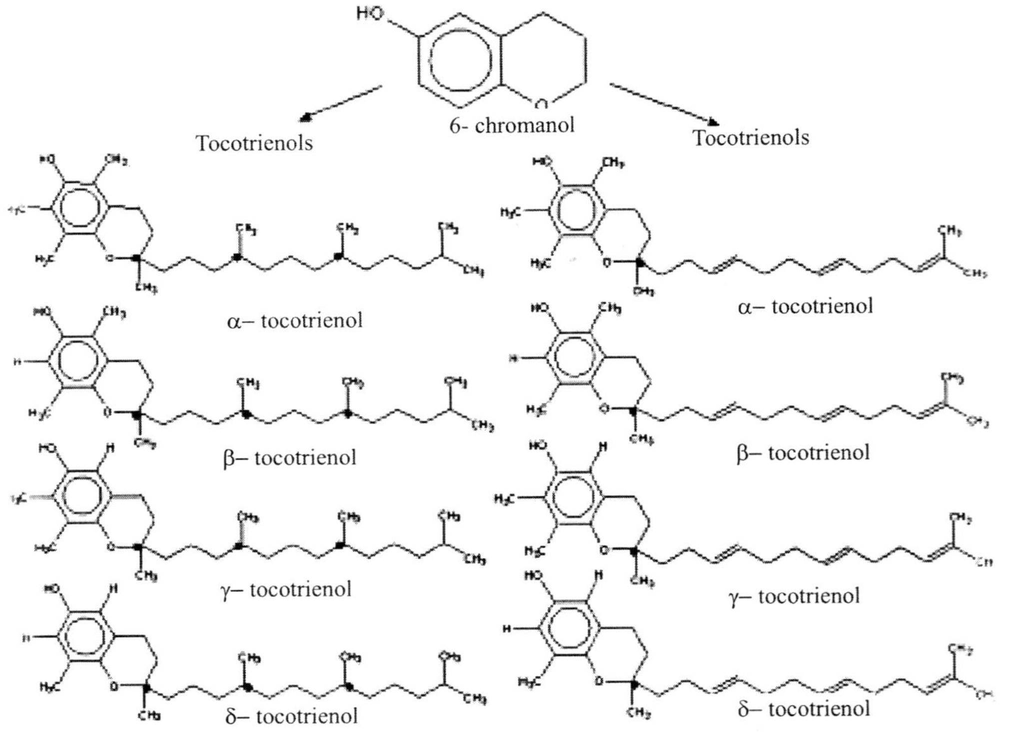

Figure 1. Molecular structure of vit E. Natural occurring components of vit E include two groups of closely related compounds, tocopherols and tocotrienols. Both types of molecules share a characteristic heterocyclic chromanol ring with an aliphatic side chain (C16) which is unsaturated for tocotrienols at positions 3', 7' and 11', and saturated for tocopherols with three chiral centres at position 2', 4' and 8'.

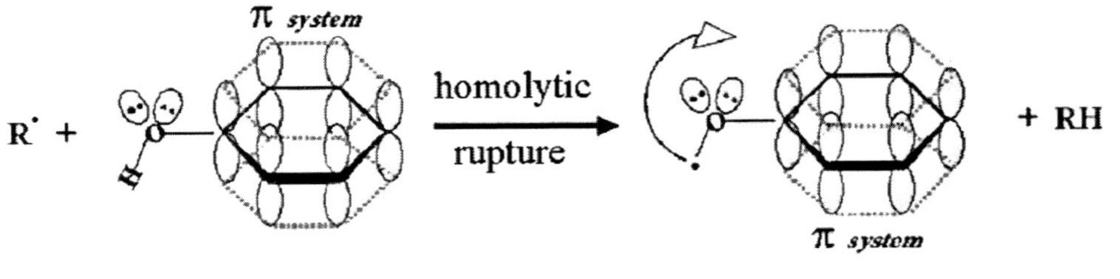

Figure 2. Antioxidant mechanism of vit E. An homolytic break of the phenolic hydroxyl leads to peroxy radical protonation and subsequent neutralization. A tocopheroxyl or a tocotrienoxyl radical is formed and its heterocyclic chromanol ring is then able to transfer the unpaired electron of the remaining oxygen throughout its π orbital system giving rise to resonance stabilization of the molecule.

Vit E Absorption and Distribution

The natural and synthetic isomers of vit E are equally absorbed, presumably, similarly to other dietary fats in the small intestinal lumen with an average efficiency of about 30%. Despite that all the vit E isomers posses equal antioxidant properties they present distinct biological activities that may depend on differential retention and distribution into the organism.

Numerous studies carried out in animals [3-5] and in humans [6, 7] concluded that the natural stereoisomer of vit E, RRR-α-tocopherol, is preferentially retained in higher organisms and accounts for the highest biological activity. This evidence strongly suggests that structural features of α-tocopherol may be very important for its specific recognition and distribution in the body and that its antioxidant capacity might not match all the possible biological activities of the molecule.

During the 80's, vit E was recognized as essential element for the maintenance of the structure and function of the human nervous system. At that time, some cases of neurodegenerative syndromes were reported in children and adults with chronic vit E deficiency caused by gastrointestinal diseases [8]. Moreover, a vit E deficiency syndrome presenting spinocerebellar ataxia and polyneuropathology, was attributed at that time to an inborn error in vit E metabolism [9, 10]. It was later described that a protein called α-tocopherol transfer protein (α-TTP) mediated selective transfer of α-tocopherol into plasma lipoproteins [11]. In 1995, it was demonstrated that the cause for the so-called ataxia with isolated vit E deficiency (AVED) was due to autosomal recessive mutations in the gene encoding for α-TTP [12].

Different isomers of α-tocopherol are equally absorbed and re-assembled together with triglycerides, cholesterol, phospholipids and apolipoproteins into chylomicrons. Chylomicrons containing vit E isoforms are secreted in the intestinal lymphatic system, and are infused in the systemic circulation via the thoracic duct. In the course of chylomicrons lipolysis, some vit E is distributed to peripheral tissues, and the liver captures the rest. Without additional mechanisms, just the systemic delivery by chylomicrons of the four tocopherols is so poor that would lead to vit E deficiency syndromes. Thus, in the liver, RRR-α-tocopherol is specifically recognized and retained by the α-TTP, which will be the main source of vit E into the body. The other isoforms of tocopherols and tocotrienols might be secreted in the bile depending on its ability to compete with RRR-α-tocopherol for α-TTP affinity. Relative affinities (RRR-α-tocopherol = 100%) calculated from the degree of competition are as follows: β-tocopherol, 38%; γ-tocopherol, 9%; δ-tocopherol, 2%; α-tocopherol acetate, 2%; α-tocopherol quinine, 2%; SRR-α-tocopherol, 11%; α-tocotrienol, 12%; trolox, 9% [13].

Probably, α-TTP is responsible for the intracellular transport and retention of α-tocopherol in hepatocytes. Subsequently, the different forms of vit E are incorporated into very low density lipoproteins (VLDLs) and secreted to the extracellular media through a non-Golgi-mediated pathway [14]. In the blood, VLDLs containing vit E are transported and delivered to peripheral tissues together with triglycerides and cholesterylesters. Lipoprotein lipase (LPL) converts VLDLs into low density lipoproteins (LDLs) and high density lipoproteins (HDLs) that contain approximately 90% of the total serum vit E in man [15].

Vit E Supply to the Brain

Another important question to address is how vit E is delivered to the brain. The distribution of vit E does not show regionalization within the CNS, although vit E uptake is considerably high in cerebellum [16]. Direct delivery of hydrophobic molecules to the brain may be less efficient compared to other peripheral tissues due to a non uniform distribution of LPL and its lower levels in certain parts of the brain [17, 18]. In a study carried out in mice, only α-tocopherol reached the brain (5.4±0.1 nmol/g) and there were no detectable levels of tocotrienols [19]. Another study demonstrated that HDLs play a major role in the supply of α-tocopherol to porcine brain capillary endothelial cells, that constitute the blood brain barrier (BBB), through the scavenger receptor class B type I (SR-BI) [20]. Moreover, SR-BI deficient mice showed a decrease of α-tocopherol levels in the bile and several tissues including ovary, testis, lung and brain but not in liver, spleen, kidney or white fat, suggesting the existence of an alternative uptake mechanisms in these tissues [21]. More recently, afamin, a 74 kDa glycoprotein member of the albumin family, was found to specifically bind α-tocopherol [22] and a physiological role in the transport of vit E in follicular and cerebrospinal fluid has been suggested [23].

All these evidences have prompted some authors to speculate about an evolutionary benefit of selecting specifically α-tocopherol for recycling in the liver. The limited dietary availability of α-tocopherol or its antioxidant function are not sufficient to explain this specific and conserved selection, as all four tocopherols could have been equally selected because of their antioxidant function. Alternatively α-tocopherol would have been specifically selected because it can exert other non-antioxidant functions. The first evidence for an *in vivo* non-antioxidant function of α-tocopherol appeared in 1991 when Angelo Azzi and co-workers found that α-tocopherol is able to regulate vascular smooth muscle cell proliferation and protein kinase C (PKC) activity [24].

Molecular Physiology of Vit E in Brain

In the last 15 years increasing evidences for an antioxidant-independent action of vit E have been reported. It involves the modulation of signaling transduction pathways and gene expression by the direct or indirect action on several enzymatic activities and transcription factors. The effects of vit E in signaling cascades and their relevance in cellular physiology and pathology, with particular interest in the CNS are reviewed in this section.

Vit E Modulates Neuronal Growth and Survival

Inhibition of PKC

PKC belongs to a diverse family of protein kinases associated with the phosphoinositide (PI) signaling pathway. In the CNS, PKC is implicated in many cellular processes, including exocytosis and endocytosis of neurotransmitter vesicles, neuronal plasticity, gene expression, regulation of cell growth and cell cycle, and activity of ion channels and receptors (Fig.3).

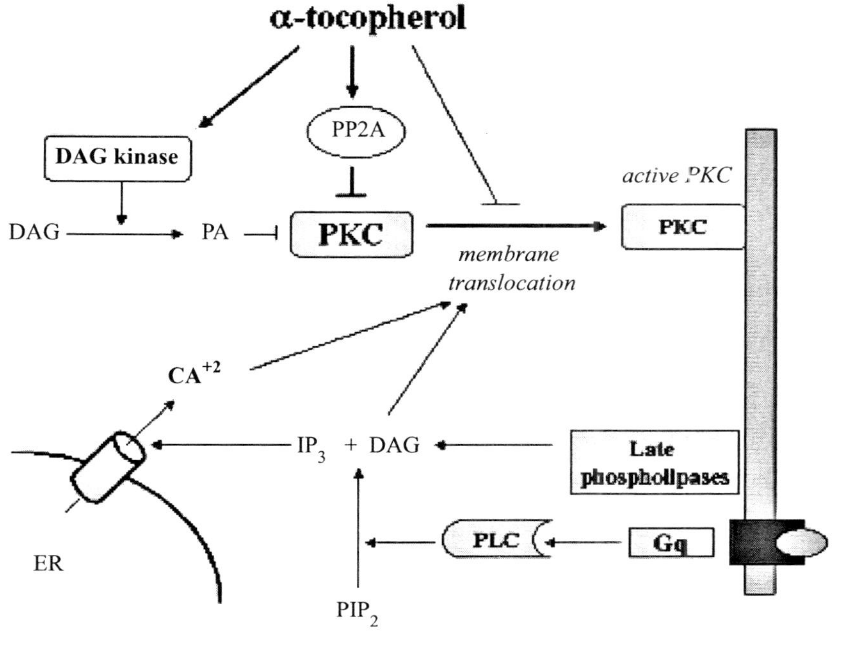

Figure 3. Inhibition of PKC by vit E. The activation of PP2A by vit E is the main mechanism to inhibit PKC but a direct effect of vit E on PKC has been also proposed. Moreover, vit E is able to activate DAG kinase, which releases phosphatidic acid and the subsequent inactivation of PKC. PKC promotes cell growth and can be activated by receptor-coupled mechanisms that involve the activation of phospholipases (i.e. PLC) or by the calcium released from the endoplasmic reticulum.

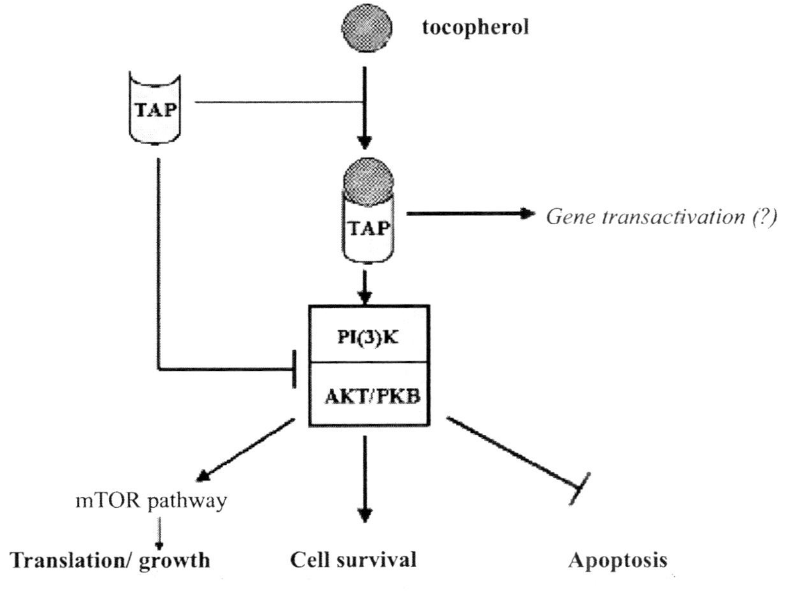

Figure 4. The interaction of vit E with TAP activates PI3K pathway. TAP is able to bind and inhibit PI3K pathway. The binding of vit E to TAP, avoids its inhibitory effect on PI3K. The activation of PI3K pathway produces an increase in cell growth and survival.

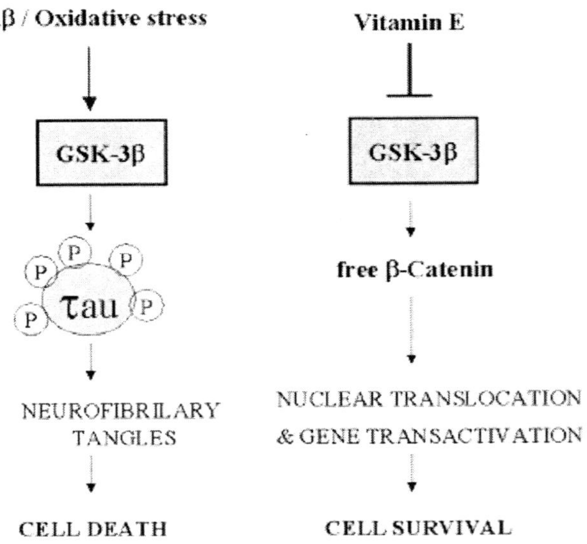

Figure 5. Inhibition of GSK-3ß by vit E. GSK-3ß is activated by oxidative stress and amyloid ß-peptide (Aß), both occurring in Alzheimer's disease (AD). The activation of GSK-3ß produces the hyperphosphorylation of protein tau, which is main component of the intracellular neurofibrillary tangles. These tangles are considered the major cause of neuronal death in AD. It has been reported that vit E avoid the activation of GSK-3ß, which involves the increase of free intracellular ß-catenin. ß-catenin is a transcription factor related with cell survival.

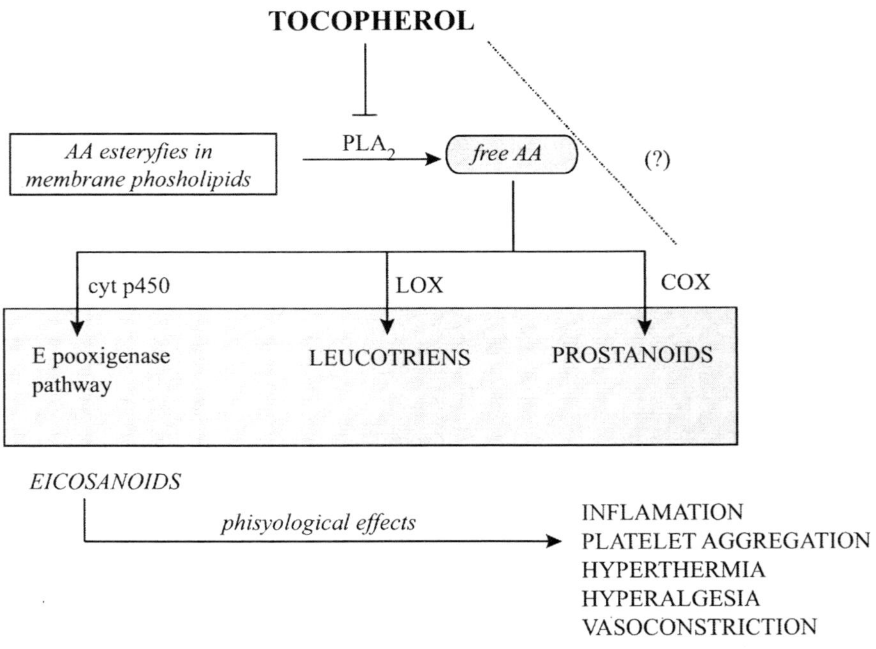

Figure 6. Inhibition of PLA_2 by vit E. An anti-inflammatory role of vit E has been proposed since it is able to inhibit PLA_2 the major source of arachidonic acid (AA). AA is the base for the production of eicosanoids that trigger the inflammatory response. A putative direct role on COX inhibition has been also proposed.

In 1988, RRR-α-tocopherol was found to inhibit *in vitro* a brain PKC enriched fraction at a concentration that can be found at the cell membrane level, the site of active PKC [25]. After this first demonstration, many reports confirmed this evidence in different cell types [24, 26-30]. In some studies, this inhibition seemed to be exclusively attributable to α-tocopherol as it could not be always confirmed when β-tocopherol or trolox, a water soluble form of α-tocopherol, were tested [31, 32].

A study in A7r5 cells (rat aortic vascular smooth-muscle cells; VSMCs) revealed that PKC inhibition was independent of a direct interaction of α-tocopherol with the enzyme or with a decrease in its expression. Instead, α-tocopherol produced dephosphorylation of the enzyme, an effect not mimicked by β-tocopherol. Moreover, the finding that α-tocopherol activated protein phosphatase type 2A (PP2A) suggested that PKC dephosphorylation and consequent inactivation is mediated by PP2A activation [33, 34].

Further studies reported alternative mechanisms for α-tocopherol-dependent PKC inactivation. A study carried out in mammary epithelial cells revealed that certain doses of both tocopherols and tocotrienols inhibited epidermal growth factor-induced PKC activation by reducing PKC translocation to the membrane [35]. Other studies revealed that vit E modulates the diacylglycerol (DAG) pathway, by enhancing the kinetics of DAG kinase. The stimulation of DAG kinase activity causes an increased conversion of DAG to phosphatidic acid (PA) subsequently contributing to the inhibition of PKC [36, 37].

In the CNS, vit E treatments against neurotoxic agents have been associated with reduced ROS production and PKC activity. However, very little is known about the possible mechanisms of PKC inhibition in neurons because the majority of reports tend to consider exclusively vit E as an antioxidant molecule regardless of the evidences of its alternative actions. In a recent study, NT2 cells (human neuroblastoma cell line) exposed to advanced glycation end products (AGEs) during 48 h presented an increase in apoptosis and/or necrosis rate. Neuronal death was associated with increased PKC_δ activity and DNA binding activity of redox-sensitive transcription factor activator protein-1 (AP-1). Pretreatments with 500 μM vit E protected neurons from the glycoxilation-dependent effects counteracting the increase in PKC_δ activity and AP-1-mediated transcriptional activity, effect that might be consistent both with the antioxidant and the non-antioxidant propertites of vit E discussed above [38]. In another study, cerebellar granule cells treated with an environmental pollutant, tetrachlorodibenzo dioxin, also showed a dose-dependent increase of total PKC activity. In this case, neurons co-treated with vit E displayed a reduction in ROS production but unfortunately the particular effects of vit E on PKC activity were not evaluated [39]. It is well-known that most of the oxidative stimuli produce a positive feedback in ROS production when interacting with membrane ion channels, membrane receptors and/or intracellular associated signaling transduction molecules [40]. This evidences suggest that under certain OS conditions, PKC activation and its downstream effectors in response to OS could be involved in the positive feed-back of ROS production. Hence, vit E might prevent ROS production by inactivating PKC.

However, the link between enhanced survival, reduced ROS production and PKC inactivation by α-tocopherol still remains unclear. How can α-tocopherol contribute to decrease OS-dependent neuronal damage by inactivating PKC and at what extent this action is entirely independent of its antioxidant capacity is a question that requires further investigation. In order to clarify this point, it would be necessary to test the ROS prevention ability of vit E isoforms with the same antioxidant capacity as α-tocopherol but unable to inhibit PKC activity.

Modulation of Phosphoinositide 3-OH Kinase (PI3K) Pathway by Vit E and its Associated Proteins

PI3K phosphorylates the D3 position of phosphoinositide (PI) to produce phosphatidylinositol-3-phosphate that acts as a second messenger. In the CNS, PI3K and one of its downstream efectors, the serine/threonine kinase Akt/protein kinase B (Akt/PKB), have been implicated in neuronal survival [41, 42] since selective PI3K inhibitors cause cerebellar granule cell death [43], and Akt/PKB phosphorylates and activates proteins implicated in survival [44], and phosphorylates and inhibits a number of pro-apoptotic proteins [45, 46].

Tocopherols are able to modulate PI3K activity through the binding to cytosolic tocopherol-associated proteins (TAPs). Using radioactively labelled α-tocopherol as tracer, a 46-kDa TAP was isolated from the cytosol of bovine liver. Sequence analysis revealed that TAP belongs to a family of conserved proteins, including cellular retinal binding protein (CRALBP), yeast Sec14p or α-TTP, which share a hydrophobic lipid binding pocket called the CRAL_TRIO [47, 48]. Proteins containing the CRAL_TRIO domain are functionally related to PI transport proteins that have been associated to intracellular transport, regulation of exocytosis, vesicular transport and composition of phospholipids in membranes. Moreover, they provide the substrates to the PI kinases and phosphatases [49, 50]. Northern analyses with the human TAP (hTAP) showed that it is ubiquitously expressed but the highest amounts of hTAP messenger are found in liver, brain and prostate [48]. Thus, TAPs might be the responsible for the intracellular distribution of α-tocopherol in human tissues and might account for its intervention into PI signaling transduction cascades.

Affinity data obtained from α-TTP suggested the recognition of the different tocopherols and tocotrienols. However, functional characterization of TAP has caused much controversy. Some authors showed a specific binding of TAP to α-tocopherol [51] while others demonstrated that it can distinguish between tocopherols and other hydrophobic ligands as well as biotinylated tocopherol [48]. Later studies, showed that the three hTAPs (hTAP1 or SEC14L2, hTAP2 and hTAP3) can bind not just tocopherols, but also PI, phosphatidylcholine (PC) and phosphatidylglycerol (PG). In addition, PC, tocopherols and tocopheryl-succinate compete with PI for the binding to hTAPs [52]. Moreover, the three hTAPs contain the Golgi dynamics (GOLD) domain predicted to mediate protein-protein interactions that is present in proteins involved in secretion, assembly of membrane-associated complexes or regulation vesicle formation [53, 54].

The fact that the hTAP1-green fluorescence protein fusion protein was able to bind and translocate α-tocopherol to the nucleus and therefore activate transcription in COS-7 cells, suggested for the first time a putative role of hTAP as an intracellular effector of α-tocopherol-dependent activation of signaling pathways and transcription [51]. Although α-tocopherol-dependent nuclear translocation of hTAP could not be further confirmed by other groups [52] hTAP immunostaining experiments in HeLa cells revealed its presence in the cytosol in association with membrane compartments and granular structures, with more intense staining surrounding the nucleus. Deletion of the carboxyterminal GOLD domain resulted in drastic changes of the intracellular localization of hTAPs suggesting an implication of this domain in the docking of hTAPs to subcellular compartments [52].

In this context, the most interesting evidence about hTAP1 and hTAP2 modulation of the PI3K pathway is that they reduce *in vitro* the activity of the catalytic subunit of PI3Kγ and stimulate it in the presence of α-tocopherol up to 5-fold whereas α-tocopherol itself can not change PI3K activity [52]. Moreover, the three hTAP proteins share similarity to a peptide fragment of the α-subunit common to G-proteins and have basal GTPase activity [52].

Then PI3K and other PI- and PC-dependent enzymes might be modulated by hTAPs and tocopherols either by facilitating enzyme-ligand bounding, transport of bound ligands to organelles, assembly of secretory granules, or even ligand-dependent signaling and transcriptional activation.

As mentioned before, PI3Kγ has been implicated in a variety of cellular responses to stimuli in the CNS, including cell survival and apoptosis [55]. In this context, modulation of PI3Ks and probably phospholipases by TAPs in a tocopherol-dependent way, could explain some of the phenotypes associated with AVED disease like axonopathy and neurodegeneration. As other authors have suggested before [52], we could hypothesize that low neuronal levels of α-tocopherol caused by AVED disease would lead to a reduction of PI3Kγ activity and the subsequent impaired neuronal survival. In this context, a microarray study established the impact of chronic vit E deficiency on rat hippocampus. Interestingly, they found that PI3Kγ was down-regulated in response to vit E deficiency [56] (Fig. 4).

Vit E Protects Against Glutamate- and Amyloid ß-Peptide (Aß)-Mediated Citotoxicity

Activation of Pp60$^{c\text{-}Src}$ Kinase and 12-Lypoxygenase

Glutamate excitotoxicity is a major event contributing to pathological cell death in the CNS. Activation of the α-amino-3-hydroxy-5-methyl-4-isoxasole-proprionic acid (AMPA), kainic acid (KA) and n-methyl-D-aspartic acid (NMDA) receptors by glutamate opens channels for Na^+ and Ca^{2+}. Under depolarizing conditions, voltage-dependent Ca^{2+} channels are activated producing enhanced intraneuronal Ca^{2+} flow that may activate phospholipase A_2 (PLA_2) initiating arachidonic acid metabolic cascade, protease activation and nitric oxide (NO) release. Depolarization also increases ATP consumption by the Na^+/K^+ ATPase, which increases ROS production [57]. As a result, an intricate crosstalk of intracellular signaling pathways may converge on neuronal degeneration. Classically, micromolar concentrations of antioxidants have been shown to protect neuronal cells against glutamate-induced excitotoxicity [58-62].

More recently, two novel non-antioxidant mechanisms of tocotrienols against glutamate-induced cell death have been reported [63]. In a first study in HT4 cells (mouse neuroblastoma cell line), the activation of pp60$^{c\text{-}Src}$ kinase and phosphorylation of extracellular signal-regulated kinase (ERK) were observed in response to glutamate treatment. Nanomolar concentrations of α-tocotrienol, but not α-tocopherol, blocked glutamate-induced early activation of c-Src kinase both in wild-type and c-Src overexpressing cells. Furthermore, rapid activation of ERK, particularly ERK2, in response to glutamate treatment was completely inhibited by α-tocotrienol suggesting that α-tocotrienol influences an early event in the glutamate-induced death pathway. The authors suggested that tocotrienol might inhibit inducible ERK activation by down-regulating Src kinase activity [63], since Src kinase activity-dependent activation of ERK has been reported [64].

Furthermore, glutamate treatment arrested growth and axo-dendritic motility of cultured neurons [63]. In this case, α-tocotrienol, but not α-tocopherol, not only protected against loss of viability as reported earlier [63], but preserved the normal growth rate and restored neurite motility even in the presence of excess glutamate. The molecular mechanisms proposed for α-tocotrienol action was the modulation of 12-lipooxygenase (12-LOX), a metabolite of arachidonic acid pathway. A central role of 12-LOX has been proposed in the execution of glutamate-induced neuronal death [65, 66]. In addition, vit E and its analogs are known to be potent inhibitors of 5-LOX and 15-LOX *in vitro* via an antioxidant-independent way [67, 68]. In cultured neurons, glutamate treatment significantly increased intracellular (*12S*)-HETE (product of 12-LOX activity) level, which was prevented in α-tocotrienol-treated cells. Moreover, thin layer chromatographic analysis of 12-LOX activity in the presence of ^{14}C arachidonic acid revealed that α-tocotrienol inhibited the activity of the pure enzyme in a dose-dependent way [63].

The concern that dietary tocotrienols may not reach the brain [13] due to its low affinity for α-TTP, has substantially dampened general interest to investigate its neuroprotective properties. However, a study performed in pregnant rats fed with a tocotrienol-rich fraction (TRF; 1.23 mmol α-tocotrienol and 0.94 mmol α-tocopherol per g weight) demonstrated that TRF feeding increased α-tocopherol and α-tocotrienol content in maternal brain 0.1- and 5-fold, respectively and a 20-fold increase of α-tocotrienol was found in the foetal brain [69, 70]. Although α-TTP has only a 12% affinity for α-tocotrienol [13] it is possible that a TRF diet increases α-TTP affinity for α-tocotrienol as α-TTP relative affinities were calculated from the degree of competition with α-tocopherol.

Inhibition of Glycogen Synthase-3β (GSK-3β)

GSK-3β is a Ser/Thr protein kinase implicated in receptor-coupled signaling systems. GSK-3β shows multiple regulatory mechanisms: phosphorylation, protein complex formation, intracellular mobilization, etc. These mechanisms are necessary for an enzyme that modifies multiple and diverse substrates, including metabolic, signaling and structural proteins, and transcription factors, therefore influencing complex cellular processes, including gene expression programs and cell survival (revised in [71, 72]).

Certain psychiatric diseases, such as bipolar mood disorder, and neurodegenerative diseases, such as AD have been extensively associated with deregulated GSK-3β activity [73-75]. Increased levels of GSK-3β have been found in the brain of AD patients. Moreover, GSK-3β has been found associated with neurofibrillary tangles and pre-tangled neurons in AD brain [76-79]. Neurofibrillary tangles are intracellular aggregates of paired helical filaments produced by the hyperphosphorylation of the microtubule-associated protein tau [80]. It has been proposed that GSK-3β is the responsible for the hyperphosphorylation of tau protein [81]. In cortical and hippocampal neurons challenged with Aβ there is an activation of GSK-3β [82, 83] and tau hyperphosphorylation [80, 84] correlating with cell death [82, 84]. Taken together, these data strongly suggests that alterations in the control of GSK-3β may occur in AD brain, a condition that could result from an impaired control of GSK-3β inhibitory signaling systems, including PI3K/Akt, PKC or *Wnt* pathway [71].

The activity of GSK-3β is negatively regulated by serine phosphorylation and positively regulated by tyrosine phosphorylation [85-88]. Several kinases are able to mediate Ser phosphorylation. Akt/PKB inactivates GSK-3β by Ser phosphorylation through the PI3K signaling pathway [89-93]. Protein-protein interactions and protein phosphorylation have been also implicated in the mechanism of *Wnt*-mediated inactivation of GSK-3β that leads to an increase in cytoplasmic β-catenin that subsequently translocates to the nucleus and activates transcription of *Wnt* target genes [94-96].

A recent study on primary rat embryo hippocampal neurons has shown attenuation Aβ- and H_2O_2-mediated neurotoxicity by 17β-estradiol (E_2) and trolox, but not vitamin C (vit C) [97]. This study demonstrated that E_2 and Trolox decrease endoperoxide production, inhibit GSK-3β and stabilize cytoplasmic β-catenin. Besides, both compounds increased the expression of *Wnt-7a* and *Wnt-5a* ligand genes and the *Wnt* target gene *en-1*, indicating a novel role in the modulation of the *Wnt* signaling pathway in hippocampal neurons by vit E [97].

The presence of a hydroxyl group in the phenolic ring of both E_2 and Trolox reveals a similar molecular feature that could give rise to a common function. Both molecules have been reported to have free radical scavenging ability as well as antioxidant-independent physiological effects [98-101]. On the one hand, some authors have demonstrated a negative modulation of *Wnt* pathway by OS [102, 103]. Thus, antioxidants through the reversion of the oxidative status of cells, could activate *Wnt* pathway and subsequently inhibit GSK-3β. On the other hand, striking evidence supports that E_2 inhibits GSK-3β and regulates interaction of estrogen receptors, GSK-3β, and β-catenin in the hippocampus either by protein complex rearrangement or through a PI3K/Akt-dependent mechanism [104]. In addition, tocopherols have been reported to interfere with Akt/PKB phosphorylation and translocation to the membrane by modulating either PI3K, the kinase that activates Akt/PKB [105]. In this case, a non-antioxidant mechanism would be the responsible for GSK-3β modulation.

In conclusion, GSK-3β down-regulation by vit E in the CNS deserves further research in order to elucidate which is the exact molecular event implicated in this action and whether it contributes to a delay in the progression of AD (Fig.5).

Vit E Decreases the Inflammatory Response in Brain

Modulation of PLA_2

OS and inflammation are major hallmarks of tissue aging. In CNS, both accumulation of pro-oxidant agents and immune dysfunction generate a positive feedback loop involved in the onset of many physiopathological processes that ultimately could lead or greatly contribute to neurological diseases.

The products of arachidonic acid (AA) metabolism are involved in the inflammatory response to different stimulus. PLA_2 is a lipolytic enzyme that hydrolyzes the acyl group from the sn-2 position of glycerophospholipids, generating free fatty acids (including AA) and lysophopholipids. AA is metabolized to eicosanoids (prostaglandins, leukotrienes, lipoxins, and tromboxanes) that serve as second messengers [106, 107] (Fig.6). Under physiological conditions, PLA_2 and its by-products may be involved in phospholipid turnover, membrane remodeling, exocytosis, detoxification of phospholipid peroxides and neurotransmitter release

[108-110]. However, under pathological situations, increased PLA_2 activity may result in altered membrane permeability, ion homeostasis, increased free fatty acid release, and accumulation of lipid peroxides [111]. An increase in PLA_2 activity has been reported in several neurodegenerative processes, including ischemia [112, 113], spinal cord injury [114], schizophrenia [115, 116] and AD [117].

Some α-tocopherol analogs have been reported to inhibit platelet and epidermal phospholipase PLA_2 [118, 119]. The shorter the phyptyl tail of the tocopherol molecule the larger the inhibition, suggesting a crucial role of the chromanol ring in its inhibitory action. Moreover, co-crystallization of α-tocopherol and PLA_2 showed a direct binding of α-tocopherol to the enzyme [120]. These data suggest that tocopherol analogs might serve as putative therapeutical drugs against inflammation-related neuronal phathologies (see Fig.6).

Inhibition of Cyclooxygenase (COX)

Activated microglia and astroglia have been found in AD and ischemic brains suggesting a contribution of inflammation in the progression of neuronal damage in these pathological situations [121-124]. In this context, several studies have shown that neurones treated with non-steroideal anti-inflamatory drugs (NSAIDs) were more resistant to amyloid β-peptide [125-127]. This type of anti-inflammatory drugs inhibit the COXs enzymes that convert arachidonic acid (AA) to prostaglandins as well as nuclear factor kappa-β and peroxisome proliferator-activated receptors. However, recent studies indicate that a subset of NSAIDs may have direct Aß-lowering properties in cell cultures as well as in transgenic models of AD-like amyloidosis [128]. Hence, the observed reduction in AD progression shown in some epidemiological studies [129-132] could be explained by a combination of traditional (anti-inflammatory) and new (anti-amyloidogenic) properties of NSAIDs.

Regarding vit E, several studies revealed that γ-tocopherol, but not α-tocopherol, inhibited COX-2 activity, the enzyme that catalyzes the synthesis of the eicosanoid prostaglandin E_2 (PGE_2)[133]. Other authors reported that the age associated increase in PGE_2 and COX-2 activity in murine macrophages was reversed by vit E (mainly the four tocopherol isomers). The effects reduction of COX-2 activity by vit E occurred at the posttranslational level [107, 134]. However, there are no direct evidences demonstrating whether vit E exerts its age-related anti-inflammatory action through direct binding to COX-2 enzyme, by inhibiting PLA_2 enzyme or via the reduction of peroxynitrite or hydroperoxide generation, which have been reported to be involved in the activation of COX-2. One the other side, it would be of much interest to evaluate if vit E also possesses anti-amyloidogenic properties.

Modulation of NADPH-Oxidase (NOX) in Activated Microglia

The NOX system in phagocytic cells, such as microglia, is an electron transport system that catalyzes the reduction of O_2 to $O_2^{\cdot-}$, by using NADPH. Under physiological conditions, this system contributes to the elimination of pathogens but under chronic inflammatory conditions it is thought to induce neurodegeneration by the massive accumulation of $O_2^{\cdot-}$ radical. The assembly of a functional NOX complex at the plasma membrane depends on the phosphorylation and subsequent translocation of several cytosolic subunits ($p40^{phox}$, $p47^{phox}$, $p67^{phox}$ and Rac1/2) [135]. Activation and assembly of these subunits occurs via complex intracellular signaling events that include activation of protein kinase A (PKA), PKC, mitogen-activated protein kinase (MAPK) [136] and PI3K [137].

Recently, the effect of α-tocopherol on $O_2^{\cdot-}$ generation by the NOX system has been studied in murine and porcine activated microglia. The results of the study demonstrated that α-tocopherol attenuates p67^{phox} translocation to the plasma membrane as a result of decreased PKC activity. This effect was partially or completely counteracted by okadaic acid and calyculin A, two potent inhibitors of protein phosphatase type 1 (PP1) and PP2A suggesting a putative mechanism for α-tocopherol-dependent on phosphatase-dependent activation and subsequent NOX inactivation [138].

In conclusion, the fact that α-tocopherol is able to modulate microglial superoxide production by a protein phosphatase-dependent pathway [138], PLA_2 activity [118, 119], and age-related increase in COX-2 activity [107, 134] might provide several feasible molecular explanations for the therapeutic role attributed to α-tocopherol in several clinical studies related to human neurodegeneration, including AD [139-142].

Vit E and the Brain Vascular System

Vit E has also direct effects on vascular cells, with protective roles in vascular diseases [143, 144].

Effects on the C-Jun N-Terminal Kinase (JNK) Pathway

Vit E has been reported to protect endothelial cells and VSMCs against hydrogen peroxide (H_2O_2) and Aß-mediated cytotoxicity [145, 146]. Although this effect has been attributed to the antioxidant properties of vit E, other non-antioxidant mechanisms can be acting. In this respect, several pieces of evidence link the protective effect of vit E with the JNK pathway. OS-mediated activation of the JNK pathway results in cell death. Vit E is able to oppose this effect by reducing JNK activity and increasing ERK activity (as seen in cardiac myocytes [147]) or inhibiting caspase-3 activation (described in endothelial cells [148]). The actual mechanism of vit E-mediated modulation of JNK still remains to be solved. An obvious possibility is that vit E antioxidant properties will revert JNK activation, as proposed in HeLa cells [149], although a direct effect of vit E on JNK pathway can not be discarded.

Inhibition of PKC and Activation of PP2A

The beneficial roles of vit E in vascular cells includes the activation of PP2A, and the inhibition of PKC□ in VSMCs [33], which should avoid the proliferation of VSMCs seen in atherosclerotic processes. This benefitial effect may contribute to delay the onset of the multi-infarct dementia, which is associated to the development of atherosclerosis in brain vessels being the second largest kind of senile dementia after AD.

Inhibition of PLA_2

Eicosanoids are related to an increased vasoconstriction, which would inhibit the blood supply to brain if inflammatory processes are triggered. Then the previously commented inhibition of PLA_2 and COX in brain by vit E would contribute to reduce the eicosanoids levels allowing a vasodilatation of the brain vessels. In fact the inhibition of eicosanoids by vit E has been reported to decrease atherosclerosis [150, 151]. Moreover, alpha-tocopherol is able to inhibit thrombin-mediated PKC activation and endothelin secretion in endothelial cells, contributing to vasodilatation [32].

Conclusion

The view that vit E protects against different pathologies has been present for quite a while, reaching even the status of common knowledge. Several studies have reported protective effects of vit E in different brain associated pathologies such as AD [139-142], cerebral amyloid angiopathy [145, 146], Parkinson's disease [152] or brain ischemia [153]. The cellular mechanism explaining its protective effects have been classically related to the antioxidant properties of vit E, although, as discussed in this chapter there is more to it than simply reducing the levels of ROS.

Acknowledgements

This work was supported by grants from FIS (Ministerio de Sanidad, Spain; grant n° PI041242; and Red HERACLES) and Generalitat de Catalunya (GSR2005-266). We acknowledge Dr. Miguel A. Valverde for his critical suggestions.

References

[1] Evans, H.M., Bishop, K.S. (1922). On the existence of a hitherto unrecognised dietary factor essential for reproduction. *Science,* 56, 650-651.

[2] Epstein, S.S., Forsyth, J., Saporoschetz, I.B. and Mantel, N. (1966). An exploratory investigation on the inhibition of selected photosensitizers by agents of varying antioxidant activity. *Radiat.Res.,* 28(2), 322-335.

[3] Ingold, K.U., Burton, G.W., Foster, D.O., Hughes, L., Lindsay, D.A. and Webb, A. (1987). Biokinetics of and discrimination between dietary RRR- and SRR-alpha-tocopherols in the male rat. *Lipids,* 22(3), 163-172.

[4] Weiser, H., Vecchi, M. and Schlachter, M. (1986). Stereoisomers of alpha-tocopheryl acetate. IV. USP units and alpha-tocopherol equivalents of all-rac-, 2-ambo- and RRR-alpha-tocopherol evaluated by simultaneous determination of resorption-gestation, myopathy and liver storage capacity in rats. *Int.J.Vitam.Nutr.Res.,* 56(1), 45-56.

[5] Fuhrmann, H., Balthazary, S.T. and Sallmann, H.P. (1994). Bioefficiency of different tocopherols in chicken as assessed by haemolysis test and microsomal pentane production. *Br.J.Nutr.,* 71(4), 605-614.

[6] Kiyose, C., Muramatsu, R., Kameyama, Y., Ueda, T. and Igarashi, O. (1997). Biodiscrimination of alpha-tocopherol stereoisomers in humans after oral administration. *Am.J Clin.Nutr.,* 65(3), 785-789.

[7] Burton, G.W., Traber, M.G., Acuff, R.V., Walters, D.N., Kayden, H., Hughes, L. and Ingold, K.U. (1998). Human plasma and tissue alpha-tocopherol concentrations in

response to supplementation with deuterated natural and synthetic vitamin E. *Am.J.Clin.Nutr.,* 67(4), 669-684.

[8] Sokol, R.J., Kayden, H.J., Bettis, D.B., Traber, M.G., Neville, H., Ringel, S., Wilson, W.B. and Stumpf, D.A. (1988). Isolated vitamin E deficiency in the absence of fat malabsorption--familial and sporadic cases: characterization and investigation of causes. *J Lab Clin.Med.,* 111(5), 548-559.

[9] Trabert, W., Stober, T., Mielke, U., Heck, F.S. and Schimrigk, K. (1989). [Isolated vitamin E deficiency]. *Fortschr.Neurol.Psychiatr.,* 57(11), 495-501.

[10] Sokol, R.J. (1989). Vitamin E and neurologic function in man. *Free Radic.Biol.Med.,* 6(2), 189-207.

[11] Arita, M., Sato, Y., Miyata, A., Tanabe, T., Takahashi, E., Kayden, H.J., Arai, H. and Inoue, K. (1995). Human alpha-tocopherol transfer protein: cDNA cloning, expression and chromosomal localization. *Biochem.J.,* 306 (Pt 2), 437-443.

[12] Ouahchi, K., Arita, M., Kayden, H., Hentati, F., Ben Hamida, M., Sokol, R., Arai, H., Inoue, K., Mandel, J.L. and Koenig, M. (1995). Ataxia with isolated vitamin E deficiency is caused by mutations in the alpha-tocopherol transfer protein. *Nat.Genet.,* 9(2), 141-145.

[13] Hosomi, A., Arita, M., Sato, Y., Kiyose, C., Ueda, T., Igarashi, O., Arai, H. and Inoue, K. (1997). Affinity for alpha-tocopherol transfer protein as a determinant of the biological activities of vitamin E analogs. *FEBS Lett.,* 409(1), 105-108.

[14] Arita, M., Nomura, K., Arai, H. and Inoue, K. (1997). alpha-tocopherol transfer protein stimulates the secretion of alpha-tocopherol from a cultured liver cell line through a brefeldin A-insensitive pathway. *Proc.Natl.Acad.Sci.U.S.A,* 94(23), 12437-12441.

[15] Behrens, W.A., Thompson, J.N. and Madere, R. (1982). Distribution of alpha-tocopherol in human plasma lipoproteins. *Am.J.Clin.Nutr.,* 35(4), 691-696.

[16] Vatassery, G.T. (1992). Vitamin E. Neurochemistry and implications for neurodegeneration in Parkinson's disease. *Ann.N.Y.Acad.Sci.,* 669, 97-109.

[17] Bessesen, D.H., Richards, C.L., Etienne, J., Goers, J.W. and Eckel, R.H. (1993). Spinal cord of the rat contains more lipoprotein lipase than other brain regions. *J.Lipid Res.,* 34(2), 229-238.

[18] Goldberg, I.J., Soprano, D.R., Wyatt, M.L., Vanni, T.M., Kirchgessner, T.G. and Schotz, M.C. (1989). Localization of lipoprotein lipase mRNA in selected rat tissues. *J.Lipid Res.,* 30(10), 1569-1577.

[19] Podda, M., Weber, C., Traber, M.G. and Packer, L. (1996). Simultaneous determination of tissue tocopherols, tocotrienols, ubiquinols, and ubiquinones. *J.Lipid Res.,* 37(4), 893-901.

[20] Goti, D., Hrzenjak, A., Levak-Frank, S., Frank, S., van der Westhuyzen, D.R., Malle, E. and Sattler, W. (2001). Scavenger receptor class B, type I is expressed in porcine brain capillary endothelial cells and contributes to selective uptake of HDL-associated vitamin E. *J.Neurochem.,* 76(2), 498-508.

[21] Goti, D., Reicher, H., Malle, E., Kostner, G.M., Panzenboeck, U. and Sattler, W. (1998). High-density lipoprotein (HDL3)-associated alpha-tocopherol is taken up by HepG2 cells via the selective uptake pathway and resecreted with endogenously synthesized apo-lipoprotein B-rich lipoprotein particles. *Biochem.J.,* 332 (Pt 1), 57-65.

[22] Voegele, A.F., Jerkovic, L., Wellenzohn, B., Eller, P., Kronenberg, F., Liedl, K.R. and Dieplinger, H. (2002). Characterization of the vitamin E-binding properties of human plasma afamin. *Biochemistry,* 41(49), 14532-14538.

[23] Jerkovic, L., Voegele, A.F., Chwatal, S., Kronenberg, F., Radcliffe, C.M., Wormald, M.R., Lobentanz, E.M., Ezeh, B., Eller, P., Dejori, N. *et al.* (2005). Afamin is a novel human vitamin E-binding glycoprotein characterization and in vitro expression. *J.Proteome.Res.,* 4(3), 889-899.

[24] Boscoboinik, D., Szewczyk, A. and Azzi, A. (1991). Alpha-tocopherol (vitamin E) regulates vascular smooth muscle cell proliferation and protein kinase C activity. *Arch.Biochem.Biophys.*, 286(1), 264-269.

[25] Mahoney, C.W., Azzi, A. (1988). Vitamin E inhibits protein kinase C activity. *Biochem.Biophys.Res.Commun.,* 154(2), 694-697.

[26] Boscoboinik, D., Szewczyk, A., Hensey, C. and Azzi, A. (1991). Inhibition of cell proliferation by alpha-tocopherol. Role of protein kinase C. *J.Biol.Chem.,* 266(10), 6188-6194.

[27] Devaraj, S., Li, D. and Jialal, I. (1996). The effects of alpha tocopherol supplementation on monocyte function. Decreased lipid oxidation, interleukin 1 beta secretion, and monocyte adhesion to endothelium. *J.Clin.Invest,* 98(3), 756-763.

[28] Devaraj, S., Adams-Huet, B., Fuller, C.J. and Jialal, I. (1997). Dose-response comparison of RRR-alpha-tocopherol and all-racemic alpha-tocopherol on LDL oxidation. *Arterioscler.Thromb.Vasc.Biol.,* 17(10), 2273-2279.

[29] Freedman, J.E., Farhat, J.H., Loscalzo, J. and Keaney, J.F., Jr. (1996). alpha-tocopherol inhibits aggregation of human platelets by a protein kinase C-dependent mechanism. *Circulation,* 94(10), 2434-2440.

[30] Tada, H., Ishii, H. and Isogai, S. (1997). Protective effect of D-alpha-tocopherol on the function of human mesangial cells exposed to high glucose concentrations. *Metabolism,* 46(7), 779-784.

[31] Fazzio, A., Marilley, D. and Azzi, A. (1997). The effect of alpha-tocopherol and beta-tocopherol on proliferation, protein kinase C activity and gene expression in different cell lines. *Biochem.Mol.Biol.Int.,* 41(1), 93-101.

[32] Martin-Nizard, F., Boullier, A., Fruchart, J.C. and Duriez, P. (1998). Alpha-tocopherol but not beta-tocopherol inhibits thrombin-induced PKC activation and endothelin secretion in endothelial cells. *J.Cardiovasc.Risk,* 5(5-6), 339-345.

[33] Ricciarelli, R., Tasinato, A., Clement, S., Ozer, N.K., Boscoboinik, D. and Azzi, A. (1998). alpha-Tocopherol specifically inactivates cellular protein kinase C alpha by changing its phosphorylation state. *Biochem.J.,* 334 (Pt 1), 243-249.

[34] Ricciarelli, R., Azzi, A. (1998). Regulation of recombinant PKC alpha activity by protein phosphatase 1 and protein phosphatase 2A. *Arch.Biochem.Biophys.,* 355(2), 197-200.

[35] Sylvester, P.W., McIntyre, B.S., Gapor, A. and Briski, K.P. (2001). Vitamin E inhibition of normal mammary epithelial cell growth is associated with a reduction in protein kinase C(alpha) activation. *Cell Prolif.,* 34(6), 347-357.

[36] Tran, K., Proulx, P.R. and Chan, A.C. (1994). Vitamin E suppresses diacylglycerol (DAG) level in thrombin-stimulated endothelial cells through an increase of DAG kinase activity. *Biochim.Biophys.Acta,* 1212(2), 193-202.

[37] Koya, D., Lee, I.K., Ishii, H., Kanoh, H. and King, G.L. (1997). Prevention of glomerular dysfunction in diabetic rats by treatment with d-alpha-tocopherol. *J.Am.Soc.Nephrol.*, 8(3), 426-435.

[38] Nitti, M., d'Abramo, C., Traverso, N., Verzola, D., Garibotto, G., Poggi, A., Odetti, P., Cottalasso, D., Marinari, U.M., Pronzato, M.A. *et al.* (2005). Central role of PKCdelta in glycoxidation-dependent apoptosis of human neurons. *Free Radic.Biol.Med.,* 38(7), 846-856.

[39] Kim, S.Y., Yang, J.H. (2005). Neurotoxic effects of 2,3,7,8-tetrachlorodibenzo-p-dioxin in cerebellar granule cells. *Exp.Mol.Med.,* 37(1), 58-64.

[40] Aarts, M., Iihara, K., Wei, W.L., Xiong, Z.G., Arundine, M., Cerwinski, W., MacDonald, J.F. and Tymianski, M. (2003). A key role for TRPM7 channels in anoxic neuronal death. *Cell,* 115(7), 863-877.

[41] Williams, E.J., Doherty, P. (1999). Evidence for and against a pivotal role of PI 3-kinase in a neuronal cell survival pathway. *Mol.Cell Neurosci.,* 13(4), 272-280.

[42] Kaplan, D.R., Miller, F.D. (2000). Neurotrophin signal transduction in the nervous system. *Curr.Opin.Neurobiol.,* 10(3), 381-391.

[43] Shimoke, K., Yamagishi, S., Yamada, M., Ikeuchi, T. and Hatanaka, H. (1999). Inhibition of phosphatidylinositol 3-kinase activity elevates c-Jun N-terminal kinase activity in apoptosis of cultured cerebellar granule neurons. *Brain Res.Dev.Brain Res.,* 112(2), 245-253.

[44] Romashkova, J.A., Makarov, S.S. (1999). NF-kappaB is a target of AKT in anti-apoptotic PDGF signalling. *Nature,* 401(6748), 86-90.

[45] Datta, S.R., Dudek, H., Tao, X., Masters, S., Fu, H., Gotoh, Y. and Greenberg, M.E. (1997). Akt phosphorylation of BAD couples survival signals to the cell-intrinsic death machinery. *Cell,* 91(2), 231-241.

[46] Brunet, A., Bonni, A., Zigmond, M.J., Lin, M.Z., Juo, P., Hu, L.S., Anderson, M.J., Arden, K.C., Blenis, J. and Greenberg, M.E. (1999). Akt promotes cell survival by phosphorylating and inhibiting a Forkhead transcription factor. *Cell,* 96(6), 857-868.

[47] Stocker, A., Zimmer, S., Spycher, S.E. and Azzi, A. (1999). Identification of a novel cytosolic tocopherol-binding protein: structure, specificity, and tissue distribution. *IUBMB.Life,* 48(1), 49-55.

[48] Zimmer, S., Stocker, A., Sarbolouki, M.N., Spycher, S.E., Sassoon, J. and Azzi, A. (2000). A novel human tocopherol-associated protein: cloning, in vitro expression, and characterization. *J Biol.Chem.,* 275(33), 25672-25680.

[49] Wirtz, K.W. (1997). Phospholipid transfer proteins revisited. *Biochem.J.,* 324 (Pt 2), 353-360.

[50] Wirtz, K.W. (1997). Phospholipid transfer proteins revisited. *Biochem.J.,* 324 (Pt 2), 353-360.

[51] Yamauchi, J., Iwamoto, T., Kida, S., Masushige, S., Yamada, K. and Esashi, T. (2001). Tocopherol-associated protein is a ligand-dependent transcriptional activator. *Biochem.Biophys.Res.Commun,* 285(2), 295-299.

[52] Kempna, P., Zingg, J.M., Ricciarelli, R., Hierl, M., Saxena, S. and Azzi, A. (2003). Cloning of novel human SEC14p-like proteins: ligand binding and functional properties. *Free Radic.Biol.Med.,* 34(11), 1458-1472.

[53] Anantharaman, V., Aravind, L. (2002). The GOLD domain, a novel protein module involved in Golgi function and secretion. *Genome Biol.,* 3(5), research0023.

[54] Sohda, M., Misumi, Y., Yamamoto, A., Yano, A., Nakamura, N. and Ikehara, Y. (2001). Identification and characterization of a novel Golgi protein, GCP60, that interacts with the integral membrane protein giantin. *J.Biol.Chem.,* 276(48), 45298-45306.

[55] Crossthwaite, A.J., Hasan, S. and Williams, R.J. (2002). Hydrogen peroxide-mediated phosphorylation of ERK1/2, Akt/PKB and JNK in cortical neurones: dependence on Ca(2+) and PI3-kinase. *J Neurochem.,* 80(1), 24-35.

[56] Rota, C., Rimbach, G., Minihane, A.M., Stoecklin, E. and Barella, L. (2005). Dietary vitamin E modulates differential gene expression in the rat hippocampus: potential implications for its neuroprotective properties. *Nutr.Neurosci.,* 8(1), 21-29.

[57] Selkoe, D.J. (2001). Alzheimer's disease: genes, proteins, and therapy. *Physiol Rev.,* 81(2), 741-766.

[58] Murphy, T.H., Schnaar, R.L. and Coyle, J.T. (1990). Immature cortical neurons are uniquely sensitive to glutamate toxicity by inhibition of cystine uptake. *FASEB J.,* 4(6), 1624-1633.

[59] Kato, S., Negishi, K., Mawatari, K. and Kuo, C.H. (1992). A mechanism for glutamate toxicity in the C6 glioma cells involving inhibition of cystine uptake leading to glutathione depletion. *Neuroscience,* 48(4), 903-914.

[60] Han, D., Sen, C.K., Roy, S., Kobayashi, M.S., Tritschler, H.J. and Packer, L. (1997). Protection against glutamate-induced cytotoxicity in C6 glial cells by thiol antioxidants. *Am.J.Physiol,* 273(5 Pt 2), R1771-R1778.

[61] Miyamoto, M., Murphy, T.H., Schnaar, R.L. and Coyle, J.T. (1989). Antioxidants protect against glutamate-induced cytotoxicity in a neuronal cell line. *J.Pharmacol.Exp.Ther.,* 250(3), 1132-1140.

[62] Murphy, T.H., Miyamoto, M., Sastre, A., Schnaar, R.L. and Coyle, J.T. (1989). Glutamate toxicity in a neuronal cell line involves inhibition of cystine transport leading to oxidative stress. *Neuron,* 2(6), 1547-1558.

[63] Sen, C.K., Khanna, S., Roy, S. and Packer, L. (2000). Molecular basis of vitamin E action. Tocotrienol potently inhibits glutamate-induced pp60(c-Src) kinase activation and death of HT4 neuronal cells. *J Biol.Chem.,* 275(17), 13049-13055.

[64] Aikawa, R., Komuro, I., Yamazaki, T., Zou, Y., Kudoh, S., Tanaka, M., Shiojima, I., Hiroi, Y. and Yazaki, Y. (1997). Oxidative stress activates extracellular signal-regulated kinases through Src and Ras in cultured cardiac myocytes of neonatal rats. *J.Clin.Invest,* 100(7), 1813-1821.

[65] Li, Y., Maher, P. and Schubert, D. (1997). A role for 12-lipoxygenase in nerve cell death caused by glutathione depletion. *Neuron,* 19(2), 453-463.

[66] Tan, S., Sagara, Y., Liu, Y., Maher, P. and Schubert, D. (1998). The regulation of reactive oxygen species production during programmed cell death. *J.Cell Biol.,* 141(6), 1423-1432.

[67] Reddanna, P., Rao, M.K. and Reddy, C.C. (1985). Inhibition of 5-lipoxygenase by vitamin E. *FEBS Lett.,* 193(1), 39-43.

[68] Grossman, S., Waksman, E.G. (1984). New aspects of the inhibition of soybean lipoxygenase by alpha-tocopherol. Evidence for the existence of a specific complex. *Int.J.Biochem.,* 16(3), 281-289.

[69] Roy, S., Lado, B.H., Khanna, S. and Sen, C.K. (2002). Vitamin E sensitive genes in the developing rat fetal brain: a high-density oligonucleotide microarray analysis. *FEBS Lett.,* 530(1-3), 17-23.

[70] Sen, C.K., Khanna, S. and Roy, S. (2004). Tocotrienol: the natural vitamin E to defend the nervous system? *Ann.N.Y.Acad.Sci.,* 1031, 127-142.

[71] Grimes, C.A., Jope, R.S. (2001). The multifaceted roles of glycogen synthase kinase 3beta in cellular signaling. *Prog.Neurobiol.,* 65(4), 391-426.

[72] Pearl, L.H., Barford, D. (2002). Regulation of protein kinases in insulin, growth factor and Wnt signalling. *Curr.Opin.Struct.Biol.,* 12(6), 761-767.

[73] Klein, P.S., Melton, D.A. (1996). A molecular mechanism for the effect of lithium on development. *Proc.Natl.Acad.Sci.U.S.A,* 93(16), 8455-8459.

[74] Stambolic, V., Ruel, L. and Woodgett, J.R. (1996). Lithium inhibits glycogen synthase kinase-3 activity and mimics wingless signalling in intact cells. *Curr.Biol.,* 6(12), 1664-1668.

[75] Woodgett, J.R. (1990). Molecular cloning and expression of glycogen synthase kinase-3/factor A. *EMBO J.,* 9(8), 2431-2438.

[76] Yamaguchi, H., Ishiguro, K., Uchida, T., Takashima, A., Lemere, C.A. and Imahori, K. (1996). Preferential labeling of Alzheimer neurofibrillary tangles with antisera for tau protein kinase (TPK) I/glycogen synthase kinase-3 beta and cyclin-dependent kinase 5, a component of TPK II. *Acta Neuropathol.*(Berl), 92(3), 232-241.

[77] Imahori, K., Uchida, T. (1997). Physiology and pathology of tau protein kinases in relation to Alzheimer's disease. *J.Biochem.*(Tokyo), 121(2), 179-188.

[78] Pei, J.J., Tanaka, T., Tung, Y.C., Braak, E., Iqbal, K. and Grundke-Iqbal, I. (1997). Distribution, levels, and activity of glycogen synthase kinase-3 in the Alzheimer disease brain. *J.Neuropathol.Exp.Neurol.,* 56(1), 70-78.

[79] Pei, J.J., Braak, E., Braak, H., Grundke-Iqbal, I., Iqbal, K., Winblad, B. and Cowburn, R.F. (1999). Distribution of active glycogen synthase kinase 3beta (GSK-3beta) in brains staged for Alzheimer disease neurofibrillary changes. *J.Neuropathol.Exp.Neurol.,* 58(9), 1010-1019.

[80] Ferreira, A., Lu, Q., Orecchio, L. and Kosik, K.S. (1997). Selective phosphorylation of adult tau isoforms in mature hippocampal neurons exposed to fibrillar A beta. *Mol.Cell Neurosci.,* 9(3), 220-234.

[81] Takashima, A., Murayama, M., Murayama, O., Kohno, T., Honda, T., Yasutake, K., Nihonmatsu, N., Mercken, M., Yamaguchi, H., Sugihara, S. *et al.* (1998). Presenilin 1 associates with glycogen synthase kinase-3beta and its substrate tau. *Proc.Natl.Acad.Sci.U.S.A,* 95(16), 9637-9641.

[82] Takashima, A., Noguchi, K., Sato, K., Hoshino, T. and Imahori, K. (1993). Tau protein kinase I is essential for amyloid beta-protein-induced neurotoxicity. *Proc.Natl.Acad.Sci.U.S.A,* 90(16), 7789-7793.

[83] Farias, G.G., Godoy, J.A., Hernandez, F., Avila, J., Fisher, A. and Inestrosa, N.C. (2004). M1 muscarinic receptor activation protects neurons from beta-amyloid toxicity. A role for Wnt signaling pathway. *Neurobiol.Dis.,* 17(2), 337-348.

[84] Busciglio, J., Lorenzo, A., Yeh, J. and Yankner, B.A. (1995). beta-amyloid fibrils induce tau phosphorylation and loss of microtubule binding. *Neuron,* 14(4), 879-888.

[85] Bhat, R.V., Shanley, J., Correll, M.P., Fieles, W.E., Keith, R.A., Scott, C.W. and Lee, C.M. (2000). Regulation and localization of tyrosine216 phosphorylation of glycogen

synthase kinase-3beta in cellular and animal models of neuronal degeneration. roc. *Natl.Acad.Sci.U.S.A*, 97(20), 11074-11079.

[86] Frame, S., Cohen, P. and Biondi, R.M. (2001). A common phosphate binding site explains the unique substrate specificity of GSK3 and its inactivation by phosphorylation. *Mol.Cell*, 7(6), 1321-1327.

[87] Cross, D.A., Alessi, D.R., Cohen, P., Andjelkovich, M. and Hemmings, B.A. (1995). Inhibition of glycogen synthase kinase-3 by insulin mediated by protein kinase B. *Nature*, 378(6559), 785-789.

[88] Plyte, S.E., Hughes, K., Nikolakaki, E., Pulverer, B.J. and Woodgett, J.R. (1992). Glycogen synthase kinase-3: functions in oncogenesis and development. *Biochim.Biophys.Acta*, 1114(2-3), 147-162.

[89] Cui, H., Meng, Y. and Bulleit, R.F. (1998). Inhibition of glycogen synthase kinase 3beta activity regulates proliferation of cultured cerebellar granule cells. *Brain Res.Dev.Brain Res.*, 111(2), 177-188.

[90] Quevedo, C., Alcazar, A. and Salinas, M. (2000). Two different signal transduction pathways are implicated in the regulation of initiation factor 2B activity in insulin-like growth factor-1-stimulated neuronal cells. *J.Biol.Chem.*, 275(25), 19192-19197.

[91] Pap, M., Cooper, G.M. (1998). Role of glycogen synthase kinase-3 in the phosphatidylinositol 3-Kinase/Akt cell survival pathway. *J.Biol.Chem.*, 273(32), 19929-19932.

[92] Haq, S., Choukroun, G., Kang, Z.B., Ranu, H., Matsui, T., Rosenzweig, A., Molkentin, J.D., Alessandrini, A., Woodgett, J., Hajjar, R. *et al.* (2000). Glycogen synthase kinase-3beta is a negative regulator of cardiomyocyte hypertrophy. *J.Cell Biol.*, 151(1), 117-130.

[93] Halse, R., Rochford, J.J., McCormack, J.G., Vandenheede, J.R., Hemmings, B.A. and Yeaman, S.J. (1999). Control of glycogen synthesis in cultured human muscle cells. *J.Biol.Chem.*, 274(2), 776-780.

[94] Behrens, J., von Kries, J.P., Kuhl, M., Bruhn, L., Wedlich, D., Grosschedl, R. and Birchmeier, W. (1996). Functional interaction of beta-catenin with the transcription factor LEF-1. *Nature*, 382(6592), 638-642.

[95] Dale, T.C. (1998). Signal transduction by the Wnt family of ligands. *Biochem.J.*, 329 (Pt 2), 209-223.

[96] Cook, D., Fry, M.J., Hughes, K., Sumathipala, R., Woodgett, J.R. and Dale, T.C. (1996). Wingless inactivates glycogen synthase kinase-3 via an intracellular signalling pathway which involves a protein kinase C. *EMBO J.*, 15(17), 4526-4536.

[97] Quintanilla, R.A., Munoz, F.J., Metcalfe, M.J., Hitschfeld, M., Godoy, J.A. and Inestrosa, N.C. (2005). Trolox and 17beta -estradiol protects from the amyloid-beta -peptide neurotoxiticy by a mechanism that involves modulation of the Wnt signaling pathway. *J.Biol.Chem.*.

[98] Shwaery, G.T., Vita, J.A. and Keaney, J.F., Jr. (1997). Antioxidant protection of LDL by physiological concentrations of 17 beta-estradiol. Requirement for estradiol modification. *Circulation*, 95(6), 1378-1385.

[99] Packer, L., Weber, S.U. and Rimbach, G. (2001). Molecular aspects of alpha-tocotrienol antioxidant action and cell signalling. *J.Nutr.*, 131(2), 369S-373S.

[100] Moosmann, B., Behl, C. (1999). The antioxidant neuroprotective effects of estrogens and phenolic compounds are independent from their estrogenic properties. *Proc.Natl.Acad.Sci.U.S.A*, 96(16), 8867-8872.

[101] Zingg, J.M., Azzi, A. (2004). Non-antioxidant activities of vitamin E. *Curr.Med.Chem.*, 11(9), 1113-1133.

[102] Essers, M.A., Vries-Smits, L.M., Barker, N., Polderman, P.E., Burgering, B.M. and Korswagen, H.C. (2005). Functional interaction between beta-catenin and FOXO in oxidative stress signaling. *Science*, 308(5725), 1181-1184.

[103] Shin, S.Y., Kim, C.G., Jho, E.H., Rho, M.S., Kim, Y.S., Kim, Y.H. and Lee, Y.H. (2004). Hydrogen peroxide negatively modulates Wnt signaling through downregulation of beta-catenin. *Cancer Lett.*, 212(2), 225-231.

[104] Cardona-Gomez, P., Perez, M., Avila, J., Garcia-Segura, L.M. and Wandosell, F. (2004). Estradiol inhibits GSK3 and regulates interaction of estrogen receptors, GSK3, and beta-catenin in the hippocampus. *Mol.Cell Neurosci.*, 25(3), 363-373.

[105] Kempna, P., Reiter, E., Arock, M., Azzi, A. and Zingg, J.M. (2004). Inhibition of HMC-1 mast cell proliferation by vitamin E: involvement of the protein kinase B pathway. *J Biol.Chem.*, 279(49), 50700-50709.

[106] Wolfe, L.S. (1982). Eicosanoids: prostaglandins, thromboxanes, leukotrienes, and other derivatives of carbon-20 unsaturated fatty acids. *J.Neurochem.*, 38(1), 1-14.

[107] Wu, D., Hayek, M.G. and Meydani, S. (2001). Vitamin E and macrophage cyclooxygenase regulation in the aged. *J.Nutr.*, 131(2), 382S-388S.

[108] Moskowitz, N., Schook, W. and Puszkin, S. (1982). Interaction of brain synaptic vesicles induced by endogenous Ca2+ -dependent phospholipase A2. *Science*, 216(4543), 305-307.

[109] Hedqvist, P., Gustafsson, L., Hjemdahl, P. and Svanborg, K. (1980). Aspects of prostaglandin action on autonomic neuroeffector transmission. *Adv.Prostaglandin Thromboxane Res.*, 8, 1245-1248.

[110] O'Regan, M.H., Perkins, L.M. and Phillis, J.W. (1995). Arachidonic acid and lysophosphatidylcholine modulate excitatory transmitter amino acid release from the rat cerebral cortex. *Neurosci.Lett.*, 193(2), 85-88.

[111] Farooqui, A.A., Yang, H.C. and Horrocks, L. (1997). Involvement of phospholipase A2 in neurodegeneration. *Neurochem.Int.*, 30(6), 517-522.

[112] Edgar, A.D., Strosznajder, J. and Horrocks, L.A. (1982). Activation of ethanolamine phospholipase A2 in Brain during ischemia. *J.Neurochem.*, 39(4), 1111-1116.

[113] Rordorf, G., Uemura, Y. and Bonventre, J.V. (1991). Characterization of phospholipase A2 (PLA2) activity in gerbil brain: enhanced activities of cytosolic, mitochondrial, and microsomal forms after ischemia and reperfusion. *J.Neurosci.*, 11(6), 1829-1836.

[114] Farooqui, A.A., Horrocks, L.A. (1991). Excitatory amino acid receptors, neural membrane phospholipid metabolism and neurological disorders. *Brain Res.Brain Res.Rev.*, 16(2), 171-191.

[115] Gattaz, W.F., Schmitt, A. and Maras, A. (1995). Increased platelet phospholipase A2 activity in schizophrenia. *Schizophr.Res.*, 16(1), 1-6.

[116] Ross, B.M., Hudson, C., Erlich, J., Warsh, J.J. and Kish, S.J. (1997). Increased phospholipid breakdown in schizophrenia. Evidence for the involvement of a calcium-independent phospholipase A2. *Arch.Gen.Psychiatry*, 54(5), 487-494.

[117] Stephenson, D.T., Lemere, C.A., Selkoe, D.J. and Clemens, J.A. (1996). Cytosolic phospholipase A2 (cPLA2) immunoreactivity is elevated in Alzheimer's disease brain. *Neurobiol.Dis.*, 3(1), 51-63.

[118] Douglas, C.E., Chan, A.C. and Choy, P.C. (1986). Vitamin E inhibits platelet phospholipase A2. *Biochim.Biophys.Acta*, 876(3), 639-645.

[119] Pentland, A.P., Morrison, A.R., Jacobs, S.C., Hruza, L.L., Hebert, J.S. and Packer, L. (1992). Tocopherol analogs suppress arachidonic acid metabolism via phospholipase inhibition. *J.Biol.Chem.*, 267(22), 15578-15584.

[120] Chandra, V., Jasti, J., Kaur, P., Betzel, C., Srinivasan, A. and Singh, T.P. (2002). First structural evidence of a specific inhibition of phospholipase A2 by alpha-tocopherol (vitamin E) and its implications in inflammation: crystal structure of the complex formed between phospholipase A2 and alpha-tocopherol at 1.8 A resolution. *J.Mol.Biol.*, 320(2), 215-222.

[121] Hensley, K., Hall, N., Subramaniam, R., Cole, P., Harris, M., Aksenov, M., Aksenova, M., Gabbita, S.P., Wu, J.F., Carney, J.M. *et al.* (1995). Brain regional correspondence between Alzheimer's disease histopathology and biomarkers of protein oxidation. *J.Neurochem.*, 65(5), 2146-2156.

[122] Pappata, S., Levasseur, M., Gunn, R.N., Myers, R., Crouzel, C., Syrota, A., Jones, T., Kreutzberg, G.W. and Banati, R.B. (2000). Thalamic microglial activation in ischemic stroke detected in vivo by PET and [11C]PK1195. *Neurology*, 55(7), 1052-1054.

[123] Cagnin, A., Brooks, D.J., Kennedy, A.M., Gunn, R.N., Myers, R., Turkheimer, F.E., Jones, T. and Banati, R.B. (2001). In-vivo measurement of activated microglia in dementia. *Lancet*, 358(9280), 461-467.

[124] Hull, M., Lieb, K. and Fiebich, B.L. (2000). Anti-inflammatory drugs: a hope for Alzheimer's disease? *Expert.Opin.Investig.Drugs*, 9(4), 671-683.

[125] Lebeau, A., Terro, F., Rostene, W. and Pelaprat, D. (2004). Blockade of 12-lipoxygenase expression protects cortical neurons from apoptosis induced by beta-amyloid peptide. *Cell Death.Differ.*, 11(8), 875-884.

[126] Ryu, J.K., Franciosi, S., Sattayaprasert, P., Kim, S.U. and McLarnon, J.G. (2004). Minocycline inhibits neuronal death and glial activation induced by beta-amyloid peptide in rat hippocampus. *Glia*, 48(1), 85-90.

[127] Bate, C., Veerhuis, R., Eikelenboom, P. and Williams, A. (2003). Neurones treated with cyclo-oxygenase-1 inhibitors are resistant to amyloid-beta1-42. *Neuroreport*, 14(16), 2099-2103.

[128] Townsend, K.P., Pratico, D. (2005). Novel therapeutic opportunities for Alzheimer's disease: focus on nonsteroidal anti-inflammatory drugs. *FASEB J.*, 19(12), 1592-1601.

[129] in, t., V, Ruitenberg, A., Hofman, A., Launer, L.J., van Duijn, C.M., Stijnen, T., Breteler, M.M. and Stricker, B.H. (2001). Nonsteroidal antiinflammatory drugs and the risk of Alzheimer's disease. *N.Engl.J.Med.*, 345(21), 1515-1521.

[130] Relkin, N.R., Reichman, W.E., Orazem, J. and McRae, T. (2003). A large, community-based, open-label trial of donepezil in the treatment of Alzheimer's disease. *Dement.Geriatr.Cogn Disord.*, 16(1), 15-24.

[131] Aisen, P.S., Schafer, K.A., Grundman, M., Pfeiffer, E., Sano, M., Davis, K.L., Farlow, M.R., Jin, S., Thomas, R.G. and Thal, L.J. (2003). Effects of rofecoxib or naproxen vs placebo on Alzheimer disease progression: a randomized controlled trial. *JAMA*, 289(21), 2819-2826.

[132] Martin, B.K., Meinert, C.L. and Breitner, J.C. (2002). Double placebo design in a prevention trial for Alzheimer's disease. *Control Clin.Trials,* 23(1), 93-99.

[133] Jiang, Q., Elson-Schwab, I., Courtemanche, C. and Ames, B.N. (2000). gamma-tocopherol and its major metabolite, in contrast to alpha-tocopherol, inhibit cyclooxygenase activity in macrophages and epithelial cells. *Proc.Natl.Acad.Sci.U.S.A,* 97(21), 11494-11499.

[134] Wu, D., Mura, C., Beharka, A.A., Han, S.N., Paulson, K.E., Hwang, D. and Meydani, S.N. (1998). Age-associated increase in PGE2 synthesis and COX activity in murine macrophages is reversed by vitamin E. *Am.J.Physiol,* 275(3 Pt 1), C661-C668.

[135] Chanock, S.J., Roesler, J., Zhan, S., Hopkins, P., Lee, P., Barrett, D.T., Christensen, B.L., Curnutte, J.T. and Gorlach, A. (2000). Genomic structure of the human p47-phox (NCF1) gene. *Blood Cells Mol.Dis.,* 26(1), 37-46.

[136] Babior, B.M. (1999). NADPH oxidase: an update. *Blood,* 93(5), 1464-1476.

[137] Parvathenani, L.K., Tertyshnikova, S., Greco, C.R., Roberts, S.B., Robertson, B. and Posmantur, R. (2003). P2X7 mediates superoxide production in primary microglia and is up-regulated in a transgenic mouse model of Alzheimer's disease. *J.Biol.Chem.,* 278(15), 13309-13317.

[138] Egger, T., Hammer, A., Wintersperger, A., Goti, D., Malle, E. and Sattler, W. (2001). Modulation of microglial superoxide production by alpha-tocopherol in vitro: attenuation of p67(phox) translocation by a protein phosphatase-dependent pathway. *J Neurochem.,* 79(6), 1169-1182.

[139] Sano, M. (2003). Noncholinergic treatment options for Alzheimer's disease. *J Clin.Psychiatry,* 64 Suppl 9, 23-28.

[140] Morris, M.C., Beckett, L.A., Scherr, P.A., Hebert, L.E., Bennett, D.A., Field, T.S. and Evans, D.A. (1998). Vitamin E and vitamin C supplement use and risk of incident Alzheimer disease. *Alzheimer Dis Assoc.Disord.,* 12(3), 121-126.

[141] Masaki, K.H., Losonczy, K.G., Izmirlian, G., Foley, D.J., Ross, G.W., Petrovitch, H., Havlik, R. and White, L.R. (2000). Association of vitamin E and C supplement use with cognitive function and dementia in elderly men. *Neurology,* 54(6), 1265-1272.

[142] Anderson, S.L., Qiu, J. and Rubin, B.Y. (2003). Tocotrienols induce IKBKAP expression: a possible therapy for familial dysautonomia. *Biochem.Biophys.Res.Commun,* 306(1), 303-309.

[143] Steinberg, D. (1995). Clinical trials of antioxidants in atherosclerosis: are we doing the right thing? *Lancet,* 346(8966), 36-38.

[144] Gotto, A.M. (2003). Antioxidants, statins, and atherosclerosis. *J.Am.Coll.Cardiol.,* 41(7), 1205-1210.

[145] Munoz, F.J., Opazo, C., Gil-Gomez, G., Tapia, G., Fernandez, V., Valverde, M.A. and Inestrosa, N.C. (2002). Vitamin E but not 17beta-estradiol protects against vascular toxicity induced by beta-amyloid wild type and the Dutch amyloid variant. *J.Neurosci.,* 22(8), 3081-3089.

[146] Coma, M., Guix, F.X., Uribesalgo, I., Espuna, G., Sole, M., Andreu, D. and Munoz, F.J. (2005). Lack of oestrogen protection in amyloid-mediated endothelial damage due to protein nitrotyrosination. *Brain,* 128(Pt 7), 1613-1621.

[147] Qin, F., Shite, J. and Liang, C.S. (2003). Antioxidants attenuate myocyte apoptosis and improve cardiac function in CHF: association with changes in MAPK pathways. *Am.J.Physiol Heart Circ.Physiol,* 285(2), H822-H832.

[148] Uemura, M., Manabe, H., Yoshida, N., Fujita, N., Ochiai, J., Matsumoto, N., Takagi, T., Naito, Y. and Yoshikawa, T. (2002). Alpha-tocopherol prevents apoptosis of vascular endothelial cells via a mechanism exceeding that of mere antioxidation. *Eur.J.Pharmacol.,* 456(1-3), 29-37.

[149] Kong, A.N., Yu, R., Lei, W., Mandlekar, S., Tan, T.H. and Ucker, D.S. (1998). Differential activation of MAPK and ICE/Ced-3 protease in chemical-induced apoptosis. The role of oxidative stress in the regulation of mitogen-activated protein kinases (MAPKs) leading to gene expression and survival or activation of caspases leading to apoptosis. *Restor.Neurol.Neurosci.,* 12(2-3), 63-70.

[150] Pratico, D., Tangirala, R.K., Rader, D.J., Rokach, J. and FitzGerald, G.A. (1998). Vitamin E suppresses isoprostane generation in vivo and reduces atherosclerosis in ApoE-deficient mice. *Nat.Med.,* 4(10), 1189-1192.

[151] Jialal, I., Devaraj, S. and Kaul, N. (2001). The effect of alpha-tocopherol on monocyte proatherogenic activity. *J.Nutr.,* 131(2), 389S-394S.

[152] Etminan, M., Gill, S.S. and Samii, A. (2005). Intake of vitamin E, vitamin C, and carotenoids and the risk of Parkinson's disease: a meta-analysis. *Lancet Neurol.,* 4(6), 362-365.

[153] Zhang, B., Tanaka, J., Yang, L., Yang, L., Sakanaka, M., Hata, R., Maeda, N. and Mitsuda, N. (2004). Protective effect of vitamin E against focal brain ischemia and neuronal death through induction of target genes of hypoxia-inducible factor-1. *Neuroscience,* 126(2), 433-440.

In: Frontiers in Atherosclerosis Research
Editor: Karin F. Kepper, pp. 93-103
ISBN 1-60021-371-5

Chapter 5

The Effect of an Alpha-Linolenic-Acid-Rich Diet on the Circadian Rhythm of Cardiac Events

Gal Dubnov, Daniel Pella **[*]** ***and Ram B. Singh*** **[1,**]**

Department of Human Nutrition & Metabolism, Hebrew University- Hadassah Medical School, Jerusalem, Israel

*Faculty of Medicine, Safaric University, Kosice, Slovakia

**Centre of Nutrition and Heart, Medical Hospital and Research Centre, Moradabad, India

Abstract

Objective

Coronary artery disease events have a circadian rhythmicity, clustering more in the second quartile of the day. n-3 fatty acid supplementation reduces the rate of cardiac events, but its effect on their circadian rhythmicity has not been tested.

Design

The Indo-Mediterranean Diet Heart Study was a single blind randomized study that assessed the effect of a diet rich in alpha-linolenic acid, the parent n-3 fatty acid, on the occurrence of myocardial infarction and sudden cardiac death.

Subjects

One thousand subjects of the Indo-Mediterranean Diet Heart Study, focusing on the 115 patients from both control and intervention groups in which cardiac events occurred.

---

[1] Corresponding author: Ram B. Singh, MD. Centre of Nutrition and Heart, Medical Hospital and Research Centre, Moradabad-10 (UP)244001, India. E-mail: icn2005@mickyonline.com

Intervention

The timing of cardiac events throughout the day was compared between the intervention and control groups. The distribution of cardiac events along the four quartiles of the day was compared between groups as well as against equal distribution.

Results

The risk ratio for a cardiac event was lowest between 4:00 and 8:00 in the morning for the intervention group. The control group had a higher rate of events in the second quartile of the day, which deviated from an equal distribution, as expected (P=0.013). In the intervention group, events were equally distributed along the day. No statistically significant difference was found in daily event distribution between the groups.

Conclusion

A diet rich in alpha-linolenic acid may abolish the higher rate of cardiac events, normally seen in the second quartile of the day. Additional studies are needed to identify the underlying mechanism.

INTRODUCTION

The classical manifestations of coronary artery disease (CAD), such as angina pectoris, silent ischemia, myocardial infarction (MI) and sudden cardiac death, have a pronounced circadian rhythmicity, tending to cluster in the second quartile of the day [1-10]. This increase in the rate of cardiovascular events in the morning may be due to a hypercoagulable state, consisted of increased platelet aggregation, increased tPA inhibitor levels, and rapid metabolism of heparin in the morning [11-13]. In addition, the morning hours are associated with a decrease in vagal tone and increase in sympathetic activity, resulting in lower levels of acetylecholine and melatonin and increased concentrations of cortisol, aldosterone, catecholamines and angiotensin, which make the atherosclerotic plaques more vulnerable to rupture and thrombosis [14-16]. These circadian manifestations are associated with a decreased heart rate variability (HRV), which is an independent risk factor for cardiovascular events [13-16].

Recent studies indicate that n-3 fatty acids may have a beneficial effect on HRV, platelet aggregation, and endothelial function, and that they are neuroprotectors and may enhance hippocampal acetylecholine levels [15-26]. In randomized controlled trials, treatment with n-3 fatty acids led to a significant reduction in cardiac events, in both patients after a MI and those with risk factors only [27-30]. To our knowledge, no study has examined the effect of n-3 fatty acids on the timing of cardiovascular events. The aim of the present study is to examine the influence of a diet rich in alpha-linolenic acid, the parent n-3 fatty acid, on the circadian rhythm of cardiac events.

METHODS

Subjects and Study Design

The Indo-Mediterranean Diet Heart Study was a randomized, single-blind study designed to assess the effect of a diet rich in n-3 fatty acids from plant sources on the occurrence of myocardial infarction and sudden cardiac death [29]. One thousand subjects were randomized to either an intervention or a control group by selection of a card from a pile. The intervention group consisted of 499 patients, and the control group 501. The ethics committee of the Medical Hospital and Research Centre at Moradabad approved the study, and written informed consent was obtained from all participants.

Participants in both groups were advised to eat food elements that would provide a dietary intake similar to that recommended at the time by the National Cholesterol Education Program (NCEP) step I prudent diet [S31], wherein less than 30% of energy comes from total fat, less than 10% from saturated fat, and less than 300 mg of cholesterol is consumed per day. Patients in the intervention group were advised to verify the intake of at least 250–300 g of fruit, 125–150 g of vegetables, and 25–50 g of nuts. They were also encouraged to eat 400–500 g of whole grains (legumes, rice, maize, wheat) daily, as well as to use mustard seed or soy bean oil in 3 to 4 servings per day, in order to ensure a high intake of alpha-linolenic acid.

Both groups were advised to exercise daily and practice yoga meditation techniques, to abstain from smoking and alcohol consumption, and to continue the use of their regular medications.

Food intake and physical activity were monitored by self-report diaries, first weekly, then monthly, and then every 3 months. Nutrient intakes were calculated using Indian foods composition tables and other sources [32,33].and reinforce adherence. Height, weight, and blood pressure were monitored by standard methods. Blood concentrations of glucose, total cholesterol (TC), high-density lipoprotein (HDL) cholesterol, low-density lipoprotein (LDL) cholesterol and triglycerides were also measured. Clinical data, drug intake, adverse events, blood pressure, blood glucose levels, blood lipid levels, hospital admission and coronary events were recorded by physicians blinded to patient grouping.

At the 2-year follow up in the original study, cardiac events had occurred in 39 subjects from the intervention group and in 76 subjects from the control group.

Cardiac Events

The principal endpoints of the original study were fatal or nonfatal MI, sudden cardiac deaths, and the combined total of these events. Owing to the relatively small number of events in each category, we did not attempt a subgroup analysis and focused only on the combined end-point of total cardiac events.

In hospitalized patients, a diagnosis of nonfatal MI was based on a diagnostic electrocardiograph at the time of the event, or the presence of ischaemic cardiac pain and diagnostic enzyme levels of at least twice the upper limit of normal, or the presence of ischaemic cardiac pain and equivocal enzyme levels and an equivocal electrocardiograph. In patients who had not been admitted to the hospital, the diagnosis of MI was considered if they complained of chest pain, breathlessness, or syncope, combined with a diagnostic electrocardiograph at the time of event or new electrocardiographic changes consistent with MI at routine check-up. The electrocardiographic coding and analysis were performed by a cardiologist blinded to patient grouping.

Fatal MI was diagnosed when a hospital record was consistent with cause of death, and there was either a preterminal hospital admission with a definite MI, or official documentation of a myocardial infarction.

Sudden cardiac death was diagnosed when coronary heart disease had been noted, and death occurred within one hour of symptom onset.

Statistical Analysis

Analyses were performed in two ways. One was determining the risk for cardiac events in specific time frames among the whole study population. Second, we determined the number of events in the four quartiles of the day among only those subjects with events in both groups.

In order to assess the effect of the ALA-rich diet on the timing of cardiac event, we constructed a Cox multivariate model, with cardiac event as outcome variable, stratified into six 4-hour periods (0:01-4:00, 4:01-8:00, 8:01-12:00, 12:01-16:00, 16:01-20:00, and 20:01-24:00). In each model, we examined the risk ratio associated with the intervention diet, with patient's age, gender and BMI as covariates. The last available values served as the final risk factors data for the subjects who had fatal events. The analyses were held using standard statistical package (SPSS 11.0).

When comparing only the subgroups in which events occurred, Student's t test with a Bonferroni adjustment was used to analyze between-group differences of the continuous variables; P values less than 0.005 were considered statistically significant. The distribution of the number of events in each quartile of the day was compared by the chi-square test. Event rates were compared between the control and intervention groups, as well as for each group against equal distribution. Thus, for the latter, the observed event rates in the control group were compared with an expected rate of 19 (76 divided by 4) events in each quartile of the day, and the observed events in the intervention group were compared with an expected rate of 9.75 (39 divided by 4) in each quartile of the day. A two-tailed P value less than 0.05 was considered statistically significant for the parametric variables.

RESULTS

Timing of Events in Total Study Population

Baseline characteristics of the Indo-Mediterranean Diet Heart study population was presented elsewhere [29]. In all strata, the ALA-rich diet was associated with protective effect for cardiac events. The lowest risk ratio (RR=0.05; 95%CI: 0.01-0.24) was calculated for cardiac events between 4:01 and 8:00, while the highest was for events between 0:01 to 4:00

(RR=0.15 (95% CI:0.03 – 0.87) as shown in Figure 1. However, differences between strata did not reach statistical significance.

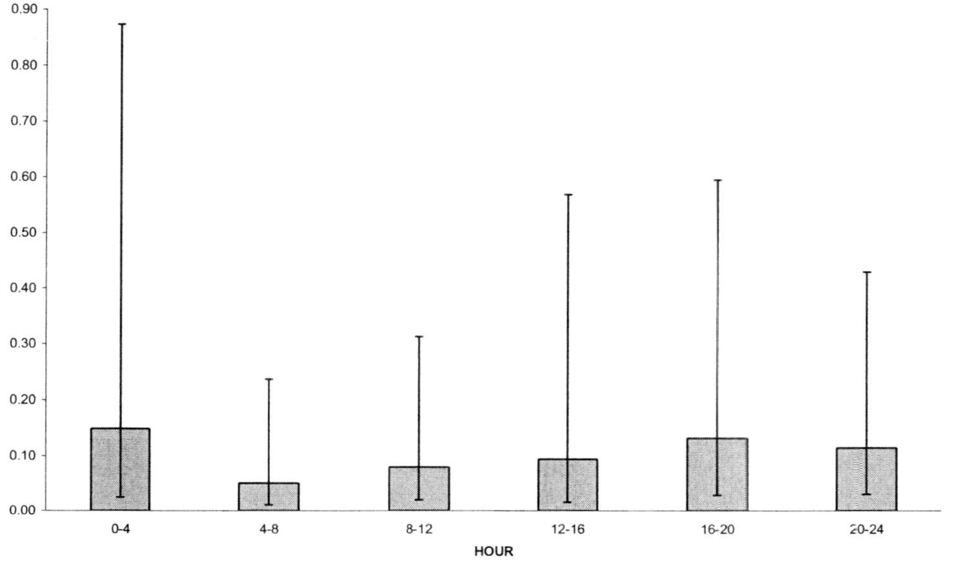

Figure 1. The risk ratio for cardiac events in the intervention group (n=499) compared with the control group (n=501) distributed into 4-hour intervals of the day.

Dispersion of Events Along Quartiles of the Day

Baseline characteristics of the subjects with cardiac events from both groups is presented in Table 1. Subjects in both groups were comparable for all major baseline variables except for body weight (borderline significance, P=0.006), yet BMIs were comparable between groups. At 2 years, only TC and LDL levels differed significantly between groups, with lower values noted in the intervention group. Nutritional data are presented in Table 2. At baseline, values of all nutrients, including fatty acids, were similar in the two groups. At 2 years, n-3 fatty acid intake was significantly higher in the intervention group, and the n-6/n-3 fatty acid ratio was lower. The number of cardiovascular events of each type in both groups is given in Table 3.

The dispersion of cardiac events along the quartiles of the day is presented in Table 4. In the control group, there was an increased rate of cardiac events clustered in the second quartile of the day, which deviated from an equal distribution (P=0.013). In the intervention group, the events were distributed equally along the day (P=0.49 when comparing observed rates and equal distribution). There was no statistically significant difference in the rate of events in each quartile of the day between the two groups (P=0.54).

Table 1. Cardiovascular risk factors at baseline and after 2 years in the intervention and control groups. Data presented as means ± SD. BMI- body mass index, BP- blood pressure, TC- total cholesterol, TG- triglyceride, FBG- fasting blood glucose.

	Intervention Group A, n = 39			Control Group B, n = 76			P value at 2 years between groups
	Baseline	2 years	P value	Baseline	2 years	P value	
Age (years)	51 ± 10	-	-	49 ± 8	-	-	-
Weight, kg	65 ± 5	62 ± 7	0.0002	68 ± 6	67 ± 6	0.0004	<0.0001
BMI, kg/m^2	24 ± 3	23 ± 3	0.0005	25 ± 2	24 ± 2	0.0005	0.0172
Systolic BP	134 ± 15	129 ± 15	0.0064	133 ± 19	132 ± 17	0.0040	0.2051
Diastolic BP	86 ± 6	84 ± 10	0.0931	88 ± 10	87 ± 10	0.0063	0.0532
Cigarettes / day	18 ± 9	19 ± 9	0.0961	21 ± 8	16 ± 5	0.0001	0.1608
TC, mmol/L	232 ± 43	220 ± 39	0.0029	245 ± 34	245 ± 32	0.7507	0.0001
LDL, mmol/L	150 ± 26	137 ± 30	0.0001	156 ± 32	157 ± 31	0.9745	0.0005
HDL, mmol/L	45 ± 15	44 ± 11	0.1319	44 ± 6	43 ± 11	0.3524	0.4414
TG, mmol/L	181 ± 51	169 ± 43	0.0259	176 ± 33	175 ± 35	0.8080	0.1881
FBG, mmol/L	112 ± 28	106 ± 25	0.0001	115 ± 33	109 ± 27	0.0029	0.2661

Table 2. Nutrient data at baseline and after 2 years in the intervention and control groups. Data presented as means ± SD.

	Intervention Group A, n = 39			**Control Group B, n = 76**			**P value at 2 years between groups**
	Baseline	**2 years**	**P value**	**Baseline**	**2 years**	**P value**	0.2589
Energy (kcal.day)	2116 ± 175	2098 241	0.3279	2167 ± 183	2123 ± 163	0.0099	<0.0001
CHO (%en)	57 ± 2	58 ± 3	0.0007	56 ± 2	55 ± 1	<0.0001	<0.0001
Protein (%en)	14 ± 1.7	14 ± 1.3	0.0112	14 ± 1.5	15 ± 0.8	0.1862	0.0241
Fat (%en)	27 ± 3	28 ± 3	0.0206	28 ± 2	30 ± 1.5	<0.0001	<0.0001
Saturated fat (%en)	13 ± 1.8	11 ± 2.3	0.0017	12 ± 1.4	13 ± 1.6	0.0003	<0.0001
MUFA (%en)	7.3 ± 1.6	9.0 ± 2.2	<0.0001	8.1 ± 2.1	8.8 ± 1.3	0.3857	0.01929
PUFA (%en)	7.0 ± 1.0	7.5±1.0	<0.0001	7.5 ± 1.0	7.9 ± 0.8	0.0111	0.0052
n-6 (%en)	6.8 ± 0.9	6.9 ± 1.0	0.4042	7.3 ± 1.0	7.6 ± 0.8	0.0001	<0.0001
n-3 (%en)	0.2 ± 0.1	0.5 ± 0.2	<0.0001	0.2 ± 0.1	0.3 ± 0.1	0.0003	<0.0001

Table 3. Distribution of cardiac events in intervention and control groups. MI – myocardial infarction.

	Intervention group (n=39)	Control group (n=76)
Nonfatal MI	21	43
Fatal MI	12	17
Sudden cardiac death	6	16

Table 4. Distribution of cardiac events along the quartiles of the day in the intervention and control groups. In the intervention group, events are near-equally distributed along the day. In the control group, quartile 2 has more events than would be expected assuming equal distribution.

Quartile (time range)	Intervention group (n=39) n (% within group)	Control group (n=76) n (% within group)
1 (00:01 – 06:00)	10 (26%)	15 (20%)
2 (06:01 – 12:00)	11 (28%)	29 (38%)
3 (12:01 – 18:00)	8 (21%)	10 (13%)
4 (18:01 – 00:00)	10 (26%)	22 (29%)

DISCUSSION

This study is the first to assess the effect of an ALA-rich diet on the circadian rhythm of cardiac events. We have found that although the intervention diet dramatically lowered the risk for events throughout the day, it nearly abolished it in the early morning hours. The increased rate of events known to occur in the second quartile of the day was eliminated by the diet.

Although n-3-rich diets have been found to be cardioprotective in several randomized controlled trials [27-30], their exact mode of action is still unknown. Our results suggest that dietary supplementation of alpha-linolenic acid may lead to a change in the circadian occurrence of cardiac events. The only major risk factors that differed significantly between the groups at the end of the trial along the trial were the lower levels of total cholesterol and LDL. However, we would expect this change to influence the total rate of events, and not just their distribution during the day, which was the focus of this study.

We are unaware of any other large-scale study that has examined the effect of n-3 fatty acids on the circadian rhythmicity of cardiac events. The Physicians Health Study recorded the number of myocardial infarctions in patients treated with aspirin or not, and found a significant decrease in the rhythmicity of myocardial infarctions in the aspirin group [34]. It is possible that this reduction was the result of the inhibitory effect of aspirin on platelet aggregation, a quality also possessed by n-3 fatty acids [25]. When these findings are combined, it appears that one of the triggers for MI in the morning hours is the increased tendency of platelets to aggregate.

Christensen and coworkers [17] reported a positive correlation between HRV and the platelet content of n-3 fatty acids (docosahexaenoic acid, DHA) in patients with post-MI left ventricular dysfunction. The increase in HRV occurred even after intake of only one fish meal per week, with an increase in standard deviation of normal-normal (SDNN) from 103 to 122ms. Further analysis revealed a negative correlation between the ratio of arachidonic acid/ DHA and the SDNN interval [18], consistent with earlier findings. In a more recent study, of 291 patients referred for coronary angiography that completed a food frequency questionnaire, researchers measured the n-3 fatty acid composition of granulocyte membranes and adipose tissue along with 24-hour HRV analysis [19]. Significant positive correlations were found between HRV indices and the levels of n-3 fatty acids in granulocytes. The positive influence of n-3 fatty acids on HRV suggests that this is indeed a major mechanism of CAD event reduction, as seen even after a few months of treatment [28].

HRV is a manifestation of sympathetic and parasympathetic activity of the heart, and a decreased HRV enhances the risk of circadian rhythmicity of cardiac events. This may well be another mechanism by which n-3 fatty acids reduce coronary events in the morning hours. In one randomized, controlled trial, of 81 patients after MI [17], treatment with n-3 fatty acids was associated with significant increase in HRV compared with controls, indicating an increased vagal cardiac tone. A retrospective analysis of a randomized, controlled intervention trial among 118 (fish oil group) and 122 (control group) patients with acute MI showed that treatment with fish oil (rich in EPA and DHA) was associated with a significant reduction in cardiac events (30% vs 56%, $P<0.02$) [27]. While the majority of cardiac events in the control group were reported in the second quartile of the day compared to first and third quartiles (35.7% vs 16.0%, 19.6%, respectively, $P<0.01$), no such association was observed in the fish oil group (unpublished data). These results are consistent with the view that fish oil administration may have a beneficial effect on circadian rhythmicity of cardiac events.

Alpha-linolenic acid is the parent n-3 fatty acid which is converted into long-chain fatty acids such as EPA and DHA in the body, to be later incorporated among phospholipids in cell membranes and adipose tissue. By using a control group which was also given dietary and exercise advice, we were able to isolate and highlight the role of the n-3 fatty acids. A detailed analysis of the role of specific nutrients in our Indo- Mediterranean diet is currently underway. Interim calculations show that the dietary intake of n-3 fatty acids had a major impact on the risk for cardiac events in the intervention group. The main sources of n-3 fatty acids in our diet were plants: walnuts, green leafy vegetables, whole grains, soy bean oil, and mustard oil. Thus, it is not necessary to consume the fish-derived long chain acids, DHA and EPA, in order to reap the benefits of n-3 fatty acids.

The exact mechanism underlying the circadian rhythmicity of cardiac events and its regulation by n-3 fatty acids remains unknown. There is consistent evidence that this rhythmicity is controlled by the suprachiasmatic nucleus [35], a tiny clump of cells in the brain which works as a biological clock and is influenced by daily changes in light and darkness. Brain neurons are rich in n-3 fatty acids, as are cell membranes of cardiomyocytes, endothelial cells and arterial smooth muscle cells. It is there fore possible that a relative deficiency of n-3 fatty acids in these cells enhances their susceptibility to excitation, causing greater neurohumoral and cardiovascular dysfunction, and resulting in a marked increase in the rhythmicity of cardiac events [36]. Increased vagal tone decreases the synthesis of tumor necrosis factor-alpha (TNF-alpha) in the liver and inhibits the release of proinflammatory cytokines such as IL-6 [20-22]. It is possible that low levels of n-3 fatty acids decrease the vagal tone, leading to increased synthesis of TNF-alpha and a greater release of proinflammatory cytokines by increased sympathetic activity. Treatment with n-3 fatty acids may break this cycle, decreasing inflammation and excitation of neurons, cardiomyocytes, endothelial and smooth muscle cells, bringing about a decreased vulnerability for cardiac events. Furthermore, n-3 fatty acids may also enhance brain acetylecholine level and parasympathetic tone, resulting in increased HRV, and hence, protection from pronounced rhythmicity of cardiac events [17-22].

One major limitation of our study is the relatively small number of events both overall and in each quartile of the day, owing to both the concomitant primary prevention arm of our original study (about half of the 1000 subjects had only risk factors for CAD, and were not post-MI patients), and the large reduction in event rate in the intervention group, brought about by the n-3 supplementation. Thus, the statistical analyses can not definitely rule out this factor as the reason for the fairly equal distribution of events in the n-3 group. Given the measured proportion of events in the high risk hours (28%), a power of 80% and 39 participants in the intervention group, allowed the minimal detection of 17% difference compared to control group; the difference observed was 10%. Nevertheless, the many mechanisms by which n-3 fatty acids may influence the circadian rhythm of CAD events cannot be overlooked, and we therefore believe that a biological explanation is plausible. A larger interventional study with more events is needed to confirm our findings.

In summary, our study suggests that an Indo-Mediterranean diet, which is rich in fruits, vegetables, nuts, whole grains, soy and mustard oils, can provide sufficient alpha-linolenic acid, to result in a modulation in the rhythmicity of cardiac events by n-3 fatty acids. Since a high n-6/n-3 ratio may blunt the beneficial effects of n-3 fatty acids, soybean oil should be replaced by more mustard oil. The exact nature of the cardioprotective action of n-3 fatty acids, whether by influencing platelet function or HRV through brain-heart connections, remains to be elucidated.

REFERENCES

[1] Pell S, D'Alonzo CA. Acute myocardial infarction in a large industrial population. *JAMA* 1963;185:831-8.

[2] Arntz HR, Willich SN, Schreiber C, et al. Diurnal, weekly and seasonal variation of sudden death. *Eur Heart J* 2000;21:315-20.

[3] Willich SN. European survey on circadian variation of angina pectoris (ESCVA): design and preliminary results. *J Cardiovasc Pharmacol* 1999;34(suppl 2):s9-13.

[4] Singh RB, Pella D, Neki NS, et al. Mechanism of acute myocardial infarction study (MAMY Study). *Biomed Pharmacother* 2004;57:in press.

[5] Rocco MB, Barry J, Campbell BAS, et al. Circadian variation of transient myocardial ischemia in patients with coronary artery disease. *Circulation* 1987;75:395-400.

[6] Muller JE, Stone PH, Turi ZG, et al. Circadian variation in the frequency of onset of acute myocardial infarction. *N Engl J Med* 1985;313:1315-22.

[7] Goldberg R, Brady P, Chen J, et al. Time of onset of acute myocardial infarction after awakening. *J Am Coll Cardiol* 1989;13:133A [abstract].

[8] Davies MJ, Thomas A. Thrombosis and acute coronary artery lesions in sudden cardiac ischemic death. *N Engl J Med* 1984;310:1137-41.

[9] Muller JE, Ludmer PL, Willich SN, et al. Circadian variation in the frequency of sudden cardiac death. *Circulation* 1987;75:131-8

[10] International Study of Infarct Survival-2 (ISIS-2) Collaborative Group. Morning peak in the incidence of myocardial infarction: experience in the ISIS-2 trial. *Eur Heart J* 1992;13:594-608.

[11] Toffler GH, Brezinski D, Schaefer A, et al. Concurrent morning increase in platelet aggregability and the risk of myocardial infarction and sudden cardiac death. *N Engl J Med* 1987;316:1514-8.

[12] Chasen C, Muller JE. Cardiovascular triggers and morning events. *Blood Pressure Monit* 1998;3:35-42.

[13] Deedwania PC. Hemodynamic changes as triggers of cardiovascular events. Cardiol Clin 1996;14:229-38.

[14] Singh RB, Cornelissen G, Siegelova J, et al. About half-weekly (circasemiseptan) pattern of blood pressure and heart rate in men and women of India. *Scripta Medica* (Brno) 2002;75:125-8.

[15] Singh RB, Weydahl A, Otsuka K, et al. Can nutrition influence circadian rhythm and heart rate variability? *Biomed Pharmacother* 2001;55 (suppl 11):s115-24.

[16] Singh RB, Niaz MA, Cornelissen GS, et al. Circadian rhythmicity of circulating vitamin concentrations. *Scripta Medica* (Brno) 2001;74:93-6.

[17] Christensen JH, Gustenhoff P, Komp E, et al. Effect of fish oil on heart rate variability in survivors of myocardial infarction. *Br Med J* 1996;312:677-8.

[18] Christensen JH, Komp E, Aaroe J, et al. Fish consumption, n-3 fatty acids in cell membranes and heart rate variability in survivors of myocardial infarction with left ventricular dysfunction. *Am J Cardiol* 1997;79:1670-2.

[19] Christensen JH, Skou HA, Fog L, et al. Marine n-3 fatty acids, wine intake, and heart rate variability in patients referred for coronary angiography. *Circulation* 2001;103:651-7.

[20] Chin JPF. Marine oils and cardiovascular reactivity. *Prostaglandins Leukot Essent Fatty Acids* 1994;50:211-22.

[21] Borovikova LV, Ivanova S, Zhang M, et al. Vagus nerve stimulation attenuates the systemic inflammatory response to endotoxin. *Nature* 2000;405:458-62.

[22] Das UN. The brain-lipid-heart connection. Nutrition 2001;17:260-3.

[23] Lauritzen I, Blondeau N, Heurteaux C, et al. Polyunsaturated fatty acids are potent neuroprotectors. *EMBO J* 2000;19:1784-93.

[24] Minami M, Kimura S, Endo T, et al. Dietary docosahexaenoic acid increases cerebral acetylcholine levels and improves passive avoidance performance in stroke-prone spontaneously hypertensive rates. *Pharmacol Biochem Behav* 1997;58:1123-9.

[25] Goodnight SH Jr, Harris WS, Connor WE. The effects of dietary omega-3 fatty acids upon platelet composition and function in man: a prospective controlled study. *Blood* 1981;58:880-5.

[26] Pella D, Singh RB, Otsuka K, et al. Nutritional predictors and modulators of insulin resistance. *J Nutr Environ Med* 2004;14:3-16

[27] Singh RB, Niaz MA, Sharma JP, et al. Randomized, double blind, placebo controlled trial of fish oil and mustard oil in patients with suspected acute myocardial infarction. The Indian Experiment of Infarct Survival. *Cardiovasc Drug Ther* 1997;11:485-91.

[28] Marchioli R, Barzi F, Bobma E, et al. Early protection against sudden death by n-3 polyunsaturated fatty acids after myocardial infarction. time-course analysis of the results of the Gruppo Italiano per lo Studio della Sopravvivenza nell'Infarto Miocardico (GISSI)-Prevenzione. *Circulation* 2002;105:1897-903.

[29] Singh RB, Dubnov G, Niaz MA, et al. Effect of an Indo-Mediterranean diet on progression of coronary artery disease in high risk patients (Indo-Mediterranean Diet Heart Study): a randomised single-blind trial. *Lancet* 2002;360:1455-61.

[30] de Lorgeril M, Salen P, Martin JL, et al. Mediterranean diet, traditional risk factors and the rate of cardiovascular complications after myocardial infarction. Final report of the Lyon Diet Heart Study. *Circulation* 1999; 99: 779–85.

[31] National Cholesterol Education Program. Second report of the expert panel on detection, evaluation, and treatment of high blood cholesterol in adults (adult treatment panel II). *Circulation* 1994;89:1333-445.

[32] Narasinga Rao BS, Deosthale YG, Pant KC. Nutrient composition of Indian foods. Hyderbad, India: National Institute of Nutrition, *Indian Council of Medical Research.* 1989.

[33] Goodhart RS, Shils ME, eds. *Modern nutrition in health and disease.* Philadelphia, PA: Lea & Febiger, 1980.

[34] Ridker PM, Manson JE, Buring JE, et al. Circadian variation of acute myocardial infarction and the effect of low dose aspirin in a randomized trial of physicians. *Circulation* 1990;82:897-902.

[35] Ralph MR, Foster RG, Davis FC, et al. Transplanted suprachiasmatic nucleus determines circadian period. *Science* 1990;247:975-8.

[36] Yehuda S. Omega-6/omega-3 ratio and brain related functions. *World Rev Nutr Diet* 2003;92:37-56.

In: Frontiers in Atherosclerosis Research
Editor: Karin F. Kepper, pp. 105-140

ISBN 1-60021-371-5

Chapter 6

CIRCADIAN CARDIOLOGY

B. Singh,[1] Ashwaria Gupta, Daniel Pella and Adarsh Kumar

Halberg Hospital and Research Institute, Moradabad, Glenmark Pharmaceuticals Limited, Mumbai; India;
Safaric University, Kosice Slovakia;
Government Medical College, Amritsar, India

ABSTRACT

A circadian cell cycle resides in every cell, and peripheral timing mechanisms are documented in molecular biologic terms at about 24-hour (circadian) and higher (ultradian) frequencies with coordination in mammals by the adrenal and the pineal-hypothalamic-pituitary network. The suprachiasmatic nuclei (SCN) and clock gene contribute to the coordination of the circadian rhythms' phase and amplitude in everyday life. The SCN are influenced by the daily alternation between light and darkness directly via the eyes and by plasma melatonin concentrations secreted by the pineal gland, which is a window to both light and geomagnetics. A clinical event occurs when the neuroendocrine time structures (chronomes) are not able to cope with the adverse effects of stimuli acting from within or from without, e. g., via the sympathetic nervous system. Triggering of the neuroendocrines by environmental factors may activate the pineal gland, pituitary functions and adrenal secretions, resulting in adverse effects on circadian variations, heart rate variability (HRV) and blood pressure variability (BPV). Circadian rhythm has been known to ancient man from the time of Homoerectus and Homosapiens who used to have intercourse in the early morning hours, prior to going hunting in the forests, causing increased secretion of testosterone in the morning. The role of time-adjusted drug intake, especially in the early morning, was also known to ancient Indian physicians. In the Ayurveda, drinking of large amounts of water in the early morning is advised, which appears to be in an attempt to increase vagal tone due to gastric distention. Frey considered the mean distribution of deaths along the scales of the day and the year. In one industrial population, Pell and D'Allonzo, discussed time-macroscopically the occurrence of a peak in the morning hours in a study of acute myocardial infarction (AMI), a proposition also ascertained and extended to the yearly pattern time-microscopically. The subsequent reports from other countries, the Soviet Union and the extensive data by WHO in the report of myocardial infarction Community Registers from 19 European centers demonstrated a peak incidence of onset of chest pain due to AMI from 8.00

[1] Correspondence: Dr R B Singh, MD Professor of Medicine, Halberg Hospital and Research Institute Civil Lines, Moradabad-10(UP)244001, Indiaicn2005@mickyonline.com

to 11.00 AM with a ratio of approximately 2 In one study from India, in 605 AMI patients, 39% of those who had Q wave infarction (n=174) had the onset between 6. 00 AM to 12. 00 noon. In a more recent Mechanism of Acute Myocardial Infarction (MAMI) study by Singh et al, among 202 AMI patients, the incidence of onset of chest pain was highest in the second quarter of the day (41. 0%), mainly between 4-8 AM, followed by the 4th quarter, usually after large meals (28. 2%). Emotion was the second most common trigger (43. 5%), which was the most common in the patients with onset of chest pain in the second quarter of the day (51. 8%). Cold weather was a predisposing factor in 29. 2% and hot temperatures (40°C) was common in 24. 7% of the patients. A large meal, especially a large breakfast in the morning was an important trigger of AMI in this study, which poses the intriguing possibility that some heart attacks could be prevented by not eating breakfast or by eating a small superfood breakfast containing walnuts, almonds, raisins and yogurt which are known to be protective against cardiovascular disease. Blood pressure is usually lower during the night, starts increasing before awakening, and remains high during the day-time, mostly in the second quarter of the day. Circadian rhythms of triggers and cardiac events and their mechanisms have been described by various workers. It is possible that circadian rhythm could be a new target for treatment with lifestyle changes, nutrient, nutraceuiticals such as w-3 fatty acids and coenzyme Q10, prayer and drug therapy in the management of cardiovascular disease.

INTRODUCTION

Many scientists believe that our universe came into existence about 20 billion years ago after an explosion of a primordial fireball of matter. Within 3 minutes of the explosion, the elementary matter particles coalesced to form the lightest elements, which were responsible for the formation of galaxies. Most of the galaxies appear to be receding from us at high velocities, which has been explained by the expansion model of the universe. Rhythm is a fundamental characteristic of the galaxies in our universe. The sun revolves around the core of the Milky Way Galaxy, rotating on its axis. The planets revolve around the sun and moon revolves around the planets. One season follows the other season, day follows night, tide-in follows tide-out. Most of the rhythms are linked to the movements of the heavenly bodies. The rotation of the earth is responsible for the day and night cycle, and the moon orbiting around the earth for the monthly cycle. The procession of the earth on its axis is responsible for the four seasons and the earth orbiting the sun for the annual cycle. Many physiological functions must adapt to these external rhythms, causing dysfunctions resulting in the development of diseases. [1-3].

The universe of living creatures appears to have similar characteristics. All living cells have life cycles and periodicity in their life function [3]. The migration of birds, the hibernation of bears, dogs and several other animals, ripening of fruits and flowering of plants, are driven by the changing seasons. Similarly, other rhythms, such as sleep and wakefulness, the opening and closing of flowers, feeding and nesting are also driven by the circadian cycle. There is substantial evidence that cardiovascular events occur in the second quarter of the day. [1-3]. The exact pathogenesis and risk factors of circadian rhythms are not known [4-9].

The Interaction of Genes and Means and Adaptation

Diet and lifestyle, tobacco, pollutants, stress, and alcohol are the most important environmental means, which interact with genes in the pathogenesis of cardiovascular disease, diabetes and cancer. The interaction of genes and environment, nature and nurture, is the foundation for the development of disease and health. It has been shown through molecular biological techniques that genetic factors determine susceptibility to disease and environmental factors determine which genetically susceptible individual will develop a disease [9]. Despite major changes in our diet and lifestyle in the last 10,000 years, our genes have not changed and hence our biological responses are unable to adapt, resulting in greater adverse effects of these factors on our circadian rhythms. The spontaneous mutation rate for nuclear DNA is estimated at 0.5% per million years. The period of 10,000 years of the agricultural revolution appears to be too short to modulate our genes, causing an approximate 0.005% alteration. It seems our genes are much similar today to our ancestors of the Paleolethic period 40,000 years ago, when our genetic profile was established [9]. It is possible to presume that humans today live in an environment that differs completely from that when our genetic constitution was selected and therefore our clock gene remains as potent as several million years ago to initiate the biorhythms of our bodies. Our clock gene does not allow us to adapt to modulate rapid changes in diet and lifestyle, which influence circadian rhythms.

Evolutionary Aspects of Biological Function Rhythmicity

Homosapiens, along with their predecessors Homo-habilis, were primarily vegetarians, although for more than a million years, they have been hunting. They became omnivorous as they moved away from other primates. Environmental influences, development of social groups and increasing demands for survival made them skillful and caused significant changes in their lifestyle. They went to the forest in the early morning for hunting animals. They were killed early in life due to accidents. It has been proposed that, in order to preserve their progeny, the Homosapiens had intercourse early in the morning resulting in one of the most important physiological adaptations of an increased release of testosterone in the morning, as a circadian rhythm. The increased release of testosterone occurred to coordinate sexual activity with the aim of conceiving the women. We suggest that since hunting used to start at about sunrise, causing enormous excitement, physical and mental exertion and increased sympathetic activity (associated with marked secretion of cortisol, catecholamines, aldosterone, angiotensin and renin in a state of low melatonin), it also became a circadian rhythm in modern men. Ancient man was able to adapt and fight the adverse effects of testosterone, cortisol and catecholamines, due to their enormous physical activity and lack of time for breakfast. Modern men is not, however, resulting in increased rhythmicity of cardiac events in the second quarter of the day. Late night falling asleep, late awakening, heavy breakfasts, no physical activity and meditation in the morning, and excitement related to rushing to the workplace, trigger a biochemical and biological atmosphere in our body that contributes to the greater cardiovascular events and deaths between 8.00-11.00 hours. [1-3].

We are comparing the diet and lifestyle as well as heart rate and blood pressures around the clock for 7 days in people in tribes living in the adverse conditions of Laddakh, with those living in Moradabad and Tokyo City to determine the pattern of circadian changes, and to provide further insight into the pathogenesis of circadian rhythms.

EVOLUTIONARY ASPECTS OF DIET AND LIFESTYLE

Recently, several scholars became interested in health and disease from an evolutionary perspective and consider whether our departure from the hunter-gatherer lifestyle may contribute to contemporary health problems [1, 2].

Foods are probably appropriate for any given species if they were regularly consumed during most of the prior evolution, as in the case of hunter gatherers. Prehistoric human hunter gatherers may have protected themselves by choosing plants that have low concentrations of xenobiotics and by avoiding dangerous plant species. The available food staples during the Palaeolithic period may have been meat, fish, shellfish, leafy vegetables, fruits, nuts, insects and larvae in varying proportions. Since tubers often require cooking for their starch to be digestible their routine consumption may have started in the later period. [6-8].

Prior to the agricultural revolution, about 10,000 years ago, humans ate an enormous variety of wild plants. Meat, fish, green leafy vegetables, fruits, nuts, berries and honey were the food items available to pre-agricultural humans which shaped modern humans' genetic nutritional requirements. Early man also managed to survive in a wide range of environments, from the tropical rainforest to near the Arctic, each of these environments offering a different and limited set of foods. However, all diets of ancient men lacked breakfast foods; milk, cheese, butter, syrups, cereals, and of course, refined carbohydrates and sugar that is sprinkled on them, which are known to have adverse effects on our metabolisms causing insulin resistance. These foods supply approximately 70% of the energy in the diets of the Western world today. Irrespective of the specific proportions of meat and vegetables, prehistoric hunter-gatherers' diets would have been very different from those of contemporary humans with regard to their nutritional value.

Hunting was the major part of the occupational physical activity of prehistoric men, which might have continued throughout the entire day. After they returned from the forest in midday or evening, they may have had a late heavy lunch, followed by dancing and eating again in the late evening. Many experts suggest that reversion to the original Palaeolithic human lifestyle (1. 5 million-10, 000 years BP) might be useful in the prevention of chronic diseases of Western populations [6-8]. The main symbols of Gods of early men were the sun, fire, sea and hills, which they worshiped to decrease their mental stress.

Several biological functions, such as temperature regulation, blood circulation in the nasal mucosa, the caliber of the tracheobronchial airway, blood pressure, heart rate, cortisol and growth hormone release exhibit an intrinsic circadian rhythm [1-5]. Most physiological rhythms may be ultradian having a duration of seconds, minutes, or at most a few hours. Circadian means 24 hours, circamensual, 30 days and circaannual, one year. The sleep phases, heart rate, respiratory rate and the functional peaks of many enzymes, receptors and endothelial nitric oxide releases show ultradian variations, depending upon triggers and clocks. (Table 1).

Table 1. Neuropsychiatric risk factors of acute myocardial infarction

Precursors	Healthy Subjects (n-595)	AMI (n=202)
Anxiety	88 (14. 8)	122 (60. 4)*
Depression	42 (7. 0)	45 (22. 3)*
Type A behaviour	103 (17. 3)	95 (47. 2)*
Emotional stress	147 (24. 2)	92 (45. 5)*
Sleep deprivation	42 (7. 0)	56 (27. 7)*
Cold Climate	-	59 (29. 2)*
Hot climate (>40 degree celsius)	-	50 (24. 7)*
Large Meals	147 (24. 7)	96 (47. 5)*
Physical Exertion	173 (29. 1)	63 (31. 2)*
Diabetes mellitus	70 (11. 7)	53 (26. 2)*

*=P<0. 05 by Chi square test

CIRCADIAN

The words circadian and chronobiology were used for the first time by Franz Halberg in 1950 and officially introduced to a nomenclature committee in Stockholm for the first time in 1955 [4, 5]. Chonobiology developed globally after 1969 when an article entitled "Chronobiology" was published in the *Annual Review of Physiology* and became a Current Contents citation classic. Body temperature shows circadian variation; it is lowest in the morning, peaks in the afternoon and falls again during the night. In contrast, cortisol release peaks in the morning. Blood pressure varies by up to 40mm Hg over the time structure of the day with a clear-cut peak in the morning.

Cholesterol is synthesized mainly in the nighttime. An annual variation has also been reported in aldosterone secretion showing a peak during the winter. The cycle of the reproductive organs is the best-known circamensual rhythm. Ultradian sleep phases (up to a few hours), heart rate, respiratory rate, circadian temperature changes in the interior of the body, all have a circadian rhythm. A circaannual rhythmicity has been observed for serum cholesterol levels with the winter values being much higher. Halberg feels that apart from circadian, circaseptan (weekly), monthly, yearly or even longer term physiological variations occur. Otsuka proposed that the physiological chronomes such as heart rate variability have counterparts in our environment and our genetic makeup over time may have evolved from our adaptation to and integration with the cosmos. There is a need to examine how these phenomena including heliomagnetics and geomagnetics, can influence physiological chronomes, especially for heart rate and blood pressure variability [10].

CLOCKS

The circadian rhythms enable the body to adapt in an optimum manner to changes in its environments including geomagnetic forces. These rhythms are set up endogenously in the body and the entire system of hormonised rhythms, the biological time structure can be influenced by external and internal factors, which are called clocks. It is very difficult to assess the internal factors that govern the circadian rhythms. Hence, we know very little about internal clocks.

It is indeed very difficult to assess the internal factors that govern biological rhythms, however. Halberg has proposed that a circadian cycle resides in every living cell and peripheral timing mechanisms are being documented in molecular biological terms at about 24 hour (circadian) and utradian frequencies, with coordination in mammals by the Adrenal, pineal-hypothalamic-pituitary network (Figure 1). Suprachiasmatic nuclei (SCN) is one known specific area of the brain that works as an internal clock and is responsible for the regulation of central nervous functions, phase and amplitude, as it receives information from the eyes. The information from the brain is transferred to the pineal gland. Melatonin released from the pituitary gland during the dark hours of the days in a circadian cycle regulates sleep and awake periods. The SCN are influenced by the daily alternation between light and darkness direcly via the eyes and melatonin levels. A cardiovascular event occurs when our neuroendocrine time structures (chronomes) are not able to cope with the adverse effects of stimuli from within or without acting eg via the sympathetic nervous system [10-13]. It appears that the two most powerful external clocks for humans are light at high intensity and social contacts. The results of initial attempts to use bright light to adapt shift workers were encouraging [14]. Most organisms from cyanobacteria to mammals are known to use circadian clocks to coordinate their metabolisms with the natural circadian light/dark cycle. The human clock gene was discovered and mapped to chromosome17p12-13. 1 in 1997 [15]. It is surprising that the clock gene is similar in all life forms on earth. In plants, several molecular components have been described for the circadian system.

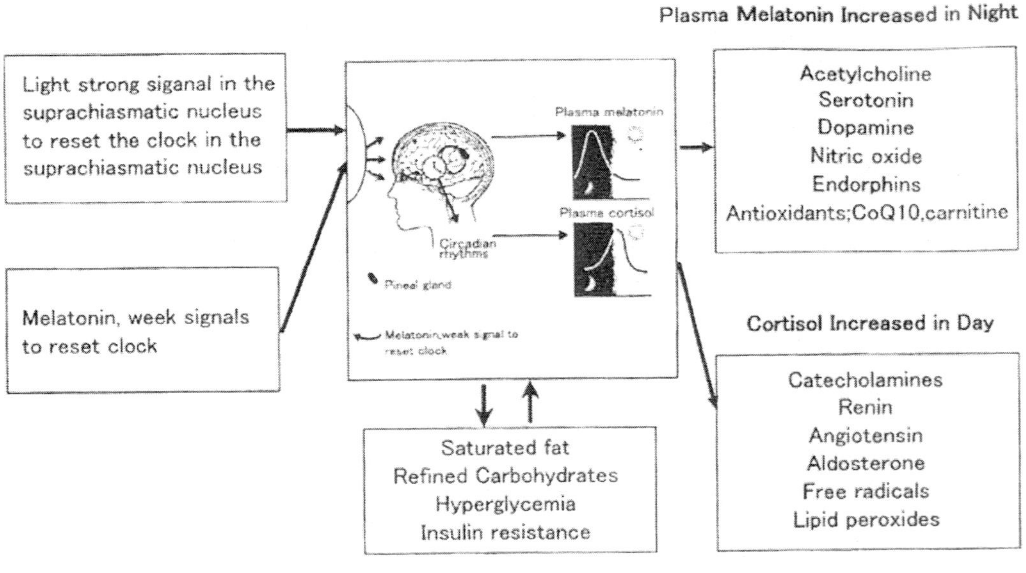

Figure 1. Control of Daily Rhythms By Molecular Clock.

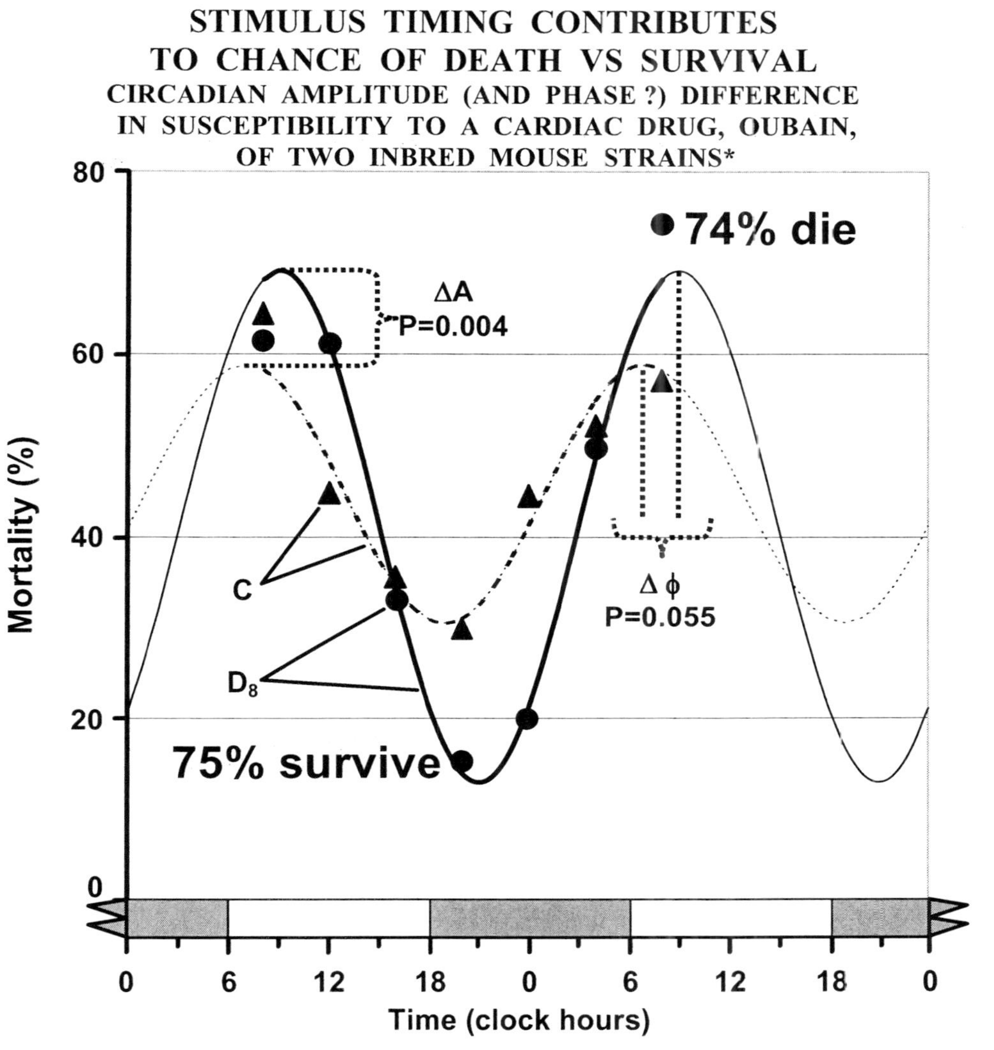

Strain	P	M	Amplitude (A)	Acrophase (ϕ**)
D_8	$P < 0.001$	40.0	28.1 (21.5; 34.8)	-135 (-119; -150)
C	$P = 0.011$	45.2	14.2 (7.3; 21.0)	-104 (- 73; -136)

*** C = Bagg albino, D_8 = subline 8 of Dilute Brown strain; oubain 0.15 or 0.5 mg/20 g of body weight, respectively. Thin lines in the graph are extrapolations of fitted cosine curves. ** In the table: 95% confidence limits in parentheses, ϕ in degrees (360° = 24 hours). M = MESOR; P from zero-A (no-rhythm) test.**
Data from F.Halberg et al., Minnesota Acad Sci Proc 1959; 27: 139-143.

Figure 2. First demonstration of the importamnce of timing with a drug, in this case > a cardiac drug and also a demonstration more generally of the importance> of statistics along the circadian scale. Feel free to use it.

TRIGGERS

Triggering of the chronomes by environmental factors may activate the pineal gland, pituitary functions and adrenal secretions, causing adverse effects on circadian rhythms, heart rate variability and blood pressure variability [10-14], resulting in cardiovascular events [11-15]. The various clinical manifestations of cardiovascular events do not occur at random times, but according to a time structure. It is possible that certain external activities known as triggers may play a major role in causing myocardial ischaemia, myocardial infarction, sudden cardiac death and stroke [11-15]. The MILIS (Multicentre Investigation of Limitation of Infarct Size) study showed that half of all myocardial infarction patients reported a temporal relationship between characteristic activities and occurrence of infarction. Emotional stress, mild and heavy physical exersion, sleep deprivation and large meals were the most frequently reported triggering activities [16].

The TRIMM (Triggers and Mechanisms of Myocardial Infarction) study showed that 76% of all infarction patients reported an unusual event shortly before the onset of infarction [17]. Emotional upset or stress was reported by 52% of the subjects and 10% reported multiple trigger activities coinciding just before the event. A morning increase in platelet aggregation appears to be one of the most important triggers for cardiovascular events in the second quarter of the day [18]. It seems that there is powerful evidence of a link between these triggers and the sequences of cellular and pathophysiological events that are proposed to be responsible for coronary artery ischaemia. In one study among 58 patents with AMI, large meals including a large breakfast, emotional stress, cold climate and hot climate (>40°C) were important triggers. A large breakfast in the morning was associated with increased concentration of proinflammatory cytokines; tumour necrosis factor-alpha and interleukin-6 as well as insulin and glucose in the blood [11] (Table 2). In the MAMI study [2], large meals, sleep deprivation, emotional stress, cold climate and hot climate were quite commonly observed (Table 3). Circadian rhythms of myocardial ischaemia, angina pectoris, myocardial infarction, sudden cardiac death and stroke have been described by several experts which are triggered by environmental factors as well as biochemical and biological triggers present in every living cell.

Table 2. Clinical Characteristics of subjects in various subgroups in relation to circadian pattern

Sub Group	1-6 hours	6-12 hours	12-18 hours	18-24 hours
Total n=202	34 (16. 8)	83 (41. 0)	28 (13. 8)	57 (28. 2)
Male (n=160)	24 (15. 0)	60 (37. 5)	25 (15. 6)	51 (31. 8)
Female (n-132)	10 (23. 8)	23 (54. 7)	3 (7. 1)	6 (14. 2)
Age>60 (n=70)	12 (17. 1)	32 (45. 7)	8 (11. 4)	18 (25. 7)
60 and less (n=132)	12 (16. 6)	51 (38. 6)	20 (15. 1)	39 (29. 5)
History of CAD	16 (30. 7)	24 (46. 1)	7 (13. 4)	5 (9. 6)
Known Diabetes (n=53)	10 (18. 8)	22 (41. 5)	8 (15. 0)	13 (24. 5)
Known Hypertension (n-75) (>140/90)	13 (17. 3)	30 (40. 0)	11 (14. 6)	21 (28. 0)

Values are number (%). P value was obtained by comparison of subgroups by chi square test. *P>0. 05m *=P<0. 02, CAD= Coronary artery disease

Circadian Rhythms in Ischemic Heart Disease

In the decade since the 1985 observation by Muller et al. that the frequency of onset of myocardial infarction peaks at 9 a. m., numerous publications have supported this observation not only for myocardial infarction, but also for sudden cardiac death, transient myocardial ischemia, and stroke. Refinement of these epidemiological observations has led to the conclusion that the morning peak in disease onset is due in part to the physical and mental stressors associated with morning awakening and activity. The observations also showed that stressors such as heavy physical activity and anger can trigger acute cardiovascular events [19].

Why Morning is so Risky?

Circadian rhythm peaking in the morning is also found for so-called silent myocardial ischaemia, which occurs in more than 20% of patients with arterial hypertension, and can be regularly detected in combined 24-h-ABPM/EKG examinations. Comparative studies have shown that hypertensives with SMI suffer more cardiac events than those with no SMI. It has further been demonstrated that an elevated blood pressure amplitude, which is considered an independent risk factor for cardiac events, is associated with an increased incidence of SMI in patients with micro- or macro-angiopathy [20].

The Possible Mechanisms Involved

Transient myocardial ischemia, detected by ambulatory ST segment monitoring, is also unevenly distributed during the day. The pathophysiology and the mechanisms underlying these variations are the focus of much investigation. Heart rate, blood pressure, neural and humoral vasoactive factors such as plasma norepinephrine levels and renin activity, and probably also contractility, are increased in the morning hours, indicating that an increase in myocardial oxygen demands contribute importantly to the increased prevalence of ischemia in the morning. A study by Li JJ found that the circadian rhythm of the ischemic threshold detected by repetitive exercise treadmill tests in patients with chronic coronary artery disease is also apparently associated with levels of plasma ET-1 [21].

Relation to Plasma Endothelin-1

Li JJ et al. demonstrated that ET-1 values were higher in the morning hours as compared to afternoon hours. Circadian variations of plasma levels of ET-1 are likely to be one of the most likely mechanisms involved of reduction of the ischemic threshold in the morning hours [22].

Table 3. Triggers observed in 202 patients of acute myocardial infarction in relation to circadian periods

Quarter of 24 hrs	1-6 hours	6-12 hours	12-18 hours	18-24hours	Total
Subjects	34	83	28	57	202
Trigger total	25 (73. 5)	70 (84. 3)	15 (53. 5)	42 (73. 7)	162 (82. 2)
Large meals	18 (52. 9)	41 (49. 4)	12 (42. 8)	26 (45. 6)	96 (47. 5)
Emotional stress	15 (44. 1)	43 (51. 8)	14 (50. 0)	20 (35. 0)	92 (45. 5)
Physical Exertion	12 (35. 3)	25 (30. 1)	8 (28. 5)	18 (31. 6)	63 (31. 2)
Sleep deprivation	8 (23. 5)	32 (38. 5)	6 (21. 4)	10 (17. 5)	56 (27. 7)
Cold climate	10 (29. 4)	35 (42. 1)	5 (17. 8)	9 (15. 5)	59 (29. 2)
Hot climate (>40 celsius)	8 (23. 5)	30 (36. 1)	5 (17. 8)	7 (12. 3)	50 (24. 7)

Values are number (%) *=P<0. 05, Pvalues were obtained by comparison of subgroups by chi square test

Fluctuation in Endothelial Function

Coronary spasms are induced by acetylcholine (ACh), which causes vasodilation when the endothelium is functioning normally. The spasms are promptly relieved by nitroglycerin (NTG), which causes vasodilation through its direct action on the smooth muscle. The frequency of ischemic attacks displays diurnal variations in patients with VA (i. e., coronary spastic angina). The number of attacks increases in the early morning and decreases in the afternoon.

Mechanism of Coronary Spasms

In patients with coronary spasms, coronary dilation caused by endothelium-dependent vasodilators is reported to be impaired. In addition, antioxidants such as vitamin C and glutathione, attenuate the constrictor response to ACh. The plasma levels of vitamin E, a natural antioxidant, are decreased. The coronary arteries of patients with VA exhibit a circadian variation in tone. As the endothelial function of the brachial artery and that of the coronary artery are closely related [22], the fluctuation of endothelium-dependent dilation in the brachial artery most likely takes place in the coronary arteries as well.

Mechanism of Diurnal Variation in Flow-Mediated Vasodilation

It is known that the day/night pattern in the intensity of physical activity causes diurnal variation of hemodynamics. In the evening and afternoon, peripheral blood flow to the skeletal muscle is increased through local regulation in proportion to its need for oxygen and nutrients. Endothelial nitric oxide synthase is known to be upregulated by increased blood flow or shear stress.

Therefore, it is possible that the variation in baseline blood flow may upregulate nitric oxide synthase and contribute to the fluctuation of the flow-mediated, endothelium dependent vasodilation in patients with VA. Diurnal fluctuations of the endothelial function may play an important role in the occurrence of ischemic episodes in patients with VA [23].

Heart Rate Variability and the Rate of Autonomic Change

The incidence of sudden cardiac death peaks during the early morning hours when there is a rapid withdrawal of vagal and an increase of sympathetic tone. The rate of autonomic change could be of prognostic importance. B. Wennerblom showed that during the night/morning hours, healthy controls demonstrated faster HF max. velocity and higher HF gradient than angina patients. The authors concluded that rapid vagal withdrawal seemed to be a sign of a healthy autonomic nervous system in the control group but was significantly slower in angina patients. IS-5-MN and metoprolol tended to normalise vagal withdrawal and metoprolol slowed down the rapid increase in sympathetic predominance in the morning in these patients [24].

Circadian Rhythm in Myocardial Infarction

Despite impressive strides in diagnosis and management over the past three decades, acute myocardial infarction (AMI) continues to be a major public health problem in the industrialized world and is becoming an increasingly important problem in developing countries. About 50 percent of the deaths associated with AMI occur within 1 hour of the event and are attributable to arrhythmias, most often ventricular fibrillation. Because AMI may strike an individual during the most productive years, it can have profoundly deleterious psychosocial and economic ramifications [25].

Circadian Periodicity

An analysis of a large number of patients hospitalized with MI, studied as a part of the Multicenter Investigation of Limitation of Infarct Size (MILIS), revealed a pronounced circadian periodicity for the time of onset of AMI, with peak incidence of events between 6 a. m. and 12 p. m. About 20% of myocardial infarctions occur between midnight and 6 AM. The circadian distribution of acute myocardial infarction has a morning peak, especially during the first few hours after awakening [26].

Pathogenesis

Circadian rhythms affect many physiological and biochemical parameters; the early morning hours are associated with rises in plasma catecholamines and cortisol as well as increases in platelet aggregability. At this time, sympathetic activation is thought to disrupt atherosclerotic plaque through vasoconstriction and an increase in blood pressure. In addition, early morning changes in hemostatic activity may lead to thrombosis. In contrast, sleep may be protective, both because of the absence of external triggers and the decline in sympathetic activity during non–rapid eye movement (REM) sleep, which accounts for about 80% of total sleep time. However, about 20% of myocardial infarctions occur between midnight and 6 AM. REM sleep, which is characterized by sympathetic surges, might be involved—as it is in vasospastic angina - but REM sleep constitutes less than 20% of total sleep time in adults [27].

Hence, the pathogenesis of nocturnal myocardial infarctions may differ from those that occur during the daytime, since they may not be related to sympathetic activation or triggering events. Other sleep-induced cardiovascular changes that affect the coronary circulation or cardiac function may be involved. For example, sleep-induced variations of flow patterns in coronary arteries might be involved, or shifts in blood volume might affect the dimensions and hemodynamic function of the right ventricle [28, 29].

Circadian Variation in Plaque Rupture

Pathologic studies have revealed that plaque rupture is one of the major causes of AMI. One large-scale multicenter study has demonstrated that AMI is 1.28 times more likely to begin between 6:00 A. M. and 12:00 P. M. than during the other three 6-hour intervals of the day[2]. Pathologic studies have revealed that plaque rupture and subsequent thrombosis is one of the major causes of AMI. Therefore, the hypothesis that increased physiologic activities in morning hours may trigger plaque disruption has been proposed [30].

A. Tanaqa et al. demonstrated that in the plaque rupture group, a morning increase (from 6:00 A. M. to 12:00 P. M) was observed, whereas in the nonrupture group there was a nocturnal nadir (from 12 to 6:00 A. M) and no significant morning increase was detected. 53% of the patients in the nonrupture group had preinfarction angina and only 31% of patients had an AMI at rest. This circadian pattern was not detectable in the nonrupture group. This morning increase in the incidence of plaque rupture accounts for the characteristic circadian rhythm of AMI [31]. Various physiologic studies have highlighted the fact that systemic physiologic processes increase in intensity in the morning, such as an arterial pressure surge accompanied by an increase in heart rate [32] and increased vascular tone [33]. Serum cortisol levels also decrease during the period of increased plaque disruption. Because the Japanese population of patients with AMI compared with whites shows a higher incidence of spasm and greater vasoconstriction of nonspastic segments after acetylcholine [34], this decrease in serum cortisol levels could enhance the sensitivity of the coronary arteries to the vasoconstrictive effects of catecholamines. Such physiologic alterations may, alone or in combination, account for the morning increase in plaque rupture. When plaque rupture occurs, the contents of the lipid core that form the most thrombogenic components of the plaque may be released into the lumen and precipitate a cascade that produces thrombosis. Increased platelet activity, increased blood viscosity, and the minimal level of fibrinolytic activity may further contribute to thrombosis in this setting during the morning hours. The efficacy of β blockers and aspirin in preventing AMI indirectly lends support to the idea that these physiological variations may play an etiologic role in plaque disruption and resultant thrombosis [31].

Several studies have shown that in many instances, MI may occur without any obvious precipitating events and may occur at rest. Grines et al [35] reported that one independent predictor of a higher frequency of onset during the morning hours was the absence of a history of angina.

Q-Wave Versus Non-Q Wave MI

V. Culic et al. [36] demonstrated that both AMI types showed a nonuniform daily distribution of onset with a night nadir (0 to 4 A. M.), and Q-wave AMI also showed a late morning peak (8 A. M. to noon). The study demonstrated that wakeful patients with Q-wave infarction were more likely to have AMI onset in the presence of a possible external trigger than those with non–Q-wave AMI. This is consistent with the hypothesis that powerful hemodynamic stresses may produce more extensive plaque rupture, often leading to complete occlusion of the coronary lumen and Q-wave infarction. Non–Q-wave infarction is more likely to result from a shorter occlusion of a major coronary artery, with earlier and more frequent reopening than from firm occlusion of a small branch.

Table 4. Circadian pattern of acute myocardial infection in relation to drug therapy

Subgroups	1-6 hours 34	6-12 hours 83	12-18 hours 28	18-24 hours 57	Total 202
Beta-blockers Calcium	10	8	6	6	30
Blockers	2	2	2	6	12
ACE-inhibitor	4	4	-	6	14
Fish Oil Coenzyme	5	2	-	2	9
Q10	8	2	12	4	26
No Drug Therapy	(4. 3)	64(54. 7)**	10(8. 5)	37(31. 6)**	117
Drug Therapy Total	29(34. 1)	19(22. 3)	18(21. 2)	20(23. 5)	85

Values are number (%) out of totals = P<0. 05, **P=P<0. 01m O value were obtained by comparison of sub-groups
by Chi square test

An acceptable explanation for a diverse circadian pattern in 2 AMI types, with late morning peak only in the Q-wave AMI, is that hemodynamic, prothrombotic, and vasoconstrictive forces resulting from a morning rise in sympathetic activity and cortisol levels contribute to the formation of sustained coronary occlusion and Q-wave infarction. A lower incidence of both infarction types during the early morning hours corresponds to the time when most patients would be expected to be asleep, so hemodynamic and other triggering forces may be reduced in patients with both types of AMI.

Table 5: Clinical characteristics of subjects

	Acute myocardial infarction (n=54)	Controls (n=85)
Sex- males	45 (83. 3)	76(89. 4)
Mean age (years)	49. 5± 4. 2	52. 1± 5. 2
Body mass index (kg/m2)	23. 7± 3. 2	22. 4±3. 4
Hypertension (>140/90 mmhg)	25(46. 3)*	25(29. 4)
Glucose intolerance	12(22. 2)*	10(11. 8)
Diabetes mellitus	14(25. 9)	--
Smoking	24(44. 4)*	28(32. 9)
Higher transfattyacids	27(50. 0)**	--
(>5g/day)	27(50. 0)**	25(29. 4)
Large meals(>1000 Kcal)	22(40. 7)**	10(11. 8)
Large breakfast(>1000 Kcal)		

*=P <0. 05 P value was obtained by z score test for proportions by comparison of two groups. Values are number (%) and mean(Standard deviation)

Table 6: Circadian rhythm of cardiac events in patients with acute myocardial infarction

Quarters of the day	Number of subjects (%)
1-6 Hours	10(18. 5)
6-12 Hours	20(40. 7)**
12-18 Hours	7(12. 9)
18-24 Hours	15(27. 7)*

*=P <0. 05, **=P>0. 02 , P value was obtained by Z score test for proportions

Table 7. Laboratory data in patients of acute myocardial infarction at baseline and after 4 weeks in relation to meal size

Data	Large breakfast, (n=22)		Small breakfast, (n=32	
	Baseline	After4	Baseline	After4
Lipoprotein(a)mg/dl	23.1+5.4	20.1+4.2*	22.5+4.6	19.7+4.1*
Triglycerides (mmol/L)	1.88+0.61	1.70+0.38*	1.81+0.60	1.64+0.32*
Blood glucose(mmol/l)	7.7+1.6	6.0+1.2*	6.6+1.4*	5.5+0.30*
Plasma insulin(mg/dl)	47.5+11.3	36.3+5.6**	43.2+8.8*	27.6+3.5*
TBARS(pmol/l)	1.87+0.46	1.32+0.33*	1.77+0.42	1.30+0.31*
MDA(pmol/l)	2.68+0.34	2.02+0.21*	2.66+0.33	2.01+0.21*
Diene conjugate(OD)	27.5+4.2	24.6+4.0*	26.2+4.1	24.2+3.5*
CoenzymeQ10(ug/ml)	0.21+0.02	0.32+0.23*	0.23+0.03	0.45+0.24*
Interleukin-6(pg/ml)	32.6+6.2	22.5+4.3*	27.5+5.2*	20.6+0.22*
TNF-alpha(ug/dl)	42.5+12.8	23.6+4.1*	38.2+10.6*	19.6+0.18*
	32.6+6.2	22.5+4.3*	27.5+5.2*	20.6+0.22*
	42.5+12.8	23.6+4.1*	38.2+10.6*	19.6+0.18*

* = P < 0.05,**=P<0.002, TNF=Tumour necrosis factor,MDA=malonaldehyde

Table 8: Circadian distribution of casEs in relation to 4 hourly period.

Periods	Men	Women	Total
0-4 hours	6(3.7)	2(4.7)	8(3.9)
4-8 hours	58(36.2)*	22(51.7)*	80(39.6)*
8-12 hours	25(15.6)	4(9.4)	29(14.3)
12-16 hours	8(5.0)	---------	8(3.9)
16-20 hours	40(25.2)*	10(23.5)*	50(24.7)*

Values are numbers (%) *=P<0.05 P values are abtained by comparison of subjects in various sub groups of periods.

Table 9: Biochemical data in patient with acute myocardial infarction compared to healthy subject.

Data	Healthy subjects (n=595)	Acute myocardial infarction (n-202)
Serum magnesium (m EQ/L)	1.64(0.25)	1.51(0.23)*
Serum potassium (m EQ/L)	4.3(0.96)	3.7(0.82)*
Vitamin C (mmol/l)	37.5(6.8)	18.6(4.3)*
Vitamin E(mmol/l)	20.1(3.7)	14.5(2.5)*
Vitamin A(mmol/l)	2.25(0.19)	1.86(0.15)*
Interleukin-6 (pg/ml)	15.6(3.2)	30.5(5.7)*
Tumour necrosis factor-alpha (pg/dl)	18.8(4.5)	41.6(8.4)*
Insulin (mg/dl)	17.6(4.2)	48.8(12.8)*

Results of a study by V. Culic suggest that pain at different body areas and other relevant symptoms more frequently follow Q-wave infarction. Both sympathetic and vagal afferent fibers can transmit cardiac pain to remote body areas due to convergence of visceral and somatic fibers on the same neurons within the central nervous system. Accordingly, a greater area of myocardial damage and more extensive stimulation of afferent fibers could induce pain sensation in a greater number of somatic regions and cause a higher frequency of other symptoms in patients with Q-wave AMI. The study also demonstrated that dyspnea was more associated with non–Q-wave infarction. A similar frequency of pulmonary congestion in 2 AMI type subsets, even in the presence of lower left ventricular ejection fraction among patients with Q-wave infarction, has been attributed to acute transient myocardial ishemia associated with non–Q-wave infarction, whereas irreversible ishemia could be the dominant mechanism of ventricular dysfunction in patients with Q-wave AMI [37].

Circadian Differences in the Site of Myocardial Infarction and in the Involved Coronary Arteries

P. Moruzzi and colleagues [27] demonstrated that 55% of the infarctions were anterior or anterolateral and 45% were inferior, including posterior or involving the right ventricle. They found that there was a slight peak in the incidence of myocardial infarction between 6 AM and noon. Anterior infarctions were more common from 6 AM to midnight, whereas inferior infarctions were more common between midnight and 6 AM.

Coronary involvement varied by the time of symptom onset among patients with inferior infarctions: right coronary artery involvement was much more common than left circumflex artery involvement among those with symptom onset from midnight to 6 AM. Among those with right coronary artery involvement, the proximal segment was more common as the site of the culprit lesion between midnight and 6 AM than between 6 AM and midnight.

The right coronary artery, which maintains its large caliber down to the crux, is characterized by slow flow velocity [38, 39]. It is possible that by decreasing the pressure gradient across a coronary artery stenosis, sleep-induced reduction in aortic pressure increases distal stasis, thereby facilitating thrombosis. This may be more of a problem in the right coronary artery than in the left coronary artery because the pressure gradient is inversely related to the fourth power of the minimum lumen diameter [27].

If the rhythmic processes that drive the circadian rhythm of myocardial-infarction onset can be identified their modification may delay or prevent the occurrence of infarction.

Circadian Rhythm and Sudden Cardiac Death

Sudden cardiac death (SCD) is natural death due to cardiac causes, heralded by abrupt loss of consciousness within 1 hour of the onset of acute symptoms in a person with or without known preexisting heart disease, but in whom the time and mode of death are unexpected. The worldwide incidence of SCD is difficult to estimate but estimates for the United States range from 300, 000 to nearly 400, 000 SCDs annually [40].

Circadian Rhythm and SCD

The biologic functions of mammals vary according to a circadian rhythm of about 24 hours, which is governed by the hypothalamus. These rhythms can be altered by disease and the actions of drugs can be affected by the time of day at which they are administered. A number of important physiological parameters such as heart rate, blood pressure, vascular reactivity, cardiac contractility, and various hemostatic factors all demonstrate a circadian pattern similar to that described for cardiovascular disorders. Circadian patterns have been observed for several supraventricular arrhythmias, premature ventricular beats, ventricular tachycardias including sudden cardiac death [41].

Sudden cardiac death has a circadian pattern, with the peak incidence occurring from 7 to 11 A. M. [42], from 7 to 9 A. M., with more sudden cardiac deaths occurring between 6 A. M. and 12 P. M. than during the other quarters of the day [43]: from 9 A. M. to 12 P. M. [44], and from 6 A. M. to 12 P. M. [45]. A study by Aronow and colleagues [46] showed that there was a circadian pattern in the number of deaths per hour in patients with CHF after prior myocardial infarction. The primary peak occurred between 6 A. M. and 12 P. M., with 39% of deaths occurring in that 6-hour period.

Flack and Yunis [47] indicate that the morning peak from 6 am to 12 noon of such occurrences as MI, thrombotic stroke, transient myocardial ischemia, and SCD is due to the high levels of coronary vasomotor tone, plasma catecholamines, and platelet aggregability, and the low levels of coronary blood flow and plasma fibrinolytic activity. At this same time, there is a rapid increase in blood pressure during the early morning hours. They also feel that it is important to maintain control of blood pressure throughout the early morning to try to avoid adverse events. A study in Auckland, New Zealand, by Van der Palen et al [48] had some slightly different findings on circadian rhythm. They report an afternoon peak in SCD (32. 5%) and a secondary morning peak (27. 6%). Also, they found a Saturday high (18. 6%) for SCD. Peckova and colleagues [49] showed a similar pattern of cardiac arrest: a low incidence at night, a sharp increase between 8 AM and noon with peaking at 10 AM, a relatively high incidence during the day, and another peak between 5 and 8 PM. Both morning and evening peaks were of a similar magnitude. Young patients had a relatively higher incidence at night than older patients and also exhibited a higher incidence in the morning than in the evening. Patients in the age category 41 to 65 years had a higher evening peak. Elderly patients maintained a rather high incidence during the daytime hours, with less pronounced peaks.

Mechanisms Underlying Sudden Cardiac Death

Cardiac arrest may have either a cardiac or a non-cardiac aetiology and may present with a variety of arrhythmias, including ventricular tachycardia, ventricular fibrillation, asystole, and electromechanical dissociation. The likelihood of a "sudden death" episode occurring and being witnessed is not constant throughout the day. Soo and colleagues [50] observed that there were three major time periods when a cardiac arrest was most likely to occur—an *early* peak in the morning around 1100 hours, a *late* peak in the evening around 2200 hours, and, for those whose arrest was from a cardiac disease, a third time period—around 1600 hours—also seemed to be critical In Seattle [51] and Berlin [52], the most important times for a cardiac arrest seemed to be around 1000 and 1800 hours. Ventricular fibrillation was most frequent around 2000 hours in the series by Peckova and colleagues[49], while Arntz and associates found that ventricular fibrillation occurred most often around 1000 hours, with the exception of ventricular fibrillation, the circadian variation of the arrest rhythm in both cardiac and non-cardiac groups appeared to be identical. The triggers for a cardiac arrest in both groups are likely to be similar when the arrhythmia is something other than ventricular fibrillation, irrespective of the aetiology of arrest [51].

Electrical Factors and Sudden Cardiac Death

The mechanisms underlying sudden cardiac death are probably multifactorial, and in some patients, primarily electrical factors or an interaction between electrical abnormalities and myocardial ischemia may be responsible for sudden cardiac death. Ambulatory recordings at the moment of sudden death have shown that ventricular tachycardia degenerating into ventricular fibrillation is a common terminal rhythm and often occurs in the absence of antecedent ischemic ST segment shifts [52]. In addition, the frequency of complex ventricular ectopy and the occurrence of sustained monomorphic ventricular tachycardia also are greatest in the early morning hours when the incidence of sudden death is greatest. Thus, a circadian variation in cardiac electrophysiological parameters may be an alternate mechanism contributing to the circadian variation in sudden death [53].

The distribution of ventricular fibrillation events followed the general pattern except that the evening peak is substantially higher than the morning peak. Peckova and colleagues [49] suggest the evening peak to be of approximately the same magnitude as the morning peak of incidence. They found that the bimodal pattern is mainly an attribute of ventricular fibrillation and that patients with asystole or pulseless electrical activity had a less pronounced evening peak. There was no difference in circadian variation between sexes, races, or days of the week. The analysis suggested that differences between the age categories are probably explicable by different rhythm distributions and thus are more likely due to sociodemographic factors than to biological differences.

Circadian Variation and Refractoriness

The circadian variation in the incidence of sudden cardiac death mainly appears to be due to variability in the time of onset of ventricular fibrillation [53]. Evidence has provided confirmation of the traditional hypothesis that ventricular fibrillation is due to multiple functional reentrant circuits, which change over time [54, 55]. Shorter refractory periods promote reentry by allowing reentrant circuits to be maintained in a smaller mass of tissue and by decreasing the length of lines of the block, leading to the variability in reentry observed during ventricular fibrillation. Experimental studies also have demonstrated that shortening of refractory periods under a variety of conditions may be proarrhythmic [56]. In the present study, maximal shortening between hourly refractory periods as well as the shortest absolute refractory periods were observed around the hour of waking, raising the possibility of a close relation between these findings and the increased morning incidence of arrhythmic sudden death. Although not measured in this study, an increased dispersion of refractoriness, which has been shown to promote ventricular arrhythmias [57], might be expected when overall ventricular refractoriness is rapidly changing. The circadian variation in refractory periods may be associated with a circadian variation in other electrophysiological properties, such as conduction velocity, which also may promote the emergence of reentrant circuits and arrhythmias. Fluctuations in sympathetic tone are mainly responsible for temporal changes in ventricular refractoriness [53].

Studies also have shown that acute cardiac events are temporally linked to waking [58]. In the Physicians' Health Study [59], 25% of myocardial infarctions occurred within 3 hours of waking, and the relative risk of infarction during this time interval was almost twice that during any other 3-hour period during the day. In the study by Kong QT et al [53], the most pronounced changes in ventricular refractoriness were also more closely linked to the hour of waking than to the absolute time of day. Results of the study therefore suggest that the time around waking is characterized by marked electrophysiological changes and possibly an increased vulnerability to arrhythmias.

Circadian Variation and Repolarization

The QT interval as measured on a surface ECG reflects global ventricular myocardial repolarization. A circadian variation in the QT interval has been described previously [61] and has been attributed to a circadian variation in ventricular repolarization. The QT interval has been found to be longest during sleep and shortest during the waking hours. However, the relevance of these observations to a potential circadian variation in ventricular refractoriness is not completely clear because the refractory period and action potential duration (as reflected globally by the QT interval) may be dissociated in some situations [62]. In addition, evaluation of the QT interval at different times of the day requires a correction for heart rate, which could limit the accuracy of the analysis of circadian changes in the QT interval. Finally, unlike refractory periods that were generally reproducible to within 4 ms with the methodology used in the study by Kong QT and colleagues [53], estimation of the QT interval may be somewhat less reproducible. Despite these potential differences, the results of the study suggest that the circadian variation in ventricular refractoriness qualitatively parallels the previously described circadian variation in the QT interval.

Yi et al [62] examined circadian variation of the QT interval in post MI patients and normal controls and its relation to SCD. They found the SCD victims did not show a significantly longer QT interval at night when compared to day as the normal subjects and MI survivors did, and the SCD victims did show a significantly longer QTc averaged over 24 hours. So, the circadian variation of the QT interval did vary when compared to normal subjects and those who survived the year following a MI.

Circadian Variation in Serum Potassium and Plasma Catecholamine Levels

Kong QT and colleagues [53] demonstrated a significant circadian variation in mean serum potassium levels, with the highest levels observed during the waking hours and the lowest levels during sleep. In eight of nine subjects, the minimum potassium levels were observed between the hours of 1:00 AM and 4:00 AM; the ninth subject had a minimum level at 2:00 PM.

A significant circadian variation was also observed in mean levels of plasma epinephrine and norepinephrine. Mean levels of each were highest during the day and lowest during sleep. A single harmonic model with a peak at 3:00 PM provided the best fit for epinephrine levels, and a double harmonic model with peaks at 9:00 AM and 9:00 PM provided the best fit for norepinephrine levels. We also observed low levels of magnesium and potassium as well as vitamine E and C and higher levels of TBARS and MDA, which are indicators of oxidative damage, in the second quarter of the day compared to evening values.

Circadian Variation in Cardiac Events

Some of the circadian variability in the incidence of sudden death may be due to a morning increase in myocardial ischemia [63, 64, 65, 66]. However, ischemic events do not account for all instances of sudden cardiac death, as autopsy studies of sudden death victims have failed to demonstrate acute coronary lesions in up to 42% of cases [67]. Furthermore, the occurrence of sustained monomorphic ventricular tachycardia, which is not generally a consequence of acute ischemia [68], also demonstrates a substantial variation [69]. Therefore, a circadian variation in cardiac electrophysiological parameters could potentially contribute to the increased morning incidence of sudden cardiac death.

Circadian Rhythm and Stroke

Monday Preference in Onset of Ischemic Stroke

The onset of stroke has a specific temporal pattern [70], characterized by a higher frequency in winter and in the mornings. According to a meta-analysis of more than 11, 000 patients, an estimated 37% of strokes occurred during morning hours [71].

A circaseptan rhythm, with a significant peak on Mondays was observed for all strokes and for ischemic strokes.

Data from a Norwegian study [72] suggested that biochemical factors associated with cardiovascular risk—such as measures of hematosis and carbohydrate and lipid metabolism—were less favorable on Mondays compared with other days of the week. Thus, similar to the association between increased thrombophilia in the mornings [73] and the circadian pattern of other thrombotic disease such as myocardial infarction [74] and limb ischemia [75], the Monday risk of ischemic stroke may reflect an increased thrombogenic condition [76].

Circadian Variation in Acute Ischemic Stroke

The existence of a circadian rhythm in ischemic stroke has been established, with a higher frequency in the early hours of the morning. The cause of this diurnal variation is uncertain. It has been related to the circadian rhythm of fibrinolysis, platelet aggregability [77] and mainly, arterial blood pressure, with its minimum value during sleep and maximum value in the early hours in the morning, in both normotensive and hypertensive patients [78]. However, it has been suggested that an increase in morning stroke onset could be due to patients awakening with neurological deficits as a result of a stroke that could have occurred during the night [79].

A. Lago et al. [79] found a higher frequency of stroke during the day and a lower frequency between 6:01 PM and 12:00 AM, obvious in all the different types of ischemic stroke viz. lacunar, thrombotic, embolic stroke.

In acute myocardial ischemia, the time of onset is easily determined [80, 81] corresponding with the onset of thoracic pain. This does not occur when the patient with ischemic stroke is discovered upon awakening; the onset may have occurred at any time during sleep. Unfortunately, at present there is no marker that indicates the time of stroke onset.

Stroke is classified within a heterogeneous group of vascular diseases, unlike myocardial ischemia, with different ethiopathogenic mechanisms. Arterial pressure, as other factors, may play an important role, favoring an increase in morning stroke onset. But these same factors, such as lower arterial pressure and heart rate during the night may contribute, through a hemodynamic mechanism, to a stroke onset during the sleeping hours, particularly in the case of thrombotic stroke. Results of study by A. Lago et al. [79] show that thrombotic and lacunar strokes have a higher onset during sleeping hours when compared with embolic stroke. The circadian rhythm of arterial blood pressure may be disturbed in patients who have suffered from stroke.

Loss of Circadian Rhythm of Blood Pressure Following Acute Stroke

Hypertension remains a dominant risk factor and prognostic indicator in patients with stroke in all communities. The risk of stroke is directly related to elevations of blood pressure.

S. Jain et al [82] showed a pathologically reduced or abolished circadian BP variation after stroke. The absence of normal dipping results in a higher 24 hour blood pressure load and may have more target organ damage than those with normal diurnal variations of blood pressure. The epidemiology of acute stroke is different in developing countries than that in the developed world. The age at stroke, risk factors, subtypes of stroke and prognosis are different in developing countries. In India, ischemic strokes constitute 70–75% while hemorrhagic strokes account for 20-25% of total cases [82]. However, hypertension remains a dominant risk factor and prognostic indicator in patients with stroke in all communities. The risk of stroke is directly related to elevations of blood pressure.

The accurate measurement of blood pressure after an acute stroke is important because antihypertensive therapy may be considered in some patients. However, blood pressure may be falsely elevated or depressed immediately after a stroke depending on the level of consciousness, severity of neurological deficit and physical activity.

The normal diurnal variation in blood pressure i. e., nighttime dipping was abolished in 88% patients in study by Jain and colleagues [82]. This nondipping was seen equally in both hemorrhagic and ischemic subgroups without any statistically significant difference.

In studies of patients with stroke, abnormal pattern of circadian rhythm of blood pressure using ambulatory blood pressure monitoring (ABPM) has been reported [83-85]. In a different study, Dawson et al[86] found a significant reduction in diurnal variation in systolic blood pressure in cortical infarct and intracerebral hemorrhage subgroups, compared with control subjects. The subcortical infarct subgroup demonstrated only minimal reduction in normal circadian variation. Fujishima et al [87] reported that blood pressure was elevated in the acute phase of a single lacunar infarction and it declined with time. No night time fall was noted in acute phase, but the circadian variation in blood pressure normalized in the subacute and chronic phase.

Circadian Variation in the Timing of Stroke Onset

Early studies of the timing of acute stroke, however, indicated that many afflicted patients reported awakening with new neurologic deficits, and several reports indicated that acute strokes tended to occur either during the evening hours or during sleep [88]. This led to the conclusion that especially because acute therapies for stroke-in-evolution were not particularly effective, there was little reason to consider acute stroke as a medical emergency because the onset of symptoms was thought to occur during sleep, when most patients would not recognize them [89].

The highest risk is found between 8:01 AM and noon; the lowest is found between midnight and 4 AM. Because there are some reports from Japan [90], especially regarding hemorrhagic stroke [91], which suggest that there may be differences in circadian variation of stroke timing according to the subtype of stroke of interest, meta-analyses of ischemic and hemorrhagic stroke (including subarachnoid and intracerebral bleeds), and transient ischemic attack were also carried out. Results of the study by WJ Elliott and colleagues [89] suggest that for each subtype of stroke studied, there is an increase in risk during the early morning hours. The data are remarkably consistent across the various subtypes of stroke, and indicate, for ischemic stroke, hemorrhagic stroke, and even transient ischemic attacks, that the excess risk during the 6 AM to noon time period is significantly higher than would be expected by chance: 89%, 52%, and 80%. Similarly, there was a significantly lower risk of stroke during the nighttime hours (midnight to 6 AM) for each stroke subtype: 30%, 54%, and 81%.

The finding that the early morning hours (and not the nighttime hours) have the highest risk for the onset of stroke symptoms has two broad implications. The first is that patients should no longer be told that stroke symptoms are not a medical emergency. Although this may have been sound public policy when acute treatments for stroke were not available, there is now some evidence that acute emergent treatments for cerebral ischemia can be delivered in a timely fashion and result in improved long-term outcomes. The results of meta-analysis contradict older conclusions that "strokes are more likely to occur during sleep". Meta-analysis indicates that irrespective of the type of stroke, most patients will be awake when the onset of stroke symptoms occurs. The recognition of new neurologic deficits should prompt afflicted patients and their families to consider these as a medical emergency (or "brain attack"). The second implication has to do with some modalities useful in stroke prevention. Blood pressure is often considered one of the most powerful risk factors for stroke and has a circadian variation that essentially parallels the circadian variation in stroke onset. Antihypertensive agents administered in the morning ought to have a long duration of action to still have an effect on the early morning rise in blood pressure. It is tempting to speculate that antihypertensive agents that specifically target the early morning rise in blood pressure and heart rate, without reducing blood pressure severely during the night, might be more advantageous in controlling the 20% rise in blood pressure during the hours around awakening. This appears also to be the time of day associated with an increased risk of stroke, myocardial infarction, and sudden cardiac death [89].

Circadian and Seasonal Occurrence of Subarachnoid and Intracerebral Hemorrhage

Subarachnoid hemorrhage (SAH) and intracerebral hemorrhage (ICH) are associated with high morbidity and mortality, and they represent about 20% of all strokes [92].

The occurrence of cerebral infarction has been reported to vary with the time of day; cerebrovascular ischemic events predominantly occur in the early morning and late afternoon [88, 93-95]. Recently, seasonal variations in the incidence of this disorder have also been detected, the peak occurrence being in the winter and autumn [96].

In some studies, the occurrence of SAH in individuals with a history of hypertension has been reported to vary with time of day [97-99].

P.A. Nyquist et al. [96] reported that the occurrence of ICH and SAH combined was increased during the winter. However, when the hemorrhage subtypes were evaluated, the main trend for seasonal differences was noted in SAH but not in ICH.

The circadian variation of blood pressure seems to mirror the time for onset of hemorrhagic stroke in that daily increases in blood pressure occur in the morning and early afternoon and lower levels occur at night [88, 98, 100]. Some investigators have hypothesized that this increase in blood pressure may be responsible for the increase in hemorrhagic stroke frequency in the early morning and afternoon. In addition, others have noted that normotensive individuals who experience SAH or ICH may have a late-afternoon locus of onset instead of an early morning locus of onset [98]. Other authors have suggested that the occurrence of SAH and ICH during the working hours may suggest an activity precipitant for SAH or ICH [101]. Factors that might contribute to an increased risk during the winter are uncertain. However, cardiovascular stresses occur during the winter, particularly in areas with extremes of seasonal climates, which may result in fluctuations in blood pressure, blood coagulability, and cardiovascular performance. These stresses include deconditioning, stress of physical activity in temperature extremes, types of activity required in a cold climate, and more specific effects of abrupt temperature changes and temperature extremes on the blood pressure and vascular system. Inflammatory factors such as cytokine levels and cortisol levels fluctuate with a circadian and circannual rhythmicity. These factors may play a role in priming the vasculature to respond in a manner predisposing the endothelium to rupture [96].

Circadian Variation in Transient Ischaemic Attack

A metaanalysis of 31 publications reporting the circadian timing of 11,816 strokes found a 49% increase in stroke of all types between 0600 and 1200 [89]. Possible explanations for the circadian pattern of cerebrovascular events have focused on circadian or postural changes in platelet aggregation, thrombolysis, blood pressure, heart rate, and catecholamine concentrations that occur after awakening with resumption of physical and mental activities. In a minority of cases, which varies in the literature from less than 10% to as much as 44%, stroke occurs at night [88, 93, 102]. This suggests that sleep, although "protective" for most cerebrovascular events, may represent a vulnerable state for a subset of patients at risk for stroke. Nocturnal blood pressure swings, cardiac arrhythmias, and sleep disordered breathing have been suggested as possible explanations for the nocturnal onset of stroke. Not only acute ischaemic stroke but also transient ischaemic attacks have a circadian pattern with a peak of onset between 0600 and 1200 and about 20% of events occurring at night time [103-105]. Furthermore, it is shown for the first time that patients with daytime and night time onset of transient ischaemic attack/stroke are similar with regard to most cardiovascular risk factors; clinical and polysomnographic sleep characteristics; and stroke parameters.

Findings by C. Bassetti et al. [106] suggest that low diastolic blood pressure values may predispose to nighttime onset of cerebrovascular events enhancing the sleep related fall in blood pressure.

Onset of Transient Ischaemic Attack/Stroke and Sleep Characteristics

Sleep disordered breathing is present in about 50% of patients with acute cerebrovascular diseases [107, 108]. Sleep apnoea—while being a risk factor for stroke [109, 110]—may only rarely represent the immediate cause of transient ischaemic attack or stroke. Rather, respiratory events during sleep may cause haemodynamic and haematological changes which increase the risk of cerebrovascular events at the transition from sleep to wakefulness and during the subsequent few hours.

It is nevertheless conceivable that in a patient with severe sleep apnoea swings in blood pressure, decreased cerebral blood flow, and cardiac arrhythmias produced by respiratory events may trigger cardiovascular and cerebrovascular events during sleep [106].

Onset of Transient Ischaemic Attack/Stroke and Stroke Characteristics

In a study of 1,233 patients, Lago et al [79] also found a higher frequency of all types of stroke during the day and a higher night time onset in macroangiopathy and microangiopathy compared with other stroke subtypes. Macroangiopathic and microangiopathic strokes may be particularly susceptible to nocturnal haemodynamic changes and decreased cerebral perfusion. Although yet to be proved, it is possible that intrathoracic pressure variations related to sleep apnoea may also predispose to cardioembolic strokes secondary to right-left shunt (for example, patent foramen ovale).

C. Bassetti et al. [106] have thus proven that [107] night time and daytime transient ischaemic attack/ stroke are similar in sleep and stroke characteristics, and [70, 71] diastolic hypotension may predispose to night time cerebrovascular events.

Nonpharmacological Treatment

Nonpharmacological management of circadian rhythm with yoga, physical activity, moderate alcohol intake, functional foods such as almonds, walnuts, rape seed oil, and neutraceuticals, eg coenzyme Q10 and w-3 fatty acids appear to be protective against circadian rhythms of cardiovascular events.

Pharmacotherapy

The concept of homeostasis in biology postulates that there is constancy of the intern milieu. Thus, it is assumed the risk and exacerbation of disease are invariable and independent of the time of day, day of month, and month of year as are the responses of patients to diagnostic tests and medications. Findings from the field of chronobiology, the study of biological rhythms, challenge the concept of homeostasis and the many assumptions and procedures of clinical medicine based on it. It is now recognized that human functions have daily, weekly, monthly and yearly biological rhythms. Plants, animals, and insects also have chronobiological rhythms. Circadian patterns have been observed for a variety of cardiovascular disorders, including cardiac arrhythmias, sudden cardiac death, cerebrovascular events, episodes of stable angina, unstable angina and acute myocardial infarction. The morning predominance of these events has been well documented in a number of large population studies. It is now recognized that circadian and other rhythms of the gastrointestinal tract and vital organs are capable of significantly affecting the pharmacokinetics and dynamics of cardiovascular and other medications. This means that the effects of therapeutic interventions administered in identical doses in the morning versus the evening may not be equivalent. The prevention and treatment of cardiovascular disease must take into account chronobiological factors [111].

Chronotherapeutics

Chronotherapeutics is the delivery of drugs at levels that match the body's needs at certain times of day or night. Chronotherapy links the effects of a disease to time, and thus the timing of drug delivery. The main objective of chronotherapy for heart disease would be to deliver needed drugs in higher concentrations during the time they are needed the most (early morning after-waking period) ; and at reduced drug levels when the need is less (during the middle of the sleep cycle) [112].

The goal of chronotherapeutics is to match the timing of treatment with the intrinsic timing of illness. Theoretically, optimum therapy is more likely to result when the right amount of drug is delivered to the correct target organ at the most appropriate time. In contrast, many side effects can be minimized if a drug is not given when it is not needed [113].

TIME-TAILORED DRUGS

Many drugs display normal, reproducible daily variations in pharmacokinetics and pharmacodynamics. Lemmer identified more than 100 drugs that display significant variation in concentrations or effects, or both, over 24 hours. Perhaps the best example is heparin. Even when it is administered at a constant infusion rate, the activated partial thromboplastin time and the risk of bleeding vary significantly according to the hour of the day and are higher at night [114]. The narrower the therapeutic window (i.e., risk-benefit ratio) for a specific drug, the more important the implication of the circadian variation in plasma levels [110].

Selected Medications Exhibiting Circadian Variations in Pharmacokinetic and Pharmacodynamic Action

Cardiovascular agents

- Enalapril
- Diltiazem HCl
- Nifedipine
- Propranolol HCl
- Verapamil

Antiasthmatic agents

- Terbutaline sulfate
- Theophylline
- Gastrointestinal agents:
- Cimetidine
- Omeprazole

Nonsteroidal anti-inflammatory drugs

- Acetylsalicylic acid
- Indomethacin
- Ketoprofen

Anticancer agents

- Cisplatin
- Doxorubicin
- Methotrexate

Other

- Diazepam
- Haloperidol

In selecting the most appropriate treatment for diseases that can be managed with chronotherapy, clinicians should understand that pharmacodynamic profiles of chronotherapeutic formulations are often different from those of traditional homeostatic formulations, even when the active drug itself is the same. Such differences may have important clinical consequences. Unlike homeostatic formulations, which provide relatively constant plasma drug levels over 24 hours, chronotherapeutic formulations may use various release mechanisms (e.g., time-delay coatings, osmotic pump mechanisms, matrix systems) that provide for varying levels throughout the day [115].

POTENTIAL ROLE OF CHRONOTHERAPY IN CARDIOVASCULAR DISEASES

Angiotensin Converting Enzyme Inhibitors

In one study, an ACE inhibitor was dosed either in the early morning or at bedtime in 18 patients with moderately high blood pressure. Palatini et al showed that nighttime dosing resulted in a greater effect on nighttime pressure than morning dosing. There was no difference in daytime pressure between the 2 groups. Measurement of ACE activity showed that nighttime dosing caused a more even, lasting reduction in blood levels of ACE.

In contrast to the ACE inhibitor study, studies with the beta-blocker atenolol, and the calcium channel blockers nifedipine and amlodipine, showed no different effects on pressure when dosed in the morning versus evening. Like many such studies, too few patients were studied to draw strong conclusions.

It is obvious, though, that drug class, formulation, and size of dose have a large influence on the effect seen [116].

Calcium Channel Blockers

In a study by Yosefy and colleagues from Israel it was found that long acting calcium channel blockers prevent the rise in blood pressure in morning hours and decreased the incidence of stroke by around 50%; thus providing a comprehensive cover during the dangerous hours in the morning [117].

Currently, preparations of verapamil hydrochloride are recommended for dosing at night to provide higher drug levels in the morning, when blood pressure, heart rate, and the risk of cardiovascular events are highest. Studies in hypertension [118] and angina pectoris [119] have demonstrated the benefits of a chronotherapeutic approach to these conditions.

Aspirin

The Physicians' Health Study, a randomized, double-blind, placebo-controlled trial of alternate-day aspirin intake (325 mg) among 22, 071 US male physicians, afforded the opportunity to assess this circadian pattern and examine whether it is altered by aspirin therapy. During a 5-year period of follow-up, 342 cases of nonfatal myocardial infarction were confirmed, of which the time of onset was available in 211 (62%). In the aspirin group, circadian variation was minimal, due primarily to a marked reduction in the morning peak of infarction. Specifically, aspirin was associated with a 59. 3% reduction in the incidence of infarction during the morning waking hours, compared with a 34. 1% reduction for the remaining hours of the day. The greater reduction was observed during the 3-hour interval immediately after awakening, a period with a risk of infarction twice that of any other comparable time interval. Aspirin intake was associated with a mean reduction in the incidence of infarction of 44. 8% over the entire 24-hour cycle. Aspirin reduces the risk of infarction by inhibiting platelet aggregation during the critical periods [118].

Beta Blockers

Drugs may suppress diurnal variation, specifically b-blockers [120, 121], antiarrhythmic drugs, and aspirin. The fact that b-blockers suppress circadian variation of myocardial infarction was already noted in several studies. If b-blockers also suppress circadian variation of cardiac arrests, we would expect that the interval between the times of day of the two arrests would widen, because the expected difference between the arrest times if no circadian variation is present is larger than in the presence of circadian variation [121].

Summary

The recognition of circadian rhythms in both normal human biologic function and disease has heightened awareness that the timing of drug regimens may have an important impact on effectiveness of treatment. Outcomes in several diseases that have predictable circadian variations have been improved by matching the timing of medication use to the circadian rhythm of the illness.

References

[1] Singh, RB;Weydahl, K;Otsuka K et al. Can nutrition influence circadian rhythm and heart rate variability? *Biomed Pharmacother* 2001, 55:(Supple)115-24.

[2] Singh, RB;Kartik, C;Otsuka K;Pella D;Pella J. Brain-heart connection and the risk of heart attack. (Editorial). *Biomed Pharmacother* 2002, 56:(Supple)257-265

[3] Otsuka, K;Cornelissen, G;Halberg, F. Circadian rhythms and clinical chronobiology. *Biomed Pharmacother* 2001, 55:(Supple)7-18.

[4] Halberg, F;Stephens, AN. Susceptibility to quabain and physiologic circadian periodicity. *Proc Minn acad Sci* 1959;27:139-43.

[5] Halberg F;Visscher MB. Regular diurnal physiological variation in eosinophil levels in five stocks of mice. *Proc Soc Exp Biol* (NY)1950, 75:846-47.

[6] Downing D. The history of man in four diets, editorial. *J Nutr Environ Med* 2003, 13:139-41.

[7] Trowell HC, Burkitt DP(eds). *Western Disease:their emergence and prevention.* London, Edward Arnold, 1981.

[8] Eaton SB, Strassman BI, Nesse RM et al. Evolutionary health promotion. *Prev Med* 2002, 34:109-18.

[9] Simopoulos AP. Genetic variation and dietary response:Nutrigenetics/nutrigenomics. *Asia Pac J Clin Nutr* 2002, 11(S6):117-128.

[10] Otsuka K, Shohgo M, Kozo M, Zi-yan Z, Weydahl A, Hansen TL. et al. Chronomes, aging and disease. In Furukawa H, Nishibuchi M, Kono Y, Kaida Y editors;*Ecological Destruction, Health and Development:Advancing Asian Paradigms*, 2004, p 367-94.

[11] Singh RB, Pella D, Rastogi S, Sharma JP, K Kartikey, Goyal VK et al. Increased concentrations of lipoprotein(a), circadian rhythms, and metabolic reactants evoked by acute myocardial infarction in relation to large breakfast. *Biomed Pharmacother* 2004, 58(Supplement):116-122.

[12] Singh RB, Pella D, Neki NS, Chandel JP, Gupta P, Rastogi S et al. Mechanism of acute myocardial infarcion(MAMI) study. *Biomed Pharmacother*, 2004, 58(Supplement):111-115.

[13] Singh RB, Cornelissen G, Weydahl A, Schwartzkopft O, Katinas G, Otsuka K et al, Circadian heart rate and blood pressure variability considered for research and patient care. *Int J Cardiol* 2003, 87:9-28.

[14] Czeisler CA, Johnson MP, Duffy JF, Brown EN, Rondo JM, Kronauer RE. Exposure to bright light and darkness to treat physiologic maladaptaion to night work. *N Engl J Med* 1990, 18:1253-59.

[15] Tei H, Okamura H, Shigeyoshi Y, Fukuhara C , Ozawa R, Hirose M, Sakaki Y. Circadian oscillation of a mammalian homologue of the Drosophila period gene. *Nature* 1997, 389, pp512-516.

[16] Tofler GH, Stone PH, Maclure M, Edelman E, Davis VG, Robertson T, Antman EM, Muller JE. Analysis of possible triggers of myocardial infarction(The MILIS Study). *Am J Cardiol* 1990, 66:22-27.

[17] Willich SN, Loewel H, Lewis M, Arntz R, Baur R, Winther K, Keil U, Shroeder R, TRIMM study group. Association of wake time and the onset of infarction. *Z Kardiol* 1991, 80(suppl 3):105-10.

[18] Tofler GH, Brezenski D, Schafer AI, Czeisler CA, Rutherford JD, Willich SN, Gleason RE, Williams GH, Mullar JE. Concurrent morning increase in platelet aggregability and the risk of myocardial infarction and sudden cardiac death. *N Engl J Med* 1987, 316:1514-18.

[19] Kozak M. Circadian rhythms in cardiovascular diseases, ischemic heart disease . *Vnitr Lek.* 2003 Apr;49(4):302-7.

[20] Un S, Baulmann J, Weisser B, Dusing R, Vetter H, Mengden T. Circadian rhythm of silent myocardial ischemia. Why morning is so risky for hypertensive patients. *MMW Fortschr Med.* 2003 Nov 20;145(47):34-8.

[21] Li JJ. Circadian variation in myocardial ischemia:the possible mechanisms involving in this phenomenon. *Med Hypotheses*. 2003 Aug;61(2):240-3.

[22] Li JJ; Huang CX; Fang CH; Chen F; Jiang H; Tang QZ; Li GS. Circadian variation in ischemic threshold in patients with stable angina: relation to plasma endothelin-1. *Angiology* - 01-Jul-2002; 53(4): 409-13.

[23] Kawano H; Motoyama T; Yasue H; Hirai N; Waly HM; Kugiyama K; Ogawa H. Endothelial function fluctuates with diurnal variation in the frequency of ischemic episodes in patients with variant angina. *J Am Coll Cardiol* - 17-Jul-2002; 40(2): 266-70

[24] Wennerblom B; Lurje L; Karlsson T; Tygesen H; Vahisalo R; Hjalmarson A. Circadian variation of heart rate variability and the rate of autonomic change in the morning hours in healthy subjects and angina patients. *Int J Cardiol* - 01-Jun-2001; 79(1): 61-9.

[25] Antman ME, Braunwald E. Acute myocardial infarction. In Braunwald (Eds.): *Heart disease: A Textbook of Cardiovascular Medicine 6th ed*; Philadelphia, W. B. Saunders Company, 2001, p. 1114.

[26] MILIS Study Group. Muller JE, Stone PH, Turi ZG, Rutherford JD, Czeisler CA, Parker C, Poole WK, Passamani E, Roberts R, Robertson T. Circadian variation in the frequency of onset of acute myocardial infarction. *N Engl J Med* 1985;313:1315-22.

[27] Moruzzi P, Marenzi G, Callegari S, Contini M. Circadian distribution of acute myocardial infarction by anatomic location and coronary artery involvement. *Am J Med*. 2004 Jan 1;116(1):24-7.

[28] Kirby DA, Verrier RL. Differential effects of sleep stage on coronary hemodynamic function. *Am J Physiol* 1989;256:H1378-83.

[29] Verrier RL, Dickerson LW. Autonomic nervous system and coronary blood flow changes related to emotional activation and sleep. *Circulation* 1991;83 (suppl II):II-81-9.

[30] Muller JE, Tofler GH, Stone PH. Circadian variation and triggers of onset of acute cardiovascular disease. *Circulation* 1989;79:733-43.

[31] Tanaka A, Kawarabayashi T, Fukuda D, Nishibori Y, Sakamoto T, Nishida Y, Shimada K, Yoshikawa J. Circadian variation of plaque rupture in acute myocardial infarction. *Am J Cardiol*. 2004 Jan 1;93(1):1-5.

[32] Millar-Craig MW, Bishop CN, Raftery EB. Circadian variation of blood-pressure. *Lancet* 1978;1:795-7.

[33] Fujita M, Franklin D. Diurnal changes in coronary blood flow in conscious dogs. *Circulation* 1987;76:488-91

[34] Pristipino C, Beltrame JF, Finocchiaro ML, Hattori R, Fujita M, Mongiardo R, Cianflone D, Sanna T, Sasayama S, Maseri A. Major racial differences in coronary constrictor response between Japanese and Caucasians with recent myocardial infarction. *Circulation* 2000;101:1102-8.

[35] Grines CL, Booth DC, Nissen SE, Gurley JC, Bennett KA, O'Connor WN, DeMaria AN. Mechanism of acute myocardial infarction in patients with prior coronary artery bypass grafting and therapeutic implications. *Am J Cardiol* 1990;65:1292-6.

[36] Culic V, Miric D, Eterovic D. Different circumstances, timing, and symptom presentation at onset of Q-wave versus non-Q-wave acute myocardial infarction. *Am J Cardiol*. 2002 Feb 15;89(4):456-60.

[37] Benhorin J., Moss A. J., Oakes D. , Marcus F. , Greenberg H. , Dwyer Jr E. M., Algeo S. , Hahn E.. Multicenter Diltiazem Post-Infarction Group. The prognostic significance of first myocardial infarction type (Q wave versus non-Q wave) and Q wave location. *J Am Coll Cardiol* 1990;15:1201-7.

[38] Ofili EO, Labovitz AJ, Kern MJ. Coronary flow velocity dynamics in normal and diseased arteries. *Am J Cardiol* 1993;71:3D-9D.

[39] Anderson HV, Stokes MJ, Leon M, Abu-Halawa SA, Stuart Y, Kirkeeide RL. Coronary artery flow velocity is related to lumen area and regional left ventricular mass. *Circulation 2000*;102:48-54.

[40] Myerburg JR, Castellanos A. Cardiac arrest and sudden cardiac death. In Braunwald (Eds.): *Heart disease: A Textbook of Cardiovascular Medicine 4th ed*; Philadelphia, W. B. Saunders Company, 2001, p. 756.

[41] Kozak M. Circadian rhythms in cardiovascular diseases—arrhythmias. *Vnitr Lek.* 2003 Apr;49(4):297-301

[42] Muller JE; Ludmer PL; Willich SN; Tofler GH; Aylmer G; Klangos I; Stone PH. Circadian variation in the frequency of sudden cardiac death. *Circulation* - 01-Jan-1987; 75(1): 131-8

[43] Willich SN; Levy D; Rocco MB; Tofler GH; Stone PH; Muller JE. Circadian variation in the incidence of sudden cardiac death in the Framingham Heart Study population. *Am J Cardiol* - 1-Oct-1987; 60(10): 801-6.

[44] Willich SN; Goldberg RJ; Maclure M; Perriello L; Muller JE. Increased onset of sudden cardiac death in the first three hours after awakening. *Am J Cardiol* - 1-Jul-1992; 70(1): 65-8

[45] Levine RL; Pepe PE; Fromm RE Jr; Curka PA; Clark PA. Prospective evidence of a circadian rhythm for out-of-hospital cardiac arrests. *JAMA* - 3-Jun-1992; 267(21):2935-7

[46] Aronow WS, Ahn C. Circadian variation of death from congestive heart failure after prior myocardial infarction in patients >60 years of age. *Am J Cardiol.* 2003 Dec 1;92 (11):1354-5.

[47] Flack JM, Yunis C. Therapeutic implications of the epidemiology and timing of myocardial infarction and other cardiovascular diseases. *J Hum Hypertens.* 1997 Jan;11(1):23-8.

[48] Van der Palen J, Doggen CJ, Beaglehole R. Variation in the time and day of onset of myocardial infarction and sudden death. *N Z Med J.* 1995 Aug 25;108 (1006):332-4.

[49] Peckova M; Fahrenbruch CE; Cobb LA; Hallstrom AP. Circadian Variations in the Occurrence of Cardiac Arrests: Initial and Repeat Episodes. *Circulation.* 1998;98:31-39.

[50] Soo L H, Gray D, Young T, Hampton JR. Circadian variation in witnessed out of hospital cardiac arrest. *Heart* 2000;84:370–376.

[51] Arntz HR, Willich SN, Oeff M, Bruggemann T, Stern R, Heinzmann A, Matenaer B, Schroder R. Circadian variation of sudden cardiac death reflects age-related variability in ventricular fibrillation. *Circulation.* 1993 Nov;88(5 Pt 1):2284-9.

[52] Leclercq JF, Maisonblanche P, Cauchemez B, Coumel P. Respective role of sympathetic tone and of cardiac pauses in the genesis of 62 cases of ventricular fibrillation recorded during Holter monitoring. *Eur Heart J.* 1988 Dec;9 (12):1276-83.

[53] Thomas Q. Kong, Jr, Jeffrey J. Goldberger, Michele Parker, RN, Ted Wang, Alan H. Kadish. Circadian Variation in Human Ventricular Refractoriness. *Circulation.* 1995;92:1507-1516.

[54] Cha YM, Birgersdotter-Green U, Wolf PL, Peters BB, Chen PS. The mechanism of termination of reentrant activity in ventricular fibrillation. *Circ Res.* 1994 Mar;74(3):495-506.

[55] Frazier DW, Wolf PD, Wharton JM, Tang AS, Smith WM, Ideker RE. Stimulus-induced critical point. Mechanism for electrical initiation of reentry in normal canine myocardium. *J Clin Invest.* 1989 Mar;83(3):1039-52.

[56] Sheridan DJ, Culling W. Electrophysiological effects of alpha-adrenoceptor stimulation in normal and ischemic myocardium. *J Cardiovasc Pharmacol.* 1985;7 Suppl 5:S55-60.

[57] Kuo CS, Atarashi H, Reddy CP, Surawicz B. Dispersion of ventricular repolarization and arrhythmia: study of two consecutive ventricular premature complexes. *Circulation.* 1985 Aug;72(2):370-6.

[58] Goldberg RJ, Brady P, Muller JE, Chen ZY, de Groot M, Zonneveld P, Dalen JE. Time of onset of symptoms of acute myocardial infarction. *Am J Cardiol.* 1990 Jul 15;66(2):140-4.

[59] Ridker PM, Manson JE, Buring JE, Muller JE, Hennekens CH. Circadian variation of acute myocardial infarction and the effect of low-dose aspirin in a randomized trial of physicians. *Circulation.* 1990 Sep;82(3):897-902.

[60] Bexton RS, Vallin HO, Camm AJ. Diurnal variation of the QT interval--influence of the autonomic nervous system. *Br Heart J.* 1986 Mar;55(3):253-8.

[61] Rozanski GJ, Jalife J, Moe GK. Determinants of postrepolarization refractoriness in depressed mammalian ventricular muscle. *Circ Res.* 1984 Oct;55(4):486-96.

[62] Yi G, Guo XH, Reardon M, Gallagher MM, Hnatkova K, Camm AJ, Malik M. Circadian variation of the QT interval in patients with sudden cardiac death after myocardial infarction. *Am J Cardiol.* 1998 Apr 15;81(8):950-6.

[63] Tofler GH, Brezinski D, Schafer AI, Czeisler CA, Rutherford JD, Willich SN, Gleason RE, Williams GH, Muller JE. Concurrent morning increase in platelet aggregability and the risk of myocardial infarction and sudden cardiac death. *N Engl J Med.* 1987 Jun 11;316(24):1514-8.

[64] Muller JE, Stone PH, Turi ZG, Rutherford JD, Czeisler CA, Parker C, Poole WK, Passamani E, Roberts R, Robertson T, et al. Circadian variation in the frequency of onset of acute myocardial infarction. *N Engl J Med.* 1985 Nov 21;313(21):1315-22.

[65] Willich SN, Linderer T, Wegscheider K, Leizorovicz A, Alamercery I, Schroder R. Increased morning incidence of myocardial infarction in the ISAM Study: absence with prior beta-adrenergic blockade. ISAM Study Group. *Circulation.* 1989 Oct;80(4):853-8.

[66] Fujita M, Franklin D. Diurnal changes in coronary blood flow in conscious dogs. *Circulation.* 1987 Aug;76(2):488-91.

[67] Roberts WC. Qualitative and quantitative comparison of amounts of narrowing by atherosclerotic plaques in the major epicardial coronary arteries at necropsy in sudden coronary death, transmural acute myocardial infarction, transmural healed myocardial infarction and unstable angina pectoris. *Am J Cardiol.* 1989 Aug 1;64(5):324-8.

[68] Davies MJ, Bland JM, Hangartner JR, Angelini A, Thomas AC. Factors influencing the presence or absence of acute coronary artery thrombi in sudden ischaemic death. *Eur Heart J.* 1989 Mar;10(3):203-8.

[69] Lampert R, Rosenfeld L, Batsford W, Lee F, McPherson C. Circadian variation of sustained ventricular tachycardia in patients with coronary artery disease and implantable cardioverter-defibrillators. *Circulation*. 1994 Jul;90(1):241-7.

[70] Manfredini R, Gallerani M, Portaluppi F, Salmi R, Fersini C. Chronobiological patterns of onset of acute cerebrovascular diseases. *Thromb Res*. 1997 Dec 15;88(6):451-63.

[71] Elliott WJ. Circadian variation in the timing of stroke onset: a meta-analysis. *Stroke*. 1998 May;29(5):992-6.

[72] Urdal P, Anderssen SA, Holme I, Hjermann I, Mundal HH, Haaland A, Torjesen P. Monday and non-Monday concentrations of lifestyle-related blood components in the Oslo Diet and Exercise Study. *J Intern Med*. 1998 Dec;244(6):507-13.

[73] Brezinski DA, Tofler GH, Muller JE, Pohjola-Sintonen S, Willich SN, Schafer AI, Czeisler CA, Williams GH. Morning increase in platelet aggregability. Association with assumption of the upright posture. *Circulation*. 1988 Jul;78(1):35-40.

[74] Cohen MC, Rohtla KM, Lavery CE, Muller JE, Mittleman MA. Meta-analysis of the morning excess of acute myocardial infarction and sudden cardiac death. *Am J Cardiol*. 1997 Jun 1;79(11):1512-6.

[75] Manfredini R, Gallerani M, Portaluppi F, Salmi R, Zamboni P, Fersini C. Circadian variation in the onset of acute critical limb ischemia. *Thromb Res*. 1998 Nov 15;92(4):163-9.

[76] Manfredini R, Casetta I, Paolino E, la Cecilia O, Boari B, Fallica E, Granieri E. Monday preference in onset of ischemic stroke. *Am J Med*. 2001 Oct 1;111(5):401-3.

[77] Kelly-Hayes M, Wolf PA, Kase CS, Brand FN, McGuirk JM, D'Agostino RB. Temporal patterns of stroke onset. The Framingham Study. *Stroke*. 1995 Aug;26(8):1343-7.

[78] Millar-Craig MW, Bishop CN, Raftery EB. Circadian variation of blood-pressure. *Lancet*. 1978 Apr 15;1(8068):795-7.

[79] Lago A, Geffner D, Tembl J, Landete L, Valero C, Baquero M. Circadian variation in acute ischemic *stroke*: a hospital-based study. *Stroke*. 1998 Sep;29(9):1873-5.

[80] Quyyumi AA. Circadian rhythms in cardiovascular disease. *Am Heart J*. 1990 Sep;120(3):726-33.

[81] Muller JE, Tofler GH, Stone PH. Circadian variation and triggers of onset of acute cardiovascular disease. *Circulation*. 1989 Apr;79(4):733-43.

[82] Jain S, Namboodri KK, Kumari S, Prabhakar S. Loss of circadian rhythm of blood pressure following acute stroke. *BMC Neurol*. 2004 Jan 6;4(1):1.

[83] Collins R, MacMahon S. Blood pressure, antihypertensive drug treatment and the risks of stroke and of coronary heart disease. *Br Med Bull*. 1994 Apr;50(2):272-98.

[84] Sander D, Klingelhofer J. Changes of circadian blood pressure patterns after hemodynamic and thromboembolic brain infarction. *Stroke*. 1994 Sep;25(9):1730-7.

[85] Yamamoto Y, Akiguchi I, Oiwa K, Satoi H, Kimura J. Diminished nocturnal blood pressure decline and lesion site in cerebrovascular disease. *Stroke*. 1995 May;26(5):829-33.

[86] Dawson SL, Evans SN, Manktelow BN, Fotherby MD, Robinson TG, Potter JF. Diurnal blood pressure change varies with stroke subtype in the acute phase. *Stroke*. 1998 Aug;29(8):1519-24.

[87] Fujishima S, Abe I, Okada Y, Saku Y, Sadoshima S, Fujishima M. Serial changes in blood pressure and neurohormone levels after the onset of lacunar stroke. *Angiology*. 1996 Jun;47(6):579-87.

[88] Marshall J. Diurnal variation in occurrence of strokes. *Stroke*. 1977 Mar-Apr;8(2):230-1.

[89] Elliott WJ. Circadian variation in the timing of stroke onset: a meta-analysis. *Stroke*. 1998 May;29(5):992-6.

[90] Hayashi S, Toyoshima H, Tanabe N, Miyanishi K. Daily peaks in the incidence of sudden cardiac death and fatal stroke in Niigata Prefecture. *Jpn Circ J*. 1996 Apr;60(4):193-200.

[91] Vermeer SE, Rinkel GJ, Algra A. Circadian fluctuations in onset of subarachnoid hemorrhage. New data on aneurysmal and perimesencephalic hemorrhage and a systematic review. *Stroke*. 1997 Apr;28(4):805-8.

[92] Brown RD, Whisnant JP, Sicks JD, O'Fallon WM, Wiebers DO. Stroke incidence, prevalence, and survival: secular trends in Rochester, Minnesota, through 1989. *Stroke*. 1996 Mar;27(3):373-80.

[93] Van der Windt C; Van Gijn J. Cerebral infarction does not occur typically at night. *J Neurol Neurosurg Psychiatry* - 01-Jan-1988; 51(1): 109-11.

[94] Wolf PA, Caplan LR, Foulkes MA. Morning increase in onset of ischemic stroke. *Stroke*. 1989 Apr;20(4):473-6.

[95] Argentino C, Toni D, Rasura M, Violi F, Sacchetti ML, Allegretta A, Balsano F, Fieschi C. Circadian variation in the frequency of ischemic stroke. *Stroke*. 1990 Mar;21(3):387-9.

[96] Nyquist PA, Brown RD Jr, Wiebers DO, Crowson CS, O'Fallon WM. Circadian and seasonal occurrence of subarachnoid and intracerebral hemorrhage. *Neurology*. 2001 Jan 23;56(2):190-3.

[97] Sloan MA, Price TR, Foulkes MA, Marler JR, Mohr JP, Hier DB, Wolf PA, Caplan LR. Circadian rhythmicity of stroke onset. Intracerebral and subarachnoid hemorrhage. *Stroke*. 1992 Oct;23(10):1420-6.

[98] Kleinpeter G, Schatzer R, Bock F. Is blood pressure really a trigger for the circadian rhythm of subarachnoid hemorrhage? *Stroke*. 1995 Oct;26(10):1805-10.

[99] Gallerani M, Manfredini R, Ricci L, Cocurullo A, Goldoni C, Bigoni M, Fersini C. Chronobiological aspects of acute cerebrovascular diseases. *Acta Neurol Scand*. 1993 Jun;87(6):482-7.

[100] Rautaharju PM, Manolio TA, Furberg CD, Siscovick D, Newman AB, Borhani NO, Gardin JM. Ischemic episodes in 24-h ambulatory electrocardiograms of elderly persons: the Cardiovascular Health Study. *Int J Cardiol*. 1995 Sep;51(2):165-75.

[101] Vermeer SE, Rinkel GJ, Algra A. Circadian fluctuations in onset of subarachnoid hemorrhage. New data on aneurysmal and perimesencephalic hemorrhage and a systematic review. *Stroke*. 1997 Apr;28(4):805-8.

[102] Chamorro A, Vila N, Ascaso C, Elices E, Schonewille W, Blanc R. Blood pressure and functional recovery in acute ischemic stroke. *Stroke*. 1998 Sep;29(9):1850-3.

[103] Marsh EE 3rd, Biller J, Adams HP Jr, Marler JR, Hulbert JR, Love BB, Gordon DL. Circadian variation in onset of acute ischemic stroke. *Arch Neurol*. 1990 Nov;47(11):1178-80.

[104] Wroe SJ, Sandercock P, Bamford J, Dennis M, Slattery J, Warlow C. Diurnal variation in incidence of stroke: Oxfordshire community stroke project. *BMJ.* 1992 Jan 18;304(6820):155-7.

[105] Haapaniemi H, Hillbom M, Juvela S. Weekend and holiday increase in the onset of ischemic stroke in young women. *Stroke.* 1996 Jun;27(6):1023-7.

[106] Bassetti C, Aldrich M. Night time versus daytime transient ischaemic attack and ischaemic stroke: a prospective study of 110 patients. *J Neurol Neurosurg Psychiatry.* 1999 Oct;67(4):463-7.

[107] Bassetti C, Aldrich MS, Chervin RD, Quint D. Sleep apnea in patients with transient ischemic attack and stroke: a prospective study of 59 patients. *Neurology.* 1996 Nov;47(5):1167-73.

[108] Dyken ME, Somers VK, Yamada T, Ren ZY, Zimmerman MB. Investigating the relationship between stroke and obstructive sleep apnea. *Stroke.* 1996 Mar;27(3):401-7.

[109] Palomaki H, Partinen M, Erkinjuntti T, Kaste M. Snoring, sleep apnea syndrome, and stroke. *Neurology.* 1992 Jul;42(7 Suppl 6):75-81; discussion 82.

[110] Partinen M. Ischaemic stroke, snoring and obstructive sleep apnoea. *J Sleep Res.* 1995 Jun;4(S1):156-159.

[111] Kozák M. Use of chronobiology findings in therapy of cardiovascular diseases. *Vnitr Lek.* 2003 Apr;49(4): 308-13.

[112] Sica DA, White W. Chronotherapeutics and Its Role in the Treatment of Hypertension and Cardiovascular Disease. *J Clin Hypertens* 2000; 2(4):279-286.

[113] Elliott WJ. Timing treatment to the rhythm of disease: a short course in chronotherapeutics. *Postgrad Med* 2001;110(2):119-29.

[114] Reinberg AE. Concepts of circadian chronopharmacology. *Ann N Y Acad Sci* 1991;618:102-15.

[115] Bhalla A, Singh R, Sachdev A, D'Cruz S, Duseja A. Circadian pattern in cerebro vascular disorders. *Neurol India* 2002;50:526-7.

[116] White WB, Black HR, Weber MA, et al. Comparison of effects of controlled onset extended release verapamil at bedtime and nifedipine gastrointestinal therapeutic system on arising on early morning blood pressure, heart rate, and the heart rate-blood pressure product. *Am J Cardiol* 1998;81:421-31

[117] Frishman WH, Glasser S, Stone P, et al. Comparison of controlled-onset extended-release verapamil with amlodipine and amlodipine plus atenolol on exercise performance and ambulatory ischemia in patients with chronic stable angina pectoris. *Am J Cardiol* 1999;83:507-14.

[118] Ridker PM, Manson JE, Buring JE, Muller JE and Hennekens CH. Circadian variation of acute myocardial infarction and the effect of low-dose aspirin in a randomized trial of physicians. *Circulation.* 1990 Sep;82(3):897-902.

[119] Willich SN, Linderer T, Wegscheider K, Leizorovicz A, Alamercery I and Schroder R. Increased morning incidence of myocardial infarction in the ISAM Study: absence with prior beta-adrenergic blockade. ISAM Study Group. *Circulation* 1989;80:853– 858.

[120] Kupari M, Koskinen P, Leinonen H. Double-peaking circadian variation in the occurrence of sustained supraventricular tachyarrhythmias. *Am Heart J.* 1990 Dec;120(6 Pt 1):1364-9.

[121] Peckova M; Fahrenbruch CE; Cobb LA; Hallstrom AP. Circadian Variations in the Occurrence of Cardiac Arrests: Initial and Repeat Episodes. *Circulation*. 1998; 98:31-39.

[122] Singh RB, Niaz MA, Cornelissen G, Otsuka K, Siegelova J, Fiser B, Halberg F. Circadian rhythmicity of circulating vitamin concentrations. *Scripta Medica (BRONO)*, 2001, 74:93-96.

In: Frontiers in Atherosclerosis Research
Editor: Karin F. Kepper, pp. 141-161

ISBN 1-60021-371-5

Chapter 7

STATINS AND ACUTE CORONARY SYNDROME

Petr Ostadal*

Department of Cardiology, Cardiocenter, Third Faculty of Medicine, Charles University in Prague and University Hospital Kralovske Vinohrady, Prague, Czech Republic

Jan Vojacek

Department of Cardiac Surgery, Second Faculty of Medicine, Charles University in Prague and University Hospital Motol, Prague, Czech Republic

ABSTRACT

It has been repeatedly shown that statins (3-hydroxy-3-methylglutaryl coenzyme A reductase inhibitors) are very effective in primary and secondary prevention of ischemic heart disease. In the settings of acute coronary syndrome (ACS), different pathological pathways are triggered that are known to be inhibited by statins, including endothelial dysfunction and activation of inflammation and coagulation; the idea to use these drugs also under conditions of ACS seems to be, therefore, fully justified. Recently, several prospective controlled clinical trials have been presented, showing safety and in some points also efficacy of statins, when administered early after ACS. An increasing number of publications demonstrates, however, that statins may express a positive effect not only in the early secondary prevention but also directly in the therapy of ACS, i.e. when statin treatment is started as a first-line care in clinically unstable patients. This therapeutic option is supported by (i) experimental studies, showing a protective effect of statins under the condition of acute ischemia, (ii) analysis of different registers and trials, demonstrating better prognosis of statin-treated patients, and (iii) small clinical trials, describing a lower peri-procedural infarction rate during coronary intervention or lower level of C-reactive protein and other inflammatory markers as a result of statin therapy. Nevertheless, confirmation of this hypothesis by large prospective controlled clinical trials will be necessary before introduction of statins as the first line therapy in unstable patients with ACS, even without knowledge of the blood cholesterol level.

3-Hydroxy-3-methylglutaryl coenzyme A (HMG-CoA) reductase inhibitors (statins), lower cholesterol level by decreasing the production of low-density lipoproteins (LDL) and up-regulating the expression of the LDL-receptor. Statins are widely used in patients with

* Address for correspondence: Petr Ostadal, MD, PhD. Dept. of Cardiology, University Hospital Kralovske Vinohrady, Srobarova 50, 100 34, Prague, Czech Republic. e-mail: ostadal@yahoo.com

hyperlipidemia and coronary artery disease (CAD) worldwide. There is strong evidence documenting their efficacy and supporting their use in both primary and secondary prevention for reduction in mortality and nonfatal cardiovascular events. This effect can be, however, only partially explained by the lipid-lowering mechanisms. During the past decade substantial effort has been expended for the investigation of non-lipid-mediated actions of statins, referred to also as "pleiotropic effects". It has been found that beyond the lipid-lowering activity, statins exert anti-inflammatory, antithrombotic, and antioxidant effects, increase nitric oxide (NO) production or improve endothelial dysfunction.

Coronary atherosclerosis has been known for a long time to be associated with lipid metabolism disorder. It has been shown, however, that "classical" risk factors, such as hypercholesterolemia, hypertension, diabetes, and cigarette smoking could not fully explain the development of coronary stenosis in all patients suffering from CAD. Intensive study of the pathogenesis of coronary plaque development and rupture led to the hypothesis of possible involvement of other mechanisms in this process. Particularly inflammation was described as an important factor in the development of CAD and the increased level of some inflammatory markers, e.g. C-reactive protein (CRP), has been shown to be one of the strongest risk factors for cardiovascular events. Activation of inflammatory pathways plays probably also the key role in coronary plaque destabilization and rupture, with subsequent thrombosis development, clinically manifested as ACS. Statins have been shown to modulate several mechanisms, involved in the pathogenesis of ACS, including inflammation or thrombosis (Table 1); the increased interest in the use of statins for the therapy of ACS is therefore fully justified.

Table 1. Possible favorable effects of statins in acute coronary syndrome

- suppression of the production of pro-inflammatory cytokines
- suppression of the expression of adhesive molecules
- inhibition of the production of metalloproteinases
- antioxidant effect
- increased production of NO
- antithrombotic effect

THE VULNERABLE PLAQUE

During the past years, marked progress has been made in the understanding of pathogenesis of ACS. Several pathways have been discovered to participate in the development of coronary instability; especially activation of inflammatory mechanisms plays probably an important role in the plaque destabilization. Simultaneously, statins have been shown to influence various factors, participating in this process. The short overview of the current knowledge of the pathogenesis of vulnerable plaque development provides, therefore, the fundamental theoretical background, essential for better understanding of possible therapeutic targets for statins.

Based on the pathological and angiographic studies, plaque fissuring or rupture was determined as a trigger of coronary thrombosis, which is the cause of the majority of ACS. Atherosclerotic plaque susceptible to disruption differs in some histological features: it usually contains a large lipid pool, accumulation of macrophages, and a thin fibrous cap (1-4). The mediators contributing to plaque vulnerability may be divided into extrinsic and intrinsic promoters (5, 6). The extrinsic factors actually trigger plaque disruption; they are represented by circumferential stress, hemodynamic shear stress, vasospasm, plaque fatigue, and prothrombotic milieu (6-9). The intrinsic factors are responsible for susceptibility to plaque rupture or directly cause that event; they include size and composition of lipid core, neovascularization, endothelial erosion/fissure, low fibrous cap thickness, inflammation, matrix degradation enzymes, decreased number of smooth muscle cells (SMC) and low collagen content, outward remodeling, and nodular calcification (6).

Several cellular types are deeply involved in the pathogenesis of vulnerable plaque development.

Macrophages

Lesional macrophages overexpress various enzymes, signaling molecules, pro-inflammatory cytokines, and other active substances. Proteinases derived from macrophages include members of the matrix metalloproteinase (MMP) family, represented by collagenases MMP-1, MMP-8, and MMP-13. Collagenases are supposed to be responsible for fibrous cap degradation (1, 10), associated with the loss of tensile stress tolerance (11). Other enzymes expressed by macrophages are myeloperoxidases, playing a major role in the release of reactive oxygen species, resulting in oxidative stress (OS). OS may activate other cell types such as endothelial cells (EC) and different MMPs (MMP-2, MMP-9, nad MMP-14) (12-14). Macrophages in atheroma secrete also (i) a number of pro-inflammatory cytokines: interleukin 1β (IL-1β), interleukin 2 (IL-2), tumor necrosis factor α (TNF-α), and interferon γ (IFN-γ) and (ii) growth factors: vascular endothelial growth factor (VEGF), macrophage-colony-stimulating factor (M-CSF), leading to activation and/or proliferation of other cell types such as SMC or EC (15). Moreover, lesional macrophages express also the tissue factor (TF), a potent initiator of coagulation cascade, and plasminogen activator inhibitor 1 (PAI-1), inhibitor of fibrinolysis (16, 17). These agents may accelerate thrombus formation after fibrous cap disruption (1).

Endothelium

Another major contributor to the coronary plaque vulnerability are EC. Expression of different surface molecules (vascular cell adhesion molecule 1 (VCAM-1), selectin E, and selectin P) and production of pro-inflammatory substances (monocyte chemoattractant protein 1 (MCP-1)) by EC lead to leukocyte recruitment and formation of macrophage-rich atheroma (18-21). In atheroma is decreased also the expression of endothelial NO synthase (eNOS), producing NO from L-arginine (22).

Smooth Muscle Cells

Proliferation of SMC similarly as production of different components of extracellular matrix by SMC is considered to be important for plaque stability (23). Advanced atherosclerotic lesions are, however, characterized by paucity of SMC proliferation and decreased collagen content (7, 10, 23).

T-lymphocytes

Different types of T-lymphocytes have been detected in atherosclerotic plaques. An important role in the unstable coronary plaque development is probably played by the interactions between various phenotypes of $CD4^+$ T-lymphocytes (Th cells). While Th_1 response, characterized by production of IFN-γ and IL-12, decreases SMC proliferation and matrix synthesis, Th_2 response (production of IL-4, IL-5, and IL-10) inhibits the development of atherosclerosis by possible inhibition of apoptosis and down-regulation of Th_1 response (6, 24, 25).

Pleiotropic Effects of Statins

As mentioned above, statins are highly effective in the treatment of dyslipidemias. They significantly reduce total cholesterol, LDL-cholesterol or triglyceride, and increase HDL-cholesterol levels already after a several-week therapy (26, 27). Statins, however, exert also other effects that seem to be independent of lipid lowering; these effects are referred to as "pleiotropic". During the past several years it has been repeatedly observed that statins could influence various mechanisms that are deeply involved in the vulnerable plaque development. Discovery of the pleiotropic effects of statins fully supports, therefore, the idea to use statins in the therapy of ACS.

Anti-inflammatory Effects of Statins

As described above, inflammation is probably deeply involved in the pathogenesis of atherosclerosis and in the development of coronary plaque vulnerability. Increased level of a variety of circulating markers of inflammation (CRP, serum amyloid A, heat-shock protein 65, IL-6, and circulating adhesion molecules ICAM-1, V-CAM-1) have been described to be related to the severity of atherosclerosis and to impaired prognosis of patients with ischemic heart disease. The level of CRP, one of the most important risk factors for cardiovascular events, has been repeatedly shown to be reduced by different statins and this reduction was independent of the lipid-lowering effect (28-36). Furthermore, statins suppressed secretion of some cytokines, such as IL-1, IL-6, IL-8, TNF-α or MCP-1 (37-44) as well as production of MMPs (39, 45-47). Moreover, reduction of circulating adhesion molecules ICAM-1, P-selectin, and E-selectin has been described after statin therapy (48-50).

Antioxidant Effects of Statins

Reactive oxygen species are directly involved in the degradation of NO and enhance endothelial dysfunction; moreover, oxidation of LDL contributes to the foam cell formation by increasing the accumulation of cholesterol in macrophages and stimulates thrombosis and inflammation (51). It has been described that fluvastatin exerts a superoxide or hydroxyl radical scavenging activity and reduces susceptibility of LDL to oxidation (52-55), cerivastatin scavenged superoxide and preserved active NO (56, 57); another member of the statin group, atorvastatin, decreased the free radical-induced lipid peroxidation in plasma and increased the total antioxidant status (58).

Statin Effects on Endothelial Dysfunction

Endothelial dysfunction can be recognized as an imbalance between mechanisms, responsible for vasoconstriction and vasodilation. Endothelium-derived vasorelaxation is mediated by NO; in contrast, potent vasoconstrictive agents are endothelin-1 (ET-1) and angiotensin (51).

Statin Effects on Nitric Oxide

NO plays a protective role in CAD by its vasodilating effect, modification of the inflammatory response, decrease of SMC proliferation, and leukocyte and platelet activation (51, 59, 60). Furthermore, NO reduces the endothelial expression of adhesion molecules, monocyte adhesion to the endothelium, and decreases production of IL-6 and IL-8 (51, 61). Increase in NO production, mediated by up-regulation of eNOS, has been observed after administration of statins in different experimental models (56, 57, 62-64); a possible explanation of this effect is the inhibition of G-proteins by statins, leading to reduced eNOS mRNA degradation and higher eNOS level and activity (51, 64-66).

Statins and Endothelin-1

ET-1 is synthesized by endothelial cells and has an action opposite to NO – it stimulates vasoconstriction and vascular cell proliferation and acts as a platelet activator (51, 67). In experimental models, the activation of ET-1 expression promotes the development of atherosclerosis (68). Administration of statins induces a down-regulation of the pre-pro ET-1-mRNA levels (69); it is not clear, however, whether this is a direct effect of statins on ET-1 synthesis or whether it is mediated by statin-induced increase of NO production that exerts a similar effect on ET-1 (51, 69).

In clinical settings, the effect of statins on endothelial dysfunction has been assessed mostly by the measurement of flow-mediated dilatation (FMD); this parameter is impaired in patients with atherosclerosis (70, 71). Administration of statins in patients with hypercholesterolemia and/or CAD significantly improved the FMD; this effect is probably independent of statin-induced changes in lipid levels (70-74).

Antithrombotic Effects of Statins

It has been repeatedly shown in cultured monocytes/macrophages, SMC or endothelial cells that statins can reduce the level and activity of TF, which initiates the coagulation cascade by activating factors IX and X (46, 75-79). This effect of statins was confirmed also *in vivo* on animal models and in human studies (46, 79-83). On the other hand, statins decrease the level of the total tissue factor pathway inhibitor (TFPI), a potent anticoagulant agent (84-87); they do not, however, influence the free TFPI (84, 86, 87). Because the anticoagulant activity of TFPI is related just to the free fraction of TFPI (87, 88), alteration of the total TFPI seems to play a relatively marginal role in the global anticoagulant activity of statins (88).

Based on the studies detecting the effect of statins on prothrombin fragment (F1+2), fibrinopeptide A (FPA), and thrombin-antithrombin III (TAT) complexes, statins significantly decrease thrombin formation (82, 89-94). It has been shown that this effect results not only from the inhibition of platelet-dependent thrombin formation but also from the decreased TF expression (76, 88).

In the clinical trials, however, there are contradictory opinions on the effect of statins on fibrinogen levels, one of the important risk factors of cardiovascular events (95-99). This discrepancy could be at least partially explained by different methods used in these studies (88). Also factor VII, factor VIII, and von Willebrand factor (vWF) have been identified as predictors of increased risk of CAD (100). Although the literature data dealing with the effect of statins on these factors are inconsistent, the majority of studies have shown favorable results (88).

Statins, however, influence not only the coagulation but also the fibrinolytic activity. It has been repeatedly described by *in vitro* studies that administration of statins results in the increased level, activity, and synthesis of tissue plasminogen activator (tPA), and simultaneously in the decreased level, activity and synthesis of PAI-1 (63, 99, 101-107). Although there is a general agreement among the *in vitro* studies concerning the fibrinolysis-stimulating role of statins, clinical trials have produced less convincing results (88). Clinical studies are, however, inconsistent in inclusion criteria, type of statin and its dosage, duration of treatment or in the methodological approaches (88).

Statins in Early Secondary Prevention

There is overwhelming evidence about the beneficial role of statins in the therapy of stable forms of CAD, arising from the large prospective trials as 4S (Scandinavian Simvastatin Survival Study) (108), CARE (Cholesterol and Recurrent Events) (109) or LIPID (Long-Term Intervention with Pravastatin in Ischaemic Disease) (110). The discovery of the non-lipid effects of statins in the recent years was, however, immediately reflected in the efforts to use statins also in less stabilized patients. Different observational studies have been published, showing the favorable effect of statin therapy started soon after ACS; furthermore, several randomized prospective trials have been carried out to evaluate the effect of statins, when administered early after ACS.

Observational Studies

A large, prospective, cohort study using data from the Swedish Register of Cardiac Intensive Care (RIKS-HIA) demonstrated that early initiation of statin therapy in patients with acute myocardial infarction was associated with a reduced 1-year mortality (RR 0.75, p=0.001) (111). Post-hoc analysis of two randomized trials – GUSTO IIb (Global Use of Strategies to Open Occluded Coronary Arteries) and PURSUIT (Platelet Glycoprotein IIb/IIIa in Unstable Angina: Receptor Suppression Using Integrilin Therapy) – showed that patients with ACS discharged on lipid-lowering drugs have a survival benefit at 6 months (RR 0.48, p<0.001) (112). In the OPUS/TIMI 16 study (Orofiban in Patients with Unstable Coronary Syndromes/Thrombolysis in Myocardial Infarction), mortality at 1 month was reduced in patients treated with lipid-lowering drugs (RR 0.30, p<0.001) (113). The analysis of SYMPHONY trial (Sibrafiban Versus Aspirin to Yield Maximum Protection from Ischemic Heart Events Post-Acute Coronary Syndromes) showed lower mortality in statin-treated patients at 3 months (RR 0.58, p<0.05) (114). Subgroup analysis of the PRISM study (Platelet Receptor Inhibition in Ischemic Syndrome Management) demonstrated better prognosis of statin-treated patients compared with patients without statin therapy; surprisingly, the worst prognosis in this analysis was described in patients in whom statin therapy was withdrawn after hospital admission for ACS (115). Early use of statin in acute myocardial infarction was associated with a reduced in-hospital mortality in MITRA registry (Maximized Individual Therapies in Acute Myocardial Ischemia) (116). It has been shown that statin therapy also improved prognosis in patients undergoing percutaneous coronary intervention (117). Moreover, analysis of the Euro Heart Survey on acute coronary syndrome showed reduced 7-day mortality in patients with ACS receiving statin therapy within 24 hours of admission (118).

Randomized Trials

Recently, several randomized trials, dealing with the statin therapy, started early after ACS, have been published. In a short survey we would like to summarize their design and results of primary endpoints (Table 2).

The Pravastatin Turkish Trial (PTT) (119) was a small study that randomized 150 patients with acute myocardial infarction (AMI) to pravastatin 40 mg or no lipid-lowering drug within 6 hours of hospital admission. All patients were treated with intravenous fibrinolytic therapy. At 6 months no difference was found in mortality; the pravastatin-treated group experienced, however, less recurrent ischemic events compared with the placebo group.

The Myocardial Ischemia Reduction with Aggressive Cholesterol Lowering (MIRACL) trial (120) randomized 3086 patients with unstable angina or non-Q-wave AMI to atorvastatin 80 mg or placebo within 24 to 96 hours after hospital admission; treatment continued for 16 weeks. The investigators showed a 16 % relative reduction in the combined endpoint of death, recurrent nonfatal AMI, resuscitated cardiac arrest, or recurrent ischemia requiring repeated hospitalization (14.8 % vs. 17.4 %; RR 0.84; p=0.048). This benefit was largely driven by a reduction in the endpoint of recurrent ischemia requiring hospitalization (6.2 % vs. 8.4 %; RR 0.74; p=0.02). Limitation of this study from the current point of view was the exclusion criterion of coronary intervention undergone or planned; only conservatively treated patients were included in this study.

Table 2. Large randomized trials concerning with the early statin therapy after acute coronary syndrome

Trial	No. of pts.	Drugs studied	Primary endpoint	Results
MIRACL	3086	atorvastatin/placebo	MACE	RR 0.84, p=0.048
FLORIDA	540	fluvastatin/placebo	ischemia	n.s.
PROVE-IT	4162	atorvastatin/pravastatin	MACE	RR 0.84, p=0.005
PACT	3408	pravastatin/placebo	MACE	n.s.
A to Z	4497	simvastatin/placebo	MACE	n.s.
PRINCESS	3600	cerivastatin/placebo	MACE	n.s.

MIRACL, the Myocardial Ischemia Reduction with Aggressive Cholesterol Lowering trial; FLORIDA, the Fluvastatin on Risk Diminishing After Acute Myocardial Infarction trial; PROVE-IT, the Pravastatin or Atorvastatin Evaluation and Infection Therapy-Thrombolysis in Myocardial Infarction 22 trial; PACT, the Pravastatin in Acute Coronary Treatment trial; PRINCESS, the Prevention of Ischemic Events by Early Treatment of Cerivastatin Study; MACE, major adverse cardiac events.

The Fluvastatin on Risk Diminishing After Acute Myocardial Infarction (FLORIDA) trial (121) randomized 540 patients with AMI to fluvastatin or placebo within 14 days of the index MI. The primary endpoint was reduction in cardiac ischemia, determined by ambulatory Holter monitoring. No differences in occurrence of ischemia were observed and, similarly, there were no differences in mortality and major adverse cardiac events (MACE) rate after 1 year.

The Lipid-Coronary Artery Disease (L-CAD) trial (122) was primarily designed to examine the effect of pravastatin on angiographic regression of atherosclerosis. In the L-CAD study, 126 patients, who had undergone percutaneous coronary intervention (PCI) for ACS, were randomized to pravastatin 20-40 mg (with or without cholestyramine and/or nicotinic acid) or to usual care determined by family physician; patients were enrolled by hospital discharge. After 2 years of follow-up, fewer patients in the pravastatin group experienced MACE as compared with the usual care group (OR 0.28, p=0.005).

The Lescol Intervention Prevention Study (LIPS) (123) enrolled 1677 patients, scheduled for a first PCI procedure for stable angina, unstable angina or silent ischemia. Patients were randomized to fluvastatin 40 mg twice daily or placebo at an average of 2.7 days after the procedure. Statin therapy resulted in a reduction of the occurrence of MACE at a median follow-up time of 3.9 years (21.4% vs. 26.7%; RR 0.78; p=0.01).

The Pravastatin or Atorvastatin Evaluation and Infection Therapy-Thrombolysis in Myocardial Infarction 22 (PROVE IT-TIMI 22) trial (124) randomized 4162 patients within 10 days of hospital admission for ACS to pravastatin 40 mg daily (standard therapy) or atorvastatin 80 mg daily (intensive therapy). After a median follow-up of 2 years, the rate of MACE was significantly lower in the intensive therapy group as compared with the standard therapy (22.4% vs. 26.3%; RR 0.84; p=0.005).

The Pravastatin in Acute Coronary Treatment (PACT) trial (125) tested the effect of pravastatin administration within 24 hours of the onset of symptoms in patients with ACS. The recruitment of 10,000 patients was planned; the study was, however, stopped early. A total of

3408 patients were randomized to pravastatin 20-40 mg or placebo. After 30 days of follow-up, no significant difference in the occurrence of MACE was observed.

Phase Z of the A to Z trial (126) compared an early intensive vs. a delayed conservative strategy of simvastatin therapy in patients with ACS. Within 5 days of the onset of symptoms, a total of 4497 patients were randomized to simvastatin 40 mg daily for 1 month followed by 80 mg daily thereafter or to placebo for 4 months followed by simvastatin 20 mg daily. The rates of MACE were not significantly different between the early intensive and the delayed conservative group either at 4 months or at 2 years.

In the Prevention of Ischemic Events by Early Treatment of Cerivastatin Study (PRINCESS) (127) patients were randomized within 48 hours of admission for ACS to cerivastatin or placebo. This trial was prematurely interrupted after cerivastatin was withdrawn from worldwide market. Data obtained from a total of 3,600 patients followed up for 4.5 months were analyzed; no significant difference in the occurrence of MACE was found between the groups.

It can be concluded that these prospective trials have shown safety and in some points also benefit of the early initiation of statin therapy after ACS (Table 2). It is, however, necessary to stress that these trials were designed for early (in some cases "very early") secondary prevention, not for the real therapy of ACS. In all of the above-mentioned studies, patients were randomized at least several hours and in most cases even several days after hospital admission (Figure 1). During such a long period of time the majority of patients are already clinically stabilized. In the context of the above described pathogenesis of vulnerable plaque development and the mechanisms of pleiotropic effects of statins it is obvious that there are relevant reasons to use these drugs not only in the secondary prevention but also directly in the therapy of ACS, when administered to really unstable patients.

Statins in the Therapy of ACS

As discussed above, pleiotropic effects of statins may affect different pathogenic pathways, participating in the development of vulnerable plaque and in the pathogenesis of ACS; expanding this suggestion, statins may significantly contribute to plaque stabilization, reduction of thrombus formation and acceleration of fibrinolysis. It is, therefore, fully justified to investigate the possible favorable effect of statin therapy at the time of coronary instability and to evaluate the shift of statin administration from hospital discharge to the first-line therapy, beside aspirin (128).

It has been repeatedly shown that treatment of animals with statins prior to the onset of myocardial ischemia reduces ischemia-reperfusion injury. Already in 1999, Lefer et al. (129) have shown in the model of isolated perfused rat heart a cardioprotective effect of simvastatin, when administered before the induction of ischemia. Simvastatin inhibited leukocyte-endothelium interactions and improved contractile parameters. Ueda et al. (130) described that pravastatin treatment decreased the infarct size after experimentally induced ischemia and ischemic preconditioning in hypercholesterolemic rabbits. In another paper Lefer et al. (131) showed reduction in the infarct size after simvastatin treatment in the model of diabetic mouse. It has been also found that this protective effect may be at least partly mediated by the stimulation of eNOS and increased production of NO (131, 132).

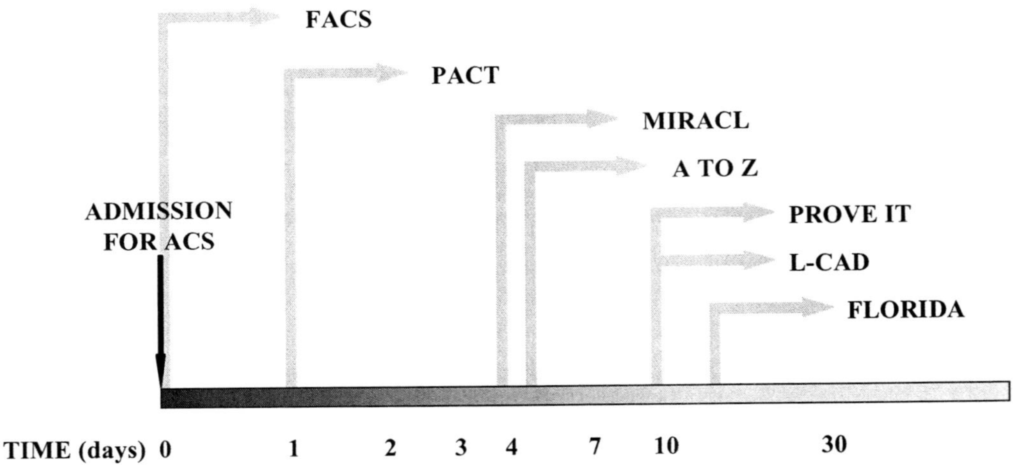

Figure 1. Relation of the randomization time to the time of admission in randomized trials with statins and ACS. In the Fluvastatin in the therapy of Acute Coronary Syndrome (FACS) trial patients are randomized at admission; in Pravastatin in Acute Coronary Treatment (PACT) trial statin therapy was initiated within 24 hours of onset of ACS; in Myocardial Ischemia Reduction With Aggressive Cholesterol Lowering (MIRACL) trial patients were randomized 24 to 96 hours after ACS; in Z-phase of the A-to-Z trial simvastatin therapy was initiated within 5 days of the onset of ACS, after clinical stabilization; in Pravastatin or Atorvastatin Evaluation and Infection Therapy (PROVE IT) trial patients were randomized up to 10 days after ACS; in Lipid-Coronary Artery Disease (L-CAD) trial statin therapy was initiated up to ten days from ACS; in Fluvastatin on Risk Diminishing After Acute Myocardial Infarction (FLORIDA) trial patients were randomized up to two weeks after ACS.

Animal Studies

While the above experimental studies demonstrate the impact of prophylactic therapy they do not address the question, whether patients with AMI might benefit from the initiation of statin therapy after the onset of ischemia or prior to reperfusion. Bauersachs et al. (133) failed to demonstrate a reduction of infarct size when the statin was administered 24 hours after onset of myocardial ischemia, similarly to the protocol of most of the randomized clinical trials. Probably the first study, showing a significant benefit of the statin therapy, started immediately after the onset of ischemia was published by Hayashidani et al. (134) They described lower mortality in mice subjected to coronary artery ligation and fluvastatin therapy, introduced just after the procedure. Furthermore, fluvastatin in this study attenuated left ventricular remodelation, decreased the incidence of heart failure, and reduced activity of MMPs. Bell and Yellon (135) demonstrated the beneficial effect of atorvastatin, administered at the time of reperfusion: in the experimental model of isolated perfused mouse heart atorvastatin reduced ischemia-reperfusion injury (infarct size), when added to the perfusion solution. Results of this *in vitro* study were recently confirmed by Wolfrum et al. (136) in their *in vivo* study of experimental infarction in rats. They have administered activated simvastatin intravenously 3 min before restoration of flow after a temporary coronary artery occlusion; simvastatin treatment decreased infarct size by 42 %. The two latest studies have shown also another important aspect of the immediate effect of statin therapy: they have demonstrated an acute increase of eNOS activity, which is probably not related to the upregulation of eNOS by stabilizing eNOS mRNA. To stabilize eNOS mRNA, several hours of statin treatment are essential as was shown in a cell culture system (62). The acute stimulation of eNOS activity is, however, at least partially mediated by PI 3-kinase/Akt pathway which is capable to phosphorylate eNOS within minutes (135, 136).

Clinical Studies

No literary data on the administration of statins as a part of the first-line therapy in patients with ACS were available. We arranged, therefore, a pilot, small, prospective trial in 44 consecutive patients with ACS without ST-elevation, randomized at admission to cerivastatin 0.3 mg or no statin therapy (137). Already 24 hours after hospital admission (and after the initiation of statin therapy), a significant reduction in the level of CRP and IL-6 was observed in the cerivastatin-treated group as compared with the untreated group. On the other hand, the level of IL-8 was not influenced by cerivastatin in this setting. A strong effect of the low dose cerivastatin therapy for only 24 hours was the main reason for organizing the Fluvastatin in the Therapy of Acute Coronary Syndrome (FACS) trial (138). This is an ongoing multicenter, randomized, double-blind, placebo-controlled study comparing the effect of 30-day 80 mg fluvastatin therapy starting at the time of hospital admission with placebo. The primary endpoint is the influence of therapy on inflammatory markers (CRP and interleukin-6) and on pregnancy-associated plasma protein A (PAPP-A), a combined secondary endpoint is 30-day and one-year occurrence of death, nonfatal myocardial infarction, recurrent symptomatic ischemia, urgent revascularization, and cardiac arrest.

Conclusion

Statins were introduced into the clinical practice as lipid-lowering drugs for treatment of high blood cholesterol. They were shown to be highly effective in hypercholesterolemic patients for primary and secondary prevention of CAD. Their efficacy in secondary prevention was demonstrated in the large prospective clinical trials in stable CAD; these studies enrolled patients at least several months after an ACS. Later, it has been observed that statins exert a favorable effect not only in hypercholesterolemia, but also in patients with normal or low cholesterol and, therefore, possible non-lipid effects of statins have been suggested. The discovery of pleiotropic effects of statins opened the new field of indication for statin treatment. Recently, several randomized trials have been published, showing safety and in some points also efficacy of statin therapy started early after ACS. Extension of knowledge of the pleiotropic effects of statins together with the increasing understanding of pathogenesis of ACS have been shifting, however, the initiation of statin therapy closer to the onset of symptoms. Recent experimental studies, similarly as the first clinical trials have brought promising results, supporting the idea of cardioprotective effect of statin administration in the first-line therapy of ACS. Confirmation of this approach by a large randomized trial is, however, needed; nevertheless, based on the currently available data, statins have a high chance of achieving a similar place in the therapy of ACS as the pillar of contemporary therapeutic strategy, aspirin.

ACKNOWLEDGEMENTS

This work was supported by the Charles University in Prague Research Project MSM 0021620817 awarded by the Ministry of Education, Youth and Physical Education of the Czech Republic and by a grant from the Ministry of Health of the Czech Republic, No. 00064203.

REFERENCES

[1] Aikawa M, Libby P. The vulnerable atherosclerotic plaque: pathogenesis and therapeutic approach. *Cardiovasc Pathol* 2004;13(3):125-38.

[2] Davies MJ. Acute coronary thrombosis--the role of plaque disruption and its initiation and prevention. *Eur Heart J* 1995;16 Suppl L:3-7.

[3] Davies MJ. Detecting vulnerable coronary plaques. *Lancet* 1996;347(9013):1422-3.

[4] Ambrose JA, Hjemdahl-Monsen CE, Borrico S, Gorlin R, Fuster V. Angiographic demonstration of a common link between unstable angina pectoris and non-Q-wave acute myocardial infarction. *Am J Cardiol* 1988;61(4):244-7.

[5] Pasterkamp G, Schoneveld AH, Hijnen DJ, de Kleijn DP, Teepen H, van der Wal AC, et al. Atherosclerotic arterial remodeling and the localization of macrophages and matrix metalloproteases 1, 2 and 9 in the human coronary artery. *Atherosclerosis* 2000;150(2):245-53.

[6] Dickson BC, Gotlieb AI. Towards understanding acute destabilization of vulnerable atherosclerotic plaques. *Cardiovasc Pathol* 2003;12(5):237-48.

[7] Falk E, Shah PK, Fuster V. Coronary plaque disruption. Circulation 1995;92(3):657-71.

[8] Rabbani R, Topol EJ. Strategies to achieve coronary arterial plaque stabilization. *Cardiovasc Res* 1999;41(2):402-17.

[9] Bank AJ, Versluis A, Dodge SM, Douglas WH. Atherosclerotic plaque rupture: a fatigue process? *Med Hypotheses* 2000;55(6):480-4.

[10] Shah PK, Falk E, Badimon JJ, Fernandez-Ortiz A, Mailhac A, Villareal-Levy G, et al. Human monocyte-derived macrophages induce collagen breakdown in fibrous caps of atherosclerotic plaques. Potential role of matrix-degrading metalloproteinases and implications for plaque rupture. *Circulation* 1995;92(6):1565-9.

[11] Loree HM, Kamm RD, Stringfellow RG, Lee RT. Effects of fibrous cap thickness on peak circumferential stress in model atherosclerotic vessels. *Circ Res* 1992;71(4):850-8.

[12] Heinecke JW. Oxidized amino acids: culprits in human atherosclerosis and indicators of oxidative stress. *Free Radic Biol Med* 2002;32(11):1090-101.

[13] Sugiyama S, Okada Y, Sukhova GK, Virmani R, Heinecke JW, Libby P. Macrophage myeloperoxidase regulation by granulocyte macrophage colony-stimulating factor in human atherosclerosis and implications in acute coronary syndromes. *Am J Pathol* 2001;158(3):879-91.

[14] Rajagopalan S, Meng XP, Ramasamy S, Harrison DG, Galis ZS. Reactive oxygen species produced by macrophage-derived foam cells regulate the activity of vascular matrix metalloproteinases in vitro. Implications for atherosclerotic plaque stability. *J Clin Invest* 1996;98(11):2572-9.

[15] Libby P. Atherosclerosis: the new view. *Sci Am* 2002;286(5):46-55.

[16] Wilcox JN, Smith KM, Schwartz SM, Gordon D. Localization of tissue factor in the normal vessel wall and in the atherosclerotic plaque. *Proc Natl Acad Sci USA* 1989;86(8):2839-43.

[17] Lupu F, Bergonzelli GE, Heim DA, Cousin E, Genton CY, Bachmann F, et al. Localization and production of plasminogen activator inhibitor-1 in human healthy and atherosclerotic arteries. *Arterioscler Thromb* 1993;13(7):1090-100.

[18] Cybulsky MI, Iiyama K, Li H, Zhu S, Chen M, Iiyama M, et al. A major role for VCAM-1, but not ICAM-1, in early atherosclerosis. *J Clin Invest* 2001;107(10):1255-62.

[19] Gu L, Okada Y, Clinton SK, Gerard C, Sukhova GK, Libby P, et al. Absence of monocyte chemoattractant protein-1 reduces atherosclerosis in low density lipoprotein receptor-deficient mice. *Mol Cell* 1998;2(2):275-81.

[20] Plutzky J. Inflammatory pathways in atherosclerosis and acute coronary syndromes. *Am J Cardiol* 2001;88(8A):10K-15K.

[21] Kadar A, Glasz T. Development of atherosclerosis and plaque biology. *Cardiovasc Surg* 2001;9(2):109-21.

[22] Oemar BS, Tschudi MR, Godoy N, Brovkovich V, Malinski T, Luscher TF. Reduced endothelial nitric oxide synthase expression and production in human atherosclerosis. *Circulation* 1998;97(25):2494-8.

[23] Braganza DM, Bennett MR. New insights into atherosclerotic plaque rupture. *Postgrad Med J* 2001;77(904):94-8.

[24] Libby P. Changing concepts of atherogenesis. *J Intern Med* 2000;247(3):349-58.

[25] Pinderski LJ, Fischbein MP, Subbanagounder G, Fishbein MC, Kubo N, Cheroutre H, et al. Overexpression of interleukin-10 by activated T lymphocytes inhibits atherosclerosis in LDL receptor-deficient Mice by altering lymphocyte and macrophage phenotypes. *Circ Res* 2002;90(10):1064-71.

[26] Jones P, Kafonek S, Laurora I, Hunninghake D. Comparative dose efficacy study of atorvastatin versus simvastatin, pravastatin, lovastatin, and fluvastatin in patients with hypercholesterolemia (the CURVES study). *Am J Cardiol* 1998;81(5):582-7.

[27] Insull W, Kafonek S, Goldner D, Zieve F. Comparison of efficacy and safety of atorvastatin (10mg) with simvastatin (10mg) at six weeks. ASSET Investigators. *Am J Cardiol* 2001;87(5):554-9.

[28] Albert MA, Danielson E, Rifai N, Ridker PM. Effect of statin therapy on C-reactive protein levels: the pravastatin inflammation/CRP evaluation (PRINCE): a randomized trial and cohort study. *Jama* 2001;286(1):64-70.

[29] Kinlay S, Schwartz GG, Olsson AG, Rifai N, Leslie SJ, Sasiela WJ, et al. High-dose atorvastatin enhances the decline in inflammatory markers in patients with acute coronary syndromes in the MIRACL study. *Circulation* 2003;108(13):1560-6.

[30] Ridker PM, Rifai N, Lowenthal SP. Rapid reduction in C-reactive protein with cerivastatin among 785 patients with primary hypercholesterolemia. *Circulation* 2001;103(9):1191-3.

[31] Jialal I, Stein D, Balis D, Grundy SM, Adams-Huet B, Devaraj S. Effect of hydroxymethyl glutaryl coenzyme a reductase inhibitor therapy on high sensitive C-reactive protein levels. *Circulation* 2001;103(15):1933-5.

[32] Riesen WF, Engler H, Risch M, Korte W, Noseda G. Short-term effects of atorvastatin on C-reactive protein. *Eur Heart J* 2002;23(10):794-9.

[33] van de Ree MA, Huisman MV, Princen HM, Meinders AE, Kluft C. Strong decrease of high sensitivity C-reactive protein with high-dose atorvastatin in patients with type 2 diabetes mellitus. *Atherosclerosis* 2003;166(1):129-35.

[34] Koh KK, Schenke WH, Waclawiw MA, Csako G, Cannon RO, 3rd. Statin attenuates increase in C-reactive protein during estrogen replacement therapy in postmenopausal women. *Circulation* 2002;105(13):1531-3.

[35] Kent SM, Flaherty PJ, Coyle LC, Markwood TT, Taylor AJ. Effect of atorvastatin and pravastatin on serum C-reactive protein. *Am Heart J* 2003;145(2):e8.

[36] Ansell BJ, Watson KE, Weiss RE, Fonarow GC. hsCRP and HDL effects of statins trial (CHEST): rapid effect of statin therapy on C-reactive protein and high-density lipoprotein levels A clinical investigation. *Heart Dis* 2003;5(1):2-7.

[37] Romano M, Diomede L, Sironi M, Massimiliano L, Sottocorno M, Polentarutti N, et al. Inhibition of monocyte chemotactic protein-1 synthesis by statins. *Lab Invest* 2000;80(7):1095-100.

[38] Blake GJ, Ridker PM. Novel clinical markers of vascular wall inflammation. *Circ Res* 2001;89(9):763-71.

[39] Koh KK, Son JW, Ahn JY, Choi YM, Jin DK, Park GS, et al. Non-lipid effects of statin on hypercholesterolemic patients established to have coronary artery disease who remained hypercholesterolemic while eating a step-II diet. *Coron Artery Dis* 2001;12(4):305-11.

[40] Rezaie-Majd A, Maca T, Bucek RA, Valent P, Muller MR, Husslein P, et al. Simvastatin reduces expression of cytokines interleukin-6, interleukin-8, and monocyte chemoattractant protein-1 in circulating monocytes from hypercholesterolemic patients. *Arterioscler Thromb Vasc Biol* 2002;22(7):1194-9.

[41] Brull DJ, Sanders J, Rumley A, Lowe GD, Humphries SE, Montgomery HE. Statin therapy and the acute inflammatory response after coronary artery bypass grafting. *Am J Cardiol* 2001;88(4):431-3.

[42] Ikeda U, Shimada K. Statins and monocytes. Lancet 1999;353(9169):2070.

[43] Ferro D, Parrotto S, Basili S, Alessandri C, Violi F. Simvastatin inhibits the monocyte expression of proinflammatory cytokines in patients with hypercholesterolemia. *J Am Coll Cardiol* 2000;36(2):427-31.

[44] Bustos C, Hernandez-Presa MA, Ortego M, Tunon J, Ortega L, Perez F, et al. HMG-CoA reductase inhibition by atorvastatin reduces neointimal inflammation in a rabbit model of atherosclerosis. *J Am Coll Cardiol* 1998;32(7):2057-64.

[45] Ikeda U, Shimpo M, Ohki R, Inaba H, Takahashi M, Yamamoto K, et al. Fluvastatin inhibits matrix metalloproteinase-1 expression in human vascular endothelial cells. *Hypertension* 2000;36(3):325-9.

[46] Aikawa M, Rabkin E, Sugiyama S, Voglic SJ, Fukumoto Y, Furukawa Y, et al. An HMG-CoA reductase inhibitor, cerivastatin, suppresses growth of macrophages expressing matrix metalloproteinases and tissue factor in vivo and in vitro. *Circulation* 2001;103(2):276-83.

[47] Crisby M, Nordin-Fredriksson G, Shah PK, Yano J, Zhu J, Nilsson J. Pravastatin treatment increases collagen content and decreases lipid content, inflammation,

metalloproteinases, and cell death in human carotid plaques: implications for plaque stabilization. *Circulation* 2001;103(7):926-33.

[48] Seljeflot I, Tonstad S, Hjermann I, Arnesen H. Reduced expression of endothelial cell markers after 1 year treatment with simvastatin and atorvastatin in patients with coronary heart disease. *Atherosclerosis* 2002;162(1):179-85.

[49] Sardo MA, Castaldo M, Cinquegrani M, Bonaiuto M, Maesano A, Versace A, et al. Effects of atorvastatin treatment on sICAM-1 and plasma nitric oxide levels in hypercholesterolemic subjects. *Clin Appl Thromb Hemost* 2002;8(3):257-63.

[50] Niwa S, Totsuka T, Hayashi S. Inhibitory effect of fluvastatin, an HMG-CoA reductase inhibitor, on the expression of adhesion molecules on human monocyte cell line. *Int J Immunopharmacol* 1996;18(11):669-75.

[51] Tsiara S, Elisaf M, Mikhailidis DP. Early vascular benefits of statin therapy. *Curr Med Res Opin* 2003;19(6):540-56.

[52] Suzumura K, Yasuhara M, Narita H. Superoxide anion scavenging properties of fluvastatin and its metabolites. *Chem Pharm Bull* (Tokyo) 1999;47(10):1477-80.

[53] Suzumura K, Yasuhara M, Tanaka K, Odawara A, Narita H, Suzuki T. An in vitro study of the hydroxyl radical scavenging property of fluvastatin, and HMG-CoA reductase inhibitor. *Chem Pharm Bull* (Tokyo) 1999;47(7):1010-2.

[54] Suzumura K, Yasuhara M, Tanaka K, Suzuki T. Protective effect of fluvastatin sodium (XU-62-320), a 3-hydroxy-3-methylglutaryl coenzyme A (HMG-CoA) reductase inhibitor, on oxidative modification of human low-density lipoprotein in vitro. *Biochem Pharmacol* 1999;57(6):697-703.

[55] Hussein O, Schlezinger S, Rosenblat M, Keidar S, Aviram M. Reduced susceptibility of low density lipoprotein (LDL) to lipid peroxidation after fluvastatin therapy is associated with the hypocholesterolemic effect of the drug and its binding to the LDL. *Atherosclerosis* 1997;128(1):11-8.

[56] Kalinowski L, Dobrucki IT, Malinski T. Cerivastatin potentiates nitric oxide release and enos expression through inhibition of isoprenoids synthesis. *J Physiol Pharmacol* 2002;53(4 Pt 1):585-95.

[57] Kalinowski L, Dobrucki LW, Brovkovych V, Malinski T. Increased nitric oxide bioavailability in endothelial cells contributes to the pleiotropic effect of cerivastatin. *Circulation* 2002;105(8):933-8.

[58] Fuhrman B, Koren L, Volkova N, Keidar S, Hayek T, Aviram M. Atorvastatin therapy in hypercholesterolemic patients suppresses cellular uptake of oxidized-LDL by differentiating monocytes. *Atherosclerosis* 2002;164(1):179-85.

[59] Vaughan CJ, Murphy MB, Buckley BM. Statins do more than just lower cholesterol. *Lancet* 1996;348(9034):1079-82.

[60] Jeremy JY, Rowe D, Emsley AM, Newby AC. Nitric oxide and the proliferation of vascular smooth muscle cells. *Cardiovasc Res* 1999;43(3):580-94.

[61] De Caterina R, Libby P, Peng HB, Thannickal VJ, Rajavashisth TB, Gimbrone MA, Jr., et al. Nitric oxide decreases cytokine-induced endothelial activation. Nitric oxide selectively reduces endothelial expression of adhesion molecules and proinflammatory cytokines. *J Clin Invest* 1995;96(1):60-8.

[62] Laufs U, La Fata V, Plutzky J, Liao JK. Upregulation of endothelial nitric oxide synthase by HMG CoA reductase inhibitors. *Circulation* 1998;97(12):1129-35.

[63] Morikawa S, Takabe W, Mataki C, Kanke T, Itoh T, Wada Y, et al. The effect of statins on mRNA levels of genes related to inflammation, coagulation, and vascular constriction in HUVEC. Human umbilical vein endothelial cells. *J Atheroscler Thromb* 2002;9(4):178-83.

[64] Laufs U, Gertz K, Dirnagl U, Bohm M, Nickenig G, Endres M. Rosuvastatin, a new HMG-CoA reductase inhibitor, upregulates endothelial nitric oxide synthase and protects from ischemic stroke in mice. *Brain Res* 2002;942(1-2):23-30.

[65] Laufs U, Endres M, Custodis F, Gertz K, Nickenig G, Liao JK, et al. Suppression of endothelial nitric oxide production after withdrawal of statin treatment is mediated by negative feedback regulation of rho GTPase gene transcription. *Circulation* 2000;102(25):3104-10.

[66] Laufs U, Liao JK. Targeting Rho in cardiovascular disease. Circ Res 2000;87(7):526-8.

[67] Jagroop IA, Mikhailidis DP. Effect of endothelin-1 on human platelet shape change: reversal of activation by naftidrofuryl. *Platelets* 2000;11(5):272-7.

[68] Barton M, Lattmann T, d'Uscio LV, Luscher TF, Shaw S. Inverse regulation of endothelin-1 and nitric oxide metabolites in tissue with aging: implications for the age-dependent increase of cardiorenal disease. *J Cardiovasc Pharmacol* 2000;36(5 Suppl 1):S153-6.

[69] Hernandez-Perera O, Perez-Sala D, Navarro-Antolin J, Sanchez-Pascuala R, Hernandez G, Diaz C, et al. Effects of the 3-hydroxy-3-methylglutaryl-CoA reductase inhibitors, atorvastatin and simvastatin, on the expression of endothelin-1 and endothelial nitric oxide synthase in vascular endothelial cells. *J Clin Invest* 1998;101(12):2711-9.

[70] Dupuis J, Tardif JC, Cernacek P, Theroux P. Cholesterol reduction rapidly improves endothelial function after acute coronary syndromes. The RECIFE (reduction of cholesterol in ischemia and function of the endothelium) trial. *Circulation* 1999;99(25):3227-33.

[71] de Jongh S, Lilien MR, op't Roodt J, Stroes ES, Bakker HD, Kastelein JJ. Early statin therapy restores endothelial function in children with familial hypercholesterolemia. *J Am Coll Cardiol* 2002;40(12):2117-21.

[72] Marchesi S, Lupattelli G, Siepi D, Schillaci G, Vaudo G, Roscini AR, et al. Short-term atorvastatin treatment improves endothelial function in hypercholesterolemic women. *J Cardiovasc Pharmacol* 2000;36(5):617-21.

[73] Tsunekawa T, Hayashi T, Kano H, Sumi D, Matsui-Hirai H, Thakur NK, et al. Cerivastatin, a hydroxymethylglutaryl coenzyme a reductase inhibitor, improves endothelial function in elderly diabetic patients within 3 days. *Circulation* 2001;104(4):376-9.

[74] Omori H, Nagashima H, Tsurumi Y, Takagi A, Ishizuka N, Hagiwara N, et al. Direct in vivo evidence of a vascular statin: a single dose of cerivastatin rapidly increases vascular endothelial responsiveness in healthy normocholesterolaemic subjects. *Br J Clin Pharmacol* 2002;54(4):395-9.

[75] Colli S, Eligini S, Lalli M, Camera M, Paoletti R, Tremoli E. Vastatins inhibit tissue factor in cultured human macrophages. A novel mechanism of protection against atherothrombosis. *Arterioscler Thromb Vasc Biol* 1997;17(2):265-72.

[76] Ferro D, Basili S, Alessandri C, Cara D, Violi F. Inhibition of tissue-factor-mediated thrombin generation by simvastatin. *Atherosclerosis* 2000;149(1):111-6.

[77] Nagata K, Ishibashi T, Sakamoto T, Ohkawara H, Shindo J, Yokoyama K, et al. Rho/Rho-kinase is involved in the synthesis of tissue factor in human monocytes. *Atherosclerosis* 2002;163(1):39-47.

[78] Eto M, Kozai T, Cosentino F, Joch H, Luscher TF. Statin prevents tissue factor expression in human endothelial cells: role of Rho/Rho-kinase and Akt pathways. *Circulation* 2002;105(15):1756-9.

[79] Camera M, Toschi V, Comparato C, Baetta R, Rossi F, Fuortes M, et al. Cholesterol-induced thrombogenicity of the vessel wall: inhibitory effect of fluvastatin. *Thromb Haemost* 2002;87(4):748-55.

[80] Baetta R, Camera M, Comparato C, Altana C, Ezekowitz MD, Tremoli E. Fluvastatin reduces tissue factor expression and macrophage accumulation in carotid lesions of cholesterol-fed rabbits in the absence of lipid lowering. *Arterioscler Thromb Vasc Biol* 2002;22(4):692-8.

[81] Ferro D, Basili S, Alessandri C, Mantovani B, Cordova C, Violi F. Simvastatin reduces monocyte-tissue-factor expression type IIa hypercholesterolaemia. *Lancet* 1997;350(9086):1222.

[82] Holschermann H, Hilgendorff A, Kemkes-Matthes B, Schonburg M, Bauer EP, Tillmanns H, et al. Simvastatin attenuates vascular hypercoagulability in cardiac transplant recipients. *Transplantation* 2000;69(9):1830-6.

[83] Cortellaro M, Cofrancesco E, Arbustini E, Rossi F, Negri A, Tremoli E, et al. Atorvastatin and thrombogenicity of the carotid atherosclerotic plaque: the ATROCAP study. *Thromb Haemost* 2002;88(1):41-7.

[84] Hansen JB, Huseby KR, Huseby NE, Sandset PM, Hanssen TA, Nordoy A. Effect of cholesterol lowering on intravascular pools of TFPI and its anticoagulant potential in type II hyperlipoproteinemia. *Arterioscler Thromb Vasc Biol* 1995;15(7):879-85.

[85] Lorena M, Perolini S, Casazza F, Milani M, Cimminiello C. Fluvastatin and tissue factor pathway inhibitor in type IIA and IIB hyperlipidemia and in acute myocardial infarction. *Thromb Res* 1997;87(4):397-403.

[86] Nordoy A, Bonaa KH, Sandset PM, Hansen JB, Nilsen H. Effect of omega-3 fatty acids and simvastatin on hemostatic risk factors and postprandial hyperlipemia in patients with combined hyperlipemia. *Arterioscler Thromb Vasc Biol* 2000;20(1):259-65.

[87] Morishita E, Asakura H, Saito M, Yamazaki M, Ontachi Y, Mizutani T, et al. Elevated plasma levels of free-form of TFPI antigen in hypercholesterolemic patients. *Atherosclerosis* 2001;154(1):203-12.

[88] Krysiak R, Okopien B, Herman Z. Effects of HMG-CoA reductase inhibitors on coagulation and fibrinolysis processes. *Drugs* 2003;63(17):1821-54.

[89] Szczeklik A, Musial J, Undas A, Gajewski P, Gora P, Swadzba J, et al. Inhibition of thrombin generation by simvastatin and lack of additive effects of aspirin in patients with marked hypercholesterolemia. *J Am Coll Cardiol* 1999;33(5):1286-93.

[90] Musial J, Undas A, Undas R, Brozek J, Szczeklik A. Treatment with simvastatin and low-dose aspirin depresses thrombin generation in patients with coronary heart disease and borderline-high cholesterol levels. *Thromb Haemost* 2001;85(2):221-5.

[91] Aoki I, Aoki N, Kawano K, Shimoyama K, Maki A, Homori M, et al. Platelet-dependent thrombin generation in patients with hyperlipidemia. *J Am Coll Cardiol* 1997;30(1):91-6.

[92] Alessandri C, Basili S, Maurelli M, Bracaglia D, Andreozzi P, Pergolini M, et al. Relationship between prothrombin activation fragment F1 + 2 and serum cholesterol. *Haemostasis* 1996;26(4):214-9.

[93] Puccetti L, Bruni F, Di Renzo M, Bova G, Cercignani M, Iadanza A, et al. Hypercoagulable state in hypercholesterolemic subjects assessed by platelet-dependent thrombin generation: in vitro effect of cerivastatin. *Eur Rev Med Pharmacol Sci* 1999;3(5):197-204.

[94] Puccetti L, Bruni F, Bova G, Cercignani M, Palazzuoli A, Console E, et al. Effect of diet and treatment with statins on platelet-dependent thrombin generation in hypercholesterolemic subjects. *Nutr Metab Cardiovasc Dis* 2001;11(6):378-87.

[95] Meade TW, Mellows S, Brozovic M, Miller GJ, Chakrabarti RR, North WR, et al. Haemostatic function and ischaemic heart disease: principal results of the Northwick Park Heart Study. *Lancet* 1986;2(8506):533-7.

[96] Wilhelmsen L, Svardsudd K, Korsan-Bengtsen K, Larsson B, Welin L, Tibblin G. Fibrinogen as a risk factor for stroke and myocardial infarction. *N Engl J Med* 1984;311(8):501-5.

[97] Kannel WB, Wolf PA, Castelli WP, D'Agostino RB. Fibrinogen and risk of cardiovascular disease. The Framingham Study. *Jama* 1987;258(9):1183-6.

[98] Davidson M, McKenney J, Stein E, Schrott H, Bakker-Arkema R, Fayyad R, et al. Comparison of one-year efficacy and safety of atorvastatin versus lovastatin in primary hypercholesterolemia. Atorvastatin Study Group I. *Am J Cardiol* 1997;79(11):1475-81.

[99] Seeger H, Wallwiener D, Mueck AO. Lipid-independent effects of an estrogen-statin combination: inhibition of expression of adhesion molecules and plasminogen activator inhibitor--I in human endothelial cell cultures. *Climacteric* 2001;4(3):209-14.

[100] Warkentin TE. Hemostasis and atherosclerosis. *Can J Cardiol* 1995;11 Suppl C:29C-34C.

[101] Essig M, Nguyen G, Prie D, Escoubet B, Sraer JD, Friedlander G. 3-Hydroxy-3-methylglutaryl coenzyme A reductase inhibitors increase fibrinolytic activity in rat aortic endothelial cells. Role of geranylgeranylation and Rho proteins. *Circ Res* 1998;83(7):683-90.

[102] Mussoni L, Banfi C, Sironi L, Arpaia M, Tremoli E. Fluvastatin inhibits basal and stimulated plasminogen activator inhibitor 1, but induces tissue type plasminogen activator in cultured human endothelial cells. *Thromb Haemost* 2000;84(1):59-64.

[103] Haslinger B, Goedde MF, Toet KH, Kooistra T. Simvastatin increases fibrinolytic activity in human peritoneal mesothelial cells independent of cholesterol lowering. *Kidney Int* 2002;62(5):1611-9.

[104] Lopez S, Peiretti F, Bonardo B, Juhan-Vague I, Nalbone G. Effect of atorvastatin and fluvastatin on the expression of plasminogen activator inhibitor type-1 in cultured human endothelial cells. *Atherosclerosis* 2000;152(2):359-66.

[105] Bourcier T, Libby P. HMG CoA reductase inhibitors reduce plasminogen activator inhibitor-1 expression by human vascular smooth muscle and endothelial cells. *Arterioscler Thromb Vasc Biol* 2000;20(2):556-62.

[106] Ishibashi T, Nagata K, Ohkawara H, Sakamoto T, Yokoyama K, Shindo J, et al. Inhibition of Rho/Rho-kinase signaling downregulates plasminogen activator inhibitor-1 synthesis in cultured human monocytes. *Biochim Biophys Acta* 2002;1590(1-3):123-30.

[107] Wiesbauer F, Kaun C, Zorn G, Maurer G, Huber K, Wojta J. HMG CoA reductase inhibitors affect the fibrinolytic system of human vascular cells in vitro: a comparative study using different statins. *Br J Pharmacol* 2002;135(1):284-92.

[108] Randomised trial of cholesterol lowering in 4444 patients with coronary heart disease: the Scandinavian Simvastatin Survival Study (4S). *Lancet* 1994;344(8934):1383-9.

[109] Sacks FM, Pfeffer MA, Moye LA, Rouleau JL, Rutherford JD, Cole TG, et al. The effect of pravastatin on coronary events after myocardial infarction in patients with average cholesterol levels. Cholesterol and Recurrent Events Trial investigators. *N Engl J Med* 1996;335(14):1001-9.

[110] Prevention of cardiovascular events and death with pravastatin in patients with coronary heart disease and a broad range of initial cholesterol levels. The Long-Term Intervention with Pravastatin in Ischaemic Disease (LIPID) Study Group. *N Engl J Med* 1998;339(19):1349-57.

[111] Stenestrand U, Wallentin L. Early statin treatment following acute myocardial infarction and 1-year survival. *Jama* 2001;285(4):430-6.

[112] Aronow HD, Topol EJ, Roe MT, Houghtaling PL, Wolski KE, Lincoff AM, et al. Effect of lipid-lowering therapy on early mortality after acute coronary syndromes: an observational study. *Lancet* 2001;357(9262):1063-8.

[113] Cannon CP, McCabe CH, Bentley J, Braunwald E. Early statin therapy is associated with markedly lower mortality in patients with acute coronary syndromes: observations from OPUS-TIMI 16 [abstract]. *J Am Coll Cardiol* 2001;37(suppl A):334A. Abstract 831-2.

[114] Newby LK, Kristinsson A, Bhapkar MV, Aylward PE, Dimas AP, Klein WW, et al. Early statin initiation and outcomes in patients with acute coronary syndromes. *Jama* 2002;287(23):3087-95.

[115] Heeschen C, Hamm CW, Laufs U, Snapinn S, Bohm M, White HD. Withdrawal of statins increases event rates in patients with acute coronary syndromes. *Circulation* 2002;105(12):1446-52.

[116] Schiele R, Gitt AK, Heer T. Early statin use in acute myocardial is associated with a reduced hospital mortality: results of the Mitra-2 [abstract]. *Circulation* 2000;102(suppl 2):II-435. Abstract 2117.

[117] Briguori C, Colombo A, Airoldi F, Violante A, Focaccio A, Balestrieri P, et al. Statin administration before percutaneous coronary intervention: impact on periprocedural myocardial infarction. *Eur Heart J* 2004;25(20):1822-8.

[118] Lenderink T, Boersma E, Gitt AK, Zeymer U, Wallentin L, Van de Werf F, et al. Patients using statin treatment within 24 h after admission for ST-elevation acute coronary syndromes had lower mortality than non-users: a report from the first Euro Heart Survey on acute coronary syndromes. *Eur Heart J* 2006;27(15):1799-1804.

[119] Kayikcioglu M, Turkoglu C, Kultursay H, Evrengul H, Can L. The short term results of combined use of pravastatin with thrombolytic therapy in acute myocardial infarction [abstract]. *Circulation* 1999;100(suppl 1):I-303. Abstract 1586.

[120] Schwartz GG, Olsson AG, Ezekowitz MD, Ganz P, Oliver MF, Waters D, et al. Effects of atorvastatin on early recurrent ischemic events in acute coronary syndromes: the MIRACL study: a randomized controlled trial. *Jama* 2001;285(13):1711-8.

[121] Liem AH, van Boven AJ, Veeger NJ, Withagen AJ, Robles de Medina RM, Tijssen JG, et al. Effect of fluvastatin on ischaemia following acute myocardial infarction: a randomized trial. *Eur Heart J* 2002;23(24):1931-7.

[122] Arntz HR, Agrawal R, Wunderlich W, Schnitzer L, Stern R, Fischer F, et al. Beneficial effects of pravastatin (+/-colestyramine/niacin) initiated immediately after a coronary event (the randomized Lipid-Coronary Artery Disease [L-CAD] Study). *Am J Cardiol* 2000;86(12):1293-8.

[123] Serruys PW, de Feyter P, Macaya C, Kokott N, Puel J, Vrolix M, et al. Fluvastatin for prevention of cardiac events following successful first percutaneous coronary intervention: a randomized controlled trial. *Jama* 2002;287(24):3215-22.

[124] Cannon CP, Braunwald E, McCabe CH, Rader DJ, Rouleau JL, Belder R, et al. Intensive versus moderate lipid lowering with statins after acute coronary syndromes. *N Engl J Med* 2004;350(15):1495-504.

[125] Thompson PL, Meredith I, Amerena J, Campbell TJ, Sloman JG, Harris PJ. Effect of pravastatin compared with placebo initiated within 24 hours of onset of acute myocardial infarction or unstable angina: the Pravastatin in Acute Coronary Treatment (PACT) trial. *Am Heart J* 2004;148(1):e2.

[126] de Lemos JA, Blazing MA, Wiviott SD, Lewis EF, Fox KA, White HD, et al. Early intensive vs a delayed conservative simvastatin strategy in patients with acute coronary syndromes: phase Z of the A to Z trial. *Jama* 2004;292(11):1307-16.

[127] LaBlanche JM, Jukema JW, Charbonneau F, Creplet J, Eldar M, Galve E, et al. PRINCESS: Prevention of ischemic events by early treatment of cerivastatin after acute myocardial infarction. In: *ESC Congress*; 2004; *Munich*; 2004.

[128] Ostadal P, Alan D, Vejvoda J. Statins in the first-line therapy of acute coronary syndromes – similar to aspirin? *Exp Clin Cardiol* 2005;10(1):9-16.

[129] Lefer AM, Campbell B, Shin YK, Scalia R, Hayward R, Lefer DJ. Simvastatin preserves the ischemic-reperfused myocardium in normocholesterolemic rat hearts. *Circulation* 1999;100(2):178-84.

[130] Ueda Y, Kitakaze M, Komamura K, Minamino T, Asanuma H, Sato H, et al. Pravastatin restored the infarct size-limiting effect of ischemic preconditioning blunted by hypercholesterolemia in the rabbit model of myocardial infarction. *J Am Coll Cardiol* 1999;34(7):2120-5.

[131] Lefer DJ, Scalia R, Jones SP, Sharp BR, Hoffmeyer MR, Farvid AR, et al. HMG-CoA reductase inhibition protects the diabetic myocardium from ischemia-reperfusion injury. *Faseb J* 2001;15(8):1454-6.

[132] Di Napoli P, Antonio Taccardi A, Grilli A, Spina R, Felaco M, Barsotti A, et al. Simvastatin reduces reperfusion injury by modulating nitric oxide synthase expression: an ex vivo study in isolated working rat hearts. *Cardiovasc Res* 2001;51(2):283-93.

[133] Bauersachs J, Galuppo P, Fraccarollo D, Christ M, Ertl G. Improvement of left ventricular remodeling and function by hydroxymethylglutaryl coenzyme a reductase inhibition with cerivastatin in rats with heart failure after myocardial infarction. *Circulation* 2001;104(9):982-5.

[134] Hayashidani S, Tsutsui H, Shiomi T, Suematsu N, Kinugawa S, Ide T, et al. Fluvastatin, a 3-hydroxy-3-methylglutaryl coenzyme a reductase inhibitor, attenuates left ventricular remodeling and failure after experimental myocardial infarction. *Circulation* 2002;105(7):868-73.

[135] Bell RM, Yellon DM. Atorvastatin, administered at the onset of reperfusion, and independent of lipid lowering, protects the myocardium by up-regulating a pro-survival pathway. *J Am Coll Cardiol* 2003;41(3):508-15.

[136] Wolfrum S, Dendorfer A, Schutt M, Weidtmann B, Heep A, Tempel K, et al. Simvastatin acutely reduces myocardial reperfusion injury in vivo by activating the phosphatidylinositide 3-kinase/Akt pathway. *J Cardiovasc Pharmacol* 2004;44(3):348-55.

[137] Ostadal P, Alan D, Hajek P, Horak D, Vejvoda J, Trefanec J, et al. The effect of early treatment by cerivastatin on the serum level of C-reactive protein, interleukin-6, and interleukin-8 in the patients with unstable angina and non-Q-wave myocardial infarction. *Mol Cell Biochem* 2003;246(1-2):45-50.

[138] Ostadal P, Alan D, Hajek P, Vejvoda J, Mates M, Blasko P, et al. Fluvastatin in the therapy of acute coronary syndrome: Rationale and design of a multicenter, randomized, double-blind, placebo-controlled trial (The FACS Trial) [ISRCTN81331696]. *Curr Control Trials Cardiovasc Med.* 2005;6(1):4.

In: Frontiers in Atherosclerosis Research
Editor: Karin F. Kepper, pp. 163-174
ISBN 1-60021-371-5

Chapter 8

Beneficial Effects of Addition of Fenofibrate to Statin Therapy in Patients with Acute Coronary Syndrome after Percutaneous Coronary Interventions

***Hetal D. Shah*[*], *Keyur H. Parikh*[**], *Milan C. Chag*[**], *Urmil G. Shah*[**], *Hemang A. Baxi*[**], *Anish H. Chandarana*[**], *Ajay M. Naik*[**], *Joyal N. Shah*[**], *Kanan J. Shah*[*], and *Ramesh K Goyal*[1*]**

[*]Department of Pharmacology, L. M. College of Pharmacy Navrangpura, Ahmedabad 380 006 Gujarat, INDIA.

[**]The Heart Care Clinic, Care Cardiology Consultants Pvt Ltd
201, Balleshwar Avenue, Opp Rajpath Club, , Ahmedabad 380 009
Gujarat, INDIA.

Abstract

Objective

The objective of the present investigation was to find out whether the addition of fenofibrate to statin monotherapy produced any synergistic or additive beneficial effects in reducing risk factors, especially plasma fibrinogen, in patients of Acute Coronary Syndromes (ACS) requiring Percutaneous Coronary Interventions (PCI).

Methods

This was a randomized, non-blind, prospective study with parallel group design, conducted in 102 patients who had angiographically documented Coronary Artery Disease (CAD). All had undergone angioplasty. The patients were randomized to atorvastatin

---

[1] Address for Correspondence and Reprints: Professor Ramesh K Goyal, Department of Pharmacology, L. M. College of Pharmacy Navrangpura, Ahmedabad 380 006 Gujarat, INDIA. Phone: 91-79-26302746. Email: goyalrk@hotmail.com, hetald_shah@yahoo.com

(20mg/day, n=25), simvastatin (40mg/day, n=27), atorvastatin(10mg/day)-fenofibrate (200mg/day) combination (n=25) and simvastatin (20mg/day)-fenofibrate(200mg/day) combination (n=25). The serum lipid profile and plasma fibrinogen were recorded before initiation of therapy and after 3 months of the respective treatments.

Results

All the patients already had desirable lipid levels as per the NCEP ATP III guidelines. The addition of fenofibrate to statin monotherapy produced additional benefits on reduction in triglyceride (TG) and very low density lipoprotein (VLDL) levels, and an increase in high density lipoprotein (HDL) levels. All the treatment groups showed a significant decrease in the plasma fibrinogen levels. This did not correlate with any of the study parameters like age, body weight, hemodynamic characteristics and lipoprotein levels. Statin monotherapy produced a significant decrease in the fibrinogen levels and the addition of fenofibrate further enhanced the reduction.

Conclusions

Addition of fenofibrate to statins seems to be beneficial in patients with ACS. Statins, contrary to various reports, were found to decrease plasma fibrinogen significantly.Furhter, in combination with fenofibrate there was enhanced reduction of the novel risk factor, fibrinogen.

Key words: Acute coronary syndromes, statins, fenofibrate, plasma fibrinogen

INTRODUCTION

The last century has seen a rapid increase in the global prevalence of Coronary artery disease (CAD). Estimates from the Global Burden of Disease Study have predicted that India faces the greatest health burden due to Coronary Artery Disease.[1] A number of inflammatory markers have been studied for their ability to predict future cardiovascular events in asymptomatic individuals and patients with established atherosclerotic disease.[2] Among the emerging novel cardiac markers, plasma fibrinogen has been identified as an important risk factor for cardiovascular diseases. Many cross-sectional, case controlled, and numerous prospective cohort studies have identified elevated plasma fibrinogen levels as an independent risk factor for coronary heart disease, stroke, and peripheral vascular disease [3]

Fibrinogen is an acute phase protein that is directly involved in coagulation. The transcription of fibrinogen is stimulated by IL-6; its synthesis is suppressed by IL-1β and TNF-α. [4,5] Fibrinogen and its metabolites strongly affect hemostasis, hemorheology, platelet aggregation and endothelial function. Infact, fibrinogen's association with increased mortality lies probably in its ability to promote thromboses, or clots, by causing platelet aggregation in blood vessels. The recognition that fibrinogen is an important factor in the promotion of various disease states has led to the search for specific therapies intended to reduce plasma fibrinogen levels.

The use of statins in the prevention of primary [6] and secondary [7,8] CAD has been demonstrated to significantly reduce cardiovascular events and total mortality. Nevertheless, the majority of patients on statin treatment still experience coronary events. [9] It is clear that a more effective reduction in the incidences of coronary events is needed. This could probably be accomplished by a further reduction in the conventional as well as novel risk factors like plasma fibrinogen, homocysteine, and C-reactive protein. Multiple small studies have reported changes in fibrinogen levels with different statins. [10, 11] While atorvastatin is claimed to increase plasma fibrinogen, simvastatin is reported to either increase or have a neutral effect. Although many different pharmacologic approaches and strategies for therapeutic modulation of fibrinogen have been tested, the efficacy of different treatments to lower plasma fibrinogen in humans is limited and the mode of action unidentified. [12, 13] Among the few compounds known to lower circulating fibrinogen levels in humans are certain fibrates.

Fibrates reportedly lower plasma fibrinogen in humans, but the regulatory mechanism of this effect remains to be clarified. Activation of the nuclear hormone receptor PPARα mediates the suppression of fibrinogen gene transcription by fibrates in rodents.[3] This establishes PPARα as a key regulatory factor in fibrinogen gene expression in rodents and may explain the suppressive effect of fibrates on plasma fibrinogen levels in humans. The fibrinogen molecule is arranged as a dimer, with each monomer composed of 3 nonidentical polypeptide chains: Aα, Bβ and γ. [14] The 3 fibrinogen chains are encoded by 3 separate, closely linked genes situated on the same chromosome and located in the sequence γ, Aα, and Bβ, with the last one in opposite transcriptional orientation to the first one.[15] Binsack et al [16] reported that in the human hepatoma cell line, HepG2, bezafibrate suppressed Aα-, Bβ- and γ- chain mRNA levels.[17] The genes encoding the 3 fibrinogen chains are negatively regulated by PPARα and since fibrates act through this receptors, it helps to explain the benefits of fibrate therapy to target a reduction in fibrinogen levels. Maison et al[18] showed that fibrinogen concentration decreased after fibrate therapy, while it increased after statin treatment. Thus this study was conducted to investigate the controversial role of statins in modifying fibrinogen levels and to study the benefits of addition of fenofibrate to statin therapy in modifying levels of plasma fibrinogen.

Research Design and Methods

The study was a controlled clinical trial. It was randomized, non blind and based on parallel group design. The protocol of the study received approval from the Institutional Review Board of the Sterling Hospital, Ahmedabad. Patients of ACS of either sex who had undergone Percutaneous Transluminal Coronary Angioplasty (PTCA) procedure irrespective of the presence of diabetes mellitus were included in the study after taking their consent. Patients with second or third degree AV (atrioventricular) block, renal or hepatic failure, recent cerebrovascular events, valve replacement surgery, or Balloon Mitral Valvuloplasty (BMV) and patients on lipid lowering therapy other than statins were excluded from the study. 102 consecutive patients meeting the eligibility criteria were randomized into four treatment groups, consisting of patients given atorvastatin, simvastatin, atorvastatin-fenofibrate combination and simvastatin-fenofibrate combination. Treatment was started after the PTCA and was continued for 3 months. Atorvastatin was given in a single dose of 20mg per day (if alone) and 10mg per day (in combination with fenofibrate), simvastatin was given in a single dose of 40mg per day (if alone) and 20mg per day (in combination with fenofibrate) and fenofibrate was given in a single dose of 200mg per day. The first blood samples were collected before beginning of the treatment and were analyzed for total cholesterol, triglycerides(TG), LDL, HDL, VLDL and plasma fibrinogen. The second blood samples were collected after 3 months of treatment for total cholesterol, triglycerides, HDL, LDL, VLDL, plasma fibrinogen and liver function tests that included SGPT, SGOT, total bilirubin and alkaline phosphatase. Total cholesterol, TG, HDL-C, SGPT, SGOT, total bilirubin and alkaline phosphatase were analyzed on automated VITROS 250 analyzer using enzymatic assay methods. LDL-C was analyzed by enzymatic method. VLDL-C was calculated using Friedewald's formula.

Plasma fibrinogen was assayed using Immunoprecipitation method using the RANDOX® kits. Many studies measure fibrinogen by the Clauss Method. However, data from the Framingham Heart Study [19] suggest that levels determined by the immunoprecipitation test have a stronger association with cardiovascular disease than those obtained by Clauss method. The results were analyzed by applying Student's t test, ANOVA and linear regression to find out degree of correlation between parameters. The probability value of less than 5% ($p<0.05$) was considered to be statistically significant.

RESULTS

We included in our study, 102 patients from the cardiology unit of Sterling hospital. All of them had angiographically documented CAD and had undergone PTCA. 25 patients each were enrolled in atorvastatin, atorvastatin-fenofibrate combination and simvastatin-fenofibrate combination treatment groups and 27 patients were enrolled in simvastatin treatment group. We had 4 dropouts in atorvastatin-fenofibrate group as well as in simvastatin monotherapy group and 3 dropouts in simvastatin-fenofibrate group, all due to non-technical reasons. So, the analysis is based on a total of 91 patients who completed the follow-up successfully. The baseline, demographic characteristics like age, sex, BMI, smoking/tobacco/ alcohol habits, past history of diabetes, hypertension, family history etc. and other hemodynamic parameters like hemoglobin, urea, creatinine, etc were recorded (Table 1). These parameters were found to be identical in all the four treatment groups indicating a symmetric study design and population.

The effects of all the treatments on lipid parameters are given in Table 2. Atorvastatin and simvastatin monotherapy reduced serum LDL-C and interestingly increased serum HDL-C significantly ($p<0.05$). Atorvastatin-fenofibrate combination produced a significant decrease in TG, VLDL ($p<0.05$) and also increased HDL-C significantly as compared to atorvastatin alone ($p<0.05$). Similar to simvastatin monotherapy, simvastatin-fenofibrate combination produced a significant increase in HDL and decrease in LDL levels ($p<0.05$). It, however, did not reduce TG significantly. All the four treatments significantly reduced total cholesterol/HDL ratio and LDL/HDL ratio ($p<0.05$). ANOVA test was applied to find if there was any difference in the effects between the four groups. The results however, indicated that the percentage change in lipoprotein levels obtained were not significantly different from each other between the four treatment groups (Figure 1).

Table 1. Baseline Demographic and Haemodynamic characteristics of the Patients

Characteristics	Atorvastatin (n=25)	Atorvastatin + Fenofibrate (n=25)	Simvastatin (n=27)	Simvastatin + Fenofibrate (n=25)
Age(years)	56.76 ± 9.4	56.44 ± 9.95	58.44 ± 11.4	58.35 ± 11.35
Females (%)	4%	12 %	7.4%	20%
Males (%)	96%	88%	92.6 %	80%
Body Mass Index(BMI)	25.79 ± 3.5	23.62 ± 1.95	25.3 ± 3.90	25.44 ± 4.25
Smokers	12%	20%	14.81 %	8%
Tobacco Chewers	12%	12%	7.4 %	4%
Diabetics	24%	36%	29.62%	48%
Hypertensives	28%	28%	51.85 %	40%
Haemoglobin (gm%)	12.61± 1.6	12.17 ± 1.75	13.16 ± 1.76	13.07 ± 1.65
Urea (mg/dl)	30.7± 18.9	26.81 ± 11.95	26.93 ± 15.46	26.91 ± 13.2
Creatinine (mg/dl)	1.23± 0.5	1.28 ± 1.1	1.10 ± 0.31	1.10 ± 0.3
Random bl. Sugar (mg/dl)	130.33± 39.25	146.73± 65.45	137.8 ± 57.45	137.48 ± 56.6
Systolic BP (mm Hg)	126.54 ± 16.05	129.52 ± 24.25	128.22 ± 22.47	128.84 ± 22.8
Diastolic BP (mm Hg)	81.29 ± 8.75	78.35 ± 9.00	80.55 ± 11.31	80.96 ± 11.55
Pulse	77.09 ± 15.4	80.55 ± 10.9	75.02 ± 15.46	75.29 ± 15.65
LVEF (%)	46.8 ± 12.35	50.94 ± 16.25	52.44 ± 12.79	52.51 ± 5.76
Single Vessel disease	68%	56%	55.55%	44%
Double vessel disease	28%	28%	29.62 %	36%
Triple vessel disease	4%	16%	14.81%	20%

Data expressed as mean ± SD; % of patients

Table 2. Effect of treatments of serum lipoprotein levels

Parameters	Time interval	Atorvastatin[1] (n=25)	Atorvastatin + Fenofibrate [2] (n=21)	Simvastatin[3] (n=23)	Simvastatin + fenofibrate [4] (n=22)
		Mean ± SD	Mean ± SD	Mean ± SD	Mean ± SD
Total cholesterol mg/dl	baseline	156.6 ± 34.15	150.9± 46.39	150.44 ± 31.1	148.9 ± 31.98
	3 months	149.68 ± 42.8	155.76± 25.42	146.42±53.65	139.74 ± 30.67
TG mg/dl	baseline	144.85±76.65	155.1±112.12	138.5 ± 78.55	136.43 ± 78.97
	3 months	133.86±61.85	108.5±47.63*	123.5±100.7	110.12±47.5
HDL-C mg/dl	baseline	37.69 ±9.1	35.34 ± 9.25	34.91 ± 8.57	34.88 ± 8.67
	3 months	41.55 ±9.2*	46.61±8.38*	43.74 ± 12.9*	43.74 ± 13.27*
LDL-C mg/dl	baseline	101.44 ± 33.5	91.11 ± 33.06	93.39± 23.33	92.10 ± 24.10
	3 months	82.49 ±34.5*	86.74 ± 18.64	76.48 ± 26.3*	76.48 ± 26.35*
VLDL-C mg/dl	baseline	28.96 ±15.2	31.0 ± 22.39	27.68 ± 15.71	27.78 ± 15.85
	3 months	26.87 ± 12.35	21.71±9.66*	24.27 ± 19.97	24.17 ± 20.02
LDL- C/HDL-C	baseline	2.87 ± 1.35	2.66 ± 0.82	2.89 ± 1.05	3.13 ± 1.92
	3 months	2.06 ±0.95*	1.91 ± 0.50*	1.92 ± 0.81*	1.92 ± 0.79*
total cholesterol/ HDL-C	baseline	4.33 ± 1.25	4.41 ± 1.42	4.42 ± 1.29	4.37 ± 1.31
	3 months	3.71 ± 1.2 *	3.42 ± 0.69	3.66 ± 1.77*	3.66 ± 1.78*

Baseline: before starting of treatment
3 months: after 3 months of treatment
* Significant change from baseline values; student's t test, $p<0.05$;
$df^1=24$, $df^2=20$, $df^3=22$, $df^4=21$ (degree of freedom)

Table 3. Effect of treatments on plasma fibrinogen levels

Plasma Fibrinogen Gm/Lt	**Atorvastatin [1] (n=25)**	**Atorvastatin + Fenofibrate [2] (n=21)**	**Simvastatin [3] (n=23)**	**Simvastatin + fenofibrate [4] (n=22)**
Initial Levels	4.44 ± 0.26	4.29 ± 0.4	4.25 ± 0.25	4.21 ± 0.27
After 3 months	3.47 ±0.18 *	3.10 ± 0.28*	3.12 ± 0.14*	3.12 ± 0.15 *

*significant change from baseline values; Paired Student's t test, $p<0.05$
$df^1 = 24$, $df^2 = 20$, $df^3 = 22$, $df^4 = 21$

Table 4. Correlation coefficient between fibrinogen and other study parameters

Parameters	Correlation coefficient (r)
Body Mass Index (BMI)	-0.02
Haemoglobin	-0.21
Urea	0.18
Creatinine	-0.21
Blood Glucose	-0.14
Cholesterol	0.05
Triglycerides	0.01
HDL-C	-0.10
LDL-C	0.07
VLDL-C	-0.02
LDL-C/HDL-C	0.10
CHO/HDL-C	0.10

Table 5. Effect of treatments of Liver Function Parameters at the end of three months

Parameters	**Atorvastatin [1] (n=25)**	**Atorvastatin + Fenofibrate [2] (n=21)**	**Simvastatin [3] (n=23)**	**Simvastatin + fenofibrate [4] (n=22)**
		Mean ± SD	Mean ± SD	Mean ± SD
Total bilirubin mg/dl	0.7 ± 0.25	0.67 ± 0.18	0.71 ± 0.28	0.71 ± 0.28
SGPT U/Lt	28.16 ± 10.9	29.62 ± 7.19	31.67 ± 7.99	31.48 ± 1.72
SGOT U/Lt	24.46 ±7.1	29.14 ± 6.59	27.62 ± 7.28	27.55 ± 1.56
Alk.Phosph-atase U/Lt	94.04 ±23.05	69.00 ± 16.48	74.51 ± 26.25	73.80 ± 5.42

Data expressed as Mean ± SD
*Significant change from baseline values; student's t test, $p<0.05$;
$df^1=24$, $df^2=20$, $df^3=22$, $df^4=21$ (degree of freedom)

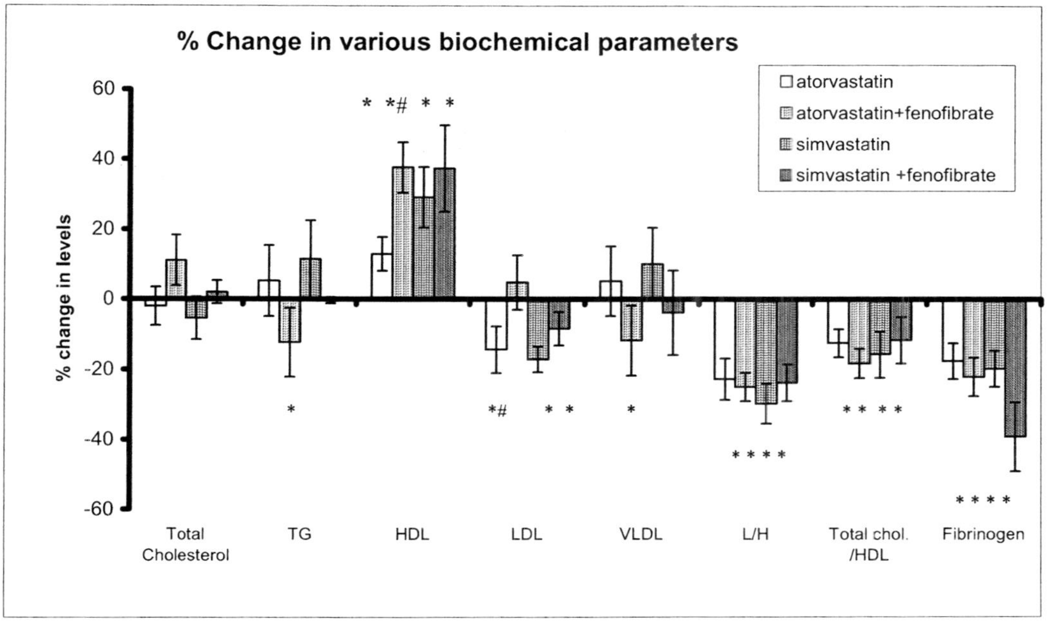

*Significant change from baseline values, Student's t test, $p<0.05$.
Significant change as compared to the respective statin monotherapy or combination, Unpaired Student's t test, $p<0.05$
ANOVA test applied on % change in levels, $P>0.05$, Changes are not significantly different from each other between the groups

Figure 1: % change in lipid levels between both the treatment group.

The effect of the treatments on plasma fibrinogen are given in Table 3. Atorvastatin as well as simvastatin was found to decrease plasma fibrinogen significantly ($p<0.01$). Combination of statins with fenofibrate also showed a significant decrease in plasma fibrinogen ($p<0.01$). However, the treatment groups were not significantly different from each other when analyzed by ANOVA test. Thus, contrary to reports, statins in our study decreased plasma fibrinogen significantly while addition of fenofibrate enhanced this effect, however significantly.

No correlation was found between fibrinogen levels and various demographical, haemodynamic and biochemical parameters (Table 4). Thus, plasma fibrinogen was found to be an independent risk factor for CAD and was lowered significantly by atorvastatin and simvastatin alone and in combination with fenofibrate.

No significant elevations in the serum bilirubin concentration, transaminases (SGPT, SGOT) and alkaline phosphatase levels were observed in any treatment group (Table 5). It thus appeared that all the treatments were safely tolerated in the given doses without any adverse hepatotoxic effects.

DISCUSSION

Statins alone as well as in combination with fenofibrate were found to produce beneficial effects in CAD patients after PTCA. Statins are potent inhibitors of HMG Co-A reductase, which decreases LDL-C by upregulating LDL receptor activity in the liver and reducing the secretion of apolipoprotein B containing lipoprotein. The latter is believed to be responsible for the TG lowering effect of atorvastatin and is profound at higher doses.[20] Various reports have indicated that atorvastatin lowers LDL-C and increases HDL.[21,22,23] The effects of atorvastatin in our study comply with such reports. On the other hand, simvastatin is reported to produce a decrease in LDL-C from 26% to 50% in various doses.[24, 25] Also, reports from Hunninghake et al [26] showed that simvastatin consistently produces a larger increase in HDL-C as compared to atorvastatin. Results from our study comply with the above findings as simvastatin in our study too produced a significant decrease in LDL-C and increase in HDL-C as compared to atorvastatin.

Fibrates activate PPAR-α which ultimately leads to their HDL raising and TG lowering effects.[27,28] Certain previous studies have suggested increased benefits of a combination of fenofibrate with statins. [29,30] Reports are available that show benefits of combining fenofibrate and simvastatin. [30, 31] A study of the literature also shows that a greater change in HDL and TG levels is obtained with fenofibrate - atorvastatin combination as compared to monotherapy [32] with either drug. Our results comply with reported findings. We observed that combining fenofibrate with statins offered a greater benefit in reducing TG and VLDL levels as well as increasing HDL levels. Thus, the combination therapy proved both safe and beneficial in our patients with ACS.

In prospective studies, plasma fibrinogen has been found to be an independent predictor of myocardial infarction in both genders. It provides information on CAD risk over and beyond that supplied by established risk factors. [33] The Framingham study has shown that for both sexes, the risk of cardiovascular diseases was correlated positively to antecedent fibrinogen values higher than 1.3 to 7.0 gm/L.[34] We found that fibrinogen in our study did not correlate with any of our study parameters including demographic characters and lipid levels. Thus, fibrinogen does appear to be an independent risk factor for CAD.

Reports from large-scale trials consistently show statins to have a neutral effect on fibrinogen. [35,36] Various studies on plasma fibrinogen indicate that fenofibrate lowers fibrinogen levels but the effects of atorvastatin and simvastatin have been variable and controversial, particularly that of atorvastatin. Wierzbicki et al [37] showed that atorvastatin increases plasma fibrinogen by 22%. Song et al [38] too found a significant increase in fibrinogen with atorvastatin treatment where as simvastatin was reported to have a neutral effect. Various reports indicated that fenofibrate decreased plasma fibrinogen significantly whereas atorvastatin produced an increase in fibrinogen levels.[39, 40,41] Otto et al [42] showed that plasma fibrinogen and other hemorheologic parameters were unchanged during atorvastatin treatment in comparison to simvastatin treatment. Athyros et al [43] reported that plasma fibrinogen was unaffected by atorvastatin and was significantly reduced by fenofibrate and combination of both. Ceska et al [44] showed that fenofibrate is a potent hypolipidemic drug with only rare side effects and reduces fibrinogen significantly. In our study, however, contrary to all above reports for statins, we observed that atorvastatin as well as simvastatin produced a significant decrease in plasma fibrinogen levels. However, our results comply with some recent findings by Kadikoylu and co- workers that show a decrease in plasma fibrinogen by atorvastatin and simvastatin. [45] Another study by Leibovitz et al [47] proved that atorvastatin reduces fibrinogen levels in patients with severe hypercholesterolemia. fibrinogen levels dropped by almost 18% in this study. Tekin et al [48] has also shown a reduction in plasma fibrinogen levels by atorvastatin in hyperlipidemic patients with angiographically proved CAD. These findings with atorvastatin are consistent with such recent data. The combination of statins with fenofibrate also produced a further decrease in fibrinogen, though not significant. These results are in agreement with the reported claims of fenofibrate to decrease plasma fibrinogen.

Previous studies have indicated an increased risk of myopathy with statin-fibrate combination. [29,46] However, no cessation of therapy was required in any patient due to such complication in our study. Liver function tests of all patients were also normal at the end of 3 months of treatments indicating no adverse hepatotoxic effects. These findings suggest that it may be safe to use fenofibrate and statins in combination contrary to reported contra-indications for the combined use of these two classes of drugs. However, we have not looked into the long-term toxicity associated with the use of these drugs in combination. Moreover, the strategy appears to be distinctly beneficial in lowering the risk factor plasma fibrinogen. Thus, the therapy offers a new method to treat patients with acute coronary syndromes.

Conclusions

Addition of fenofibrate to statins seems to be beneficial in patients with ACS. Statins, contrary to various reports, were found to decrease plasma fibrinogen significantly. Also, in combination with fenofibrate there was enhanced reduction of the novel risk factor, fibrinogen.

References

[1] Murray JL, Lopez AL. Alternative projections of mortality and disability by cause 1990-2020. Global Burden of Disease Study. *Lancet* 1997; 349:1498-1504.

[2] Tsimihodimos V, Kostoula A, Kakafika A, Bairaktari E, Tselepis AD, Mikhailidis DP, Elisaf M. Effect of fenofibrate on serum inflammatory markers in patients with high triglyceride values. *J Cardiovasc Pharmacol Ther* 2004; 9:27-33.

[3] Kockx M, Gervois PP, Poulain P, Derudas B, Peters JM, Gonzalez FJ, Princen HM, Kooistra T, Staels B. Fibrates suppress fibrinogen gene expression in rodents via activation of the peroxisome proliferators-activated receptor-alpha. *Blood* 1999; 93: 2991-8.

[4] Green F, Humphries S. Control of plasma fibrinogen levels. *Baillieres Clin Haematol* 1989;2: 945-59.

[5] Woods A, Brull DJ, Humphries SE, Montgomery HE. Genetics of inflammation and risk of coronary artery disease: the central role of interleukin-6. *Eur Heart J* 2002; 21: 1574-83.

[6] Shepherd, J., Cobbe, S. M., Ford, I. Prevention of coronary heart disease with pravastatin in men with hypercholesterolemia. *N Engl J Med* 1995; 333: 1301-7.

[7] Sacks, F. M., Pfeffer, M. A., Moye, L. A. The effect of pravastatin on coronary events after myocardial infarction in patients with average cholesterol levels. *N Engl J Med* 1996 335:1001-9

[8] The Scandinavian Simvastatin Survival Group. Randomized trial of cholesterol lowering in 4444 patients with coronary heart disease: The Scandinavian Simvastatin Survival Study (4S*). Lancet* 1994; 344: 1383-9.

[9] Athyros, V. G., Papageorgiou, A. A., Hatzikonstandinou, H. A., Athyrou, V. V., Kontopoulos, A. G.Effect of atorvastatin versus simvastatin on lipid profile and plasma fibrinogen in patients with hypercholesterolemia. *Clin Drug Inves* 1998; 16: 219-27.

[10] Rosenson RS, Tangney CC, Casey LC. Inhibition of proinflammatory cytokine production by pravastatin. *Lancet* 1999; 353: 983-4.

[11] Rosenson RS, Tangney CC. Anti-atherothrombotic properties of statins: implications for cardiovascular event reduction. *JAMA* 1998; 279:1643-50.

[12] Handley DA, Hughes TE. Pharmacological approaches and strategies for therapeutic modulation of fibrinogen. *Thromb Res* 1997: 87:1-5.

[13] Ernst E, Resch KL. Therapeutic interventions to lower plasma fibrinogen concentration. *Eur Heart J* 1995; 16:47-51.

[14] Fuller GM. Fibrinogen: a multifunctional acute phase protein, in Mackiewicz A, Kushner I, Baumann H (eds): Acute phase proteins: Molecular Biology, biochemistry and clinical applications, New York, NY, Doubleday, 1993,p 169.

[15] Kant JA, Fornace AJ, Saxe D, Simon MI, McBride OW, Crabtree GR. Evolution and organization of the fibrinogen locus on chromosome 4: Gene duplication accompanied by transposition and inversion. *Proc Natl Acad Sci* USA 1985: 82: 2344-50

[16] Binsack R, Stegmeier K, Dorge L, Volkl A. Bezafibrate down-regulates fibrinogen biosynthesis in human hepatoma HepG2 cells. *Eur J Clin Invest* 1998; 28:151-5.

[17] Roy SN, Mukhopadhyay G, Redman CM. Regulation of fibrinogen assembly. Transfection of Hep G2 cells with B beta cDNA specifically enhances synthesis of the 3 component chains of fibrinogen. *J Biol Chem* 1990; 265:6389-93.

[18] Maison, P., Mennon, L., Sapinho, D., Balkau, B., Sigalas, J., Chesnier, M. C., Eschwege, E. D.E.S.I.R. Study group. A pharmacoepidemiological assessment of the effect of statins and fibrates on fibrinogen concentration. *Atheroscler* 2002; 160:155-60

[19] Stec JJ, Silbershatz H, Tofler GH, Matheney TH, Sutherland P,Lipinska I, Massaro JM, Wilson PF, Muller JE, D'Agostino RB Sr. Association of fibrinogen with cardiovascular risk factors and cardiovascular disease in the Framingham Offspring Population. *Circ* 2000; 102: 1634-8.

[20] Burnett JR, Wilcox LT, Telford DE, Kleinstiver SJ, Barrett PHR, Newton RS, Huff MW. Inhibition of HMG Co A reductase by atorvastatin decreases both VLDL and LDL, apoB productionin miniature pigs. *Arterioscler Thromb Vasc Biol* 1997;17:2489-2500.

[21] Haw N, Fowler G, Patel H, Eminton Z, Maton S. An assessment of the efficacy of atorvastatin in achieving LDL cholesterol target levels in patients with coronary heart disease: a general practice study. *Int J Clin Prac* 1999;53:422-6.

[22] Marais AD, Firth JC, Bateman M, Jones J, Mountney J. Atorvastatin is a powerful and safe agent for lowering plasma cholesterol concentration in heterozygous familial hypercholesterolemia. *Atheroscler* 1994;109:316-20.

[23] Frost R, Otto C, Geiss C, Schwandt P, Parhofer KG. Effects of atorvastatin versus fenofibrate on lipoprotein profiles, low density lipoprotein subfraction distribution, and hemorheologic parameters in type 2 diabetes mellitus with mixed hyperlipoproteinemia. *Am J Cardiol* 2001;87:44-8.

[24] Jones, P., Kafonek, S., Laurova, I. Comparative dose efficacy study of atorvastatin versus simvastatin, pravastatin, lovastatin and fluvastatin in patients with hypercholesterolemia. (The CURVES Study). *Am J Cardiol* 1998; 81: 582-7.

[25] Crouse JR III, Frolich J, Ose L, Mercuri M, Tobert JA. Effects of high doses of simvastatin and atorvastatin on high-density lipoprotein cholesterol and apolipoprotein A-1. *Am J Cardiol* 1999;83:1476-7.

[26] Hunninghake DB, Ballantyne CM, Maccubbin DL, Shah AK, Gumbiner B, Mitchel YB. Comparative effects of simvastatin and atorvastatin in hypercholesterolemic patients with characteristics of metabolic syndrome. *Clin Ther* 2003;25:1670-86.

[27] Staels B, Dallongvile J, Auwerx J, Schoonjans K, Leitersdorf E, Fruchart JC. Mechanism of action of fibrates on lipid and lipoprotein metabolism. *Circ* 1998;98:2088-93.

[28] Watts GF, Dimmit SB. Fibrates, dyslipoproteinemia and cardiovascular disease. *Curr Opin Lipid* 1999;10:561-74.

[29] Athyros VG, Papageorgiou AA, Hatziknonstandinou HA, Didangelos TP, Carina MV, Kranitsas DF, Kontupoulos AG. Safety and efficacy of long term statin-fibrate combination in patients with refractory familial combined hyperlipidemia. *Amer J Cardiol* 1997; 80: 608-13.

[30] Ruth LBE and Ruth McPherson. Long term efficacy and safety of fenofibrate and statin in treatment of combined hyperlipidemia. *Amer J Cardiol* 1998; 81: 60B-65B.

[31] Vega GL, Ma PT, Cater NB, Fillipchuk N, Megura S, Garcia AB, Grundy SM. Effects of adding fenofibrate (200mg/day) in patients with combined hyperlipidemia and metabolic syndrome. *Amer J Cardiol* 2003; 91: 956-60.

[32] Keating GM, Ormod D. Micronised fenofibrate: an updated review of its clinical efficacy in the management of dyslipidaemia. *Drugs* 2002; 62:1909-44.

[33] Heinrich, J., Assmann, G. Fibrinogen and cardiovascular risk. *J Cardiovasc Risk* 1995;2: 197-205.

[34] Kannel, W. B., Neaton, J. D., Wentworth, D., Thomas, H. E., Stamler, J., Hulley, S. B. For the MRFIT Research group. Overall and coronary heart disease mortality rates in relation to major risk factors in 325,348 men screened for the MRFIT trial. Multiple Risk Factor Intervention Trial. *Am Heart J* 1987; 112:825-36.

[35] Rosenson RS, Koenig W. Utility of inflammatory markers in the management of Coronary artery disease. *Amer J Cardiol* 2003; 92:10i-18i.

[36] Lowe G, Rumley A, Norrie J, Ford I, Shepherd J, Cobbe S, Macfarlane P, Packard C, on behalf of the West of Scotland Coronary Prevention Study Group. Blood Rheology, cardiovascular risk factors and cardiovascular disease: the west of Scotland Coronary Prevention Study. *Thromb Haemost* 2000; 84: 553-8.

[37] Wierzbicki, A. S., Lumb, P. J., Semra, Y. K. Effect of atorvastatin on plasma fibrinogen. *Lancet* 1998; 351:569-70.

[38] Song, J. C., White, C. M. Do HMG CoA reductase inhibitors affect fibrinogen? *Ann Pharmacother* 2001; 35:236-41.

[39] Bairaktari, E. T., Tzallas, C. S., Tsimihodimos, V. K., Liberopoulos, E. N., Miltiadous, G. A., Elisaf, M. S. Comparison of the efficacy of atorvastatin and micronized fenofibrate in the treatment of mixed hyperlipidemia. *J Cardiovasc Risk* 1999; 6:113-6.

[40] Frost, R., Otto, C., Geiss, C., Schwandt, P., Parhofer, K. G. Effects of atorvastatin versus fenofibrate on lipoprotein profiles, low density lipoprotein subfraction distribution, and hemorheologic parameters in type 2 diabetes mellitus with mixed hyperlipoproteinemia. *Am J Cardiol* 2001; 87:44-8.

[41] Serna, G., Cadarso, C. Fenofibrate decreases plasma fibrinogen, improves lipid profile, and reduces uricemia. *Clin Pharmacol Ther* 1999; 66:166-72.

[42] Otto, C., Geiss, H. C., Donner, M. G., Parhofer, K. G., Schwandt, P. Influence of atorvastatin versus simvastatin on fibrinogen and other hemorheological parameters in patients with severe hypercholesterolemia treated with regular low density lipoprotein immunoadsorption apheresis. *Ther Apher* 2000; 4:244-8.

[43] Athyros, V. G., Papageorgiou, A. A., Athyrou, V. V., Demitriadis, D. S., Kontopoulos, A. G. Atorvastatin and micronized fenofibrate alone and in combination in type 2 diabetes with combined hyperlipidemia. *Diab Care* 2002; 25:1198-1202.

[44] Ceska R, Sobra J, Kvasnicka J, Prochazkova R, Kvasilova M, Haas T. The effect of micronized fenofibrate on lipid parameters and fibrinogen in heterozygous familial hypercholesterolemia and familial combined hyperlipidemia. *Cas Lek Cesk* 1996;135: 413-6.

[45] Kadikoylu, G., Yukselen, V., Yavasoglu, I., Bolaman, Z. Hemostatic effects of atorvastatin versus simvastatin. *Ann Pharmacother* 2003; 37:478-84.

[46] Tikkanen MJ. Statins within-group comparisons, statin escape and combination therapy. *Curr Opin Lipidol* 1996; 7: 385-8.

[47] Leibovitz E, Hazanov N, Frieman A, Elly I, Gavish D. Atorvastatin reduces fibrinogen levels in patients with severe hypercholesterolemia: additional evidence to support the anti-inflammatory effects of statins. *Isr Med Assoc J* 2004;6:456-9.

[48] Tekin A, Tekin G, Guzelsoy D, Kaya A, Gurel CV, Yigit Z, Ulutin T. Effects of atorvastatin (10 mg) on hemostatic and inflammatory parameters in hyperlipidemic patients with angiographically proven coronary artery disease. *Am J Cardiol.* 2004;94:206-9.

In: Frontiers in Atherosclerosis Research
Editor: Karin F. Kepper, pp. 175-190

ISBN 1-60021-371-5

Chapter 9

MYOCARDIUM VIABILITY ASSESSED BY DELAYED CONTRAST-ENHANCED MAGNETIC RESONANCE IMAGING IN PATIENTS WITH SEVERE ISCHEMIC HEART FAILURE: A COMPARISON WITH THALLIUM SPECT AND DOBUTAMINE ECHOCARDIOGRAPHY

Yen-Wen Wu,[1,2] Por-Jau Huang,[2] Mao-Yuan Su,[3] Lung-Chun Lin,[2] Ruoh-Fang Yen,[1] Yih-Sharng Chen,[4] Chii-Ming Lee,[2] Hsi-Yu Yu,[4] Yi-Ting Wang,[3] Kai-Yuan Tzen[1] and Wen-Yih I. Tseng[3*]

Departments of [1]Nuclear Medicine
[2]Internal Medicine
[3]Medical Imaging
[4]Surgery, National Taiwan University Hospital and National Taiwan University College of Medicine, Taipei, Taiwan

ABSTRACT

Purpose

Functional recovery of ischemic cardiomyopathy depends on accurate identification of viable myocardium. We evaluated the value of delayed contrast-enhanced magnetic resonance imaging (MRI) in the assessment of myocardial viability.

---

*Reprints requests: Wen-Yih I. Tseng, MD, PhD. Department of Medical Imaging, National Taiwan University Hospital and Center of Optoelectronic Biomedicine, National Taiwan University College of Medicine. No.7, Chung-Shan South Road, Taipei, Taiwan. Tel: 886-2-23123456, ext 8758; Fax: 886-2-23926922; E-mail: wytseng@ha.mc.ntu.edu.tw

Materials and Methods

Forty patients with significant coronary artery disease and severe left ventricular (LV) dysfunction received delayed contrast-enhanced MRI and ^{201}Tl single-photon emission computed tomography (SPECT) within one month. Ten of them received simultaneous ^{201}Tl SPECT and dobutamine stress echocardiography (DSE). Three imaging modalities were compared based on a standardized 17-segment model. Improved regional wall thickening on follow-up MRI was used as an index of functional recovery in patients received revascularization.

Results

Of 680 segments, MRI hyperenhancement showed positive correlation with ^{201}Tl reduction (r =0.61, $p < 0.0001$). The viability concordance was 75.3% between DSE and MRI, 80.5% between ^{201}Tl SPECT and MRI, and 66.5% among all tests. Contrast-enhanced MRI detected more myocardial viability than ^{201}Tl SPECT, especially in the inferior wall and apex ($p < 0.0001$). Eight patients underwent revascularization. Comparing with functional recovery in the follow-up results, the diagnostic accuracy, sensitivity, specificity, positive predictive value, and negative predictive value of delayed contrast-enhanced MRI were 64%, 95%, 24%, 62% and 77%, respectively. For ^{201}Tl SPECT, these values were 55%, 75%, 29%, 58% and 54%, respectively. Areas under the ROC curves by MRI and ^{201}Tl SPECT were 0.59 ± 0.04, 0.52 ± 0.05, respectively (p=0.07). Of 16 segments viable on MRI but nonviable on ^{201}Tl SPECT, 12 (75%) recovered function after revascularization, while only one of 3 segments classified as nonviable on MRI but viable on ^{201}Tl SPECT recovered function ($p < 0.05$). Of 10 segments classified as scar by both tests, none recovered function after revascularization.

Conclusion

Delayed contrast-enhanced MRI detects viability better than ^{201}Tl SPECT, especially in the inferior wall and apex. Myocardial viability detected by MRI may predict functional recovery after revascularization in ischemic cardiomyopathy, even in patients with severe LV dysfunction.

Keywords: myocardial viability, magnetic resonance imaging, ^{201}Tl SPECT, dobutamine stress, echocardiography

INTRODUCTION

Improved ejection fraction (EF) after revascularization shows positive impact on prognosis in chronic ischemic cardiomyopathy [1,2]. Measurement of regional wall thickening of dysfunctional myocardium offers quantitative assessment of functional recovery after revascularization [3-5]. Determination of the viability of dysfunctional myocardium, however, remains a problem. The sensitivity of the dobutamine stress echo (DSE) is poor. Although the positron-emitting and single photon-emitting scintigraphic imaging techniques are known to assess myocardial viability, these modalities display rather lower specificity [1,2,5-8]. Cardiac MRI was reported to offer reliable and accurate assessment of myocardial scar burden [9], coronary perfusion [10] and contractile reserve [11]. The technique of delayed contrast-enhanced MRI using an inversion-recovery prepared T_1-weighted gradient-echo sequence was shown to provide exquisite contrast and spatial resolution of myocardial fibrosis [12,13]. While the infarct areas in the myocardium appeared cold regions on ^{201}Tl single-photon emission tomography (^{201}Tl SPECT) [12], it was vividly enhanced on MRI [13]. In addition, superior resolution of MRI made it more sensitive than other techniques to differentiate transmural from non-transmural infarction [14]. Larger transmural extent of contrast enhancement was found to correlate with less functional recovery after revascularization of dysfunctional myocardium [15]. To date, reports on comparing cardiac MRI, ^{201}Tl SPECT and DSE in the assessment of chronic ischemic cardiomyopathy are limited. The present study aimed to compare the delayed contrast-enhanced MRI with ^{201}Tl SPECT and DSE in the assessment of myocardial viability, and to evaluate its predictive power of functional recovery after revascularization in patients with chronic ischemic heart failure.

Materials and Methods

Patients

Between February, 2002 and September, 2004, forty consecutive patients (36 male; age, 59.4 ± 12.5 years) with angiographically significant coronary artery disease (CAD) (≥ 70% diameter stenosis) and symptoms of heart failure (New York Heart Association functional class ≥ II) for more than three months were prospectively enrolled for the evaluation of myocardial viability as shown in Table 1. All patients had a LVEF ≤ 40% and dysfunctional myocardium identified by resting echocardiography. All patients were excluded for recent myocardial infarction (MI) or unstable angina pectoris for < six weeks, valvular disease or contraindications to MRI as criteria laid down elsewhere. All patients consented under the approval of the Institutional Review Board of the National Taiwan University Hospital. All the imaging studies on myocardial viability received by each patient were performed within the duration of one month. Eight patients underwent revascularization within one month after viability study, and another cardiac MRI study was followed at least 3 months after the intervention. A flow chart of viability study and treatment of these patients is shown in the Figure 1.

Table 1. Patient Demographics

	Patients	N = 40
Male gender	36	90 %
Age, yrs	59.4 ± 12.5	37 – 83
Risk factors		
Hypertension	25	63%
Diabetes	14	35%
Hyperlipidemia	14	35%
History of MI (> 6 weeks)	20	50%
Previous interventions	23	58%
PCI	20	

Table 1. Continued

	Patients	N = 40
CABG	3	
NYHA functional class		
II	20	50%
III	14	35%
IV	6	15%
Mean	2.7 ± 0.7	
CAD		
1-VD	4	10%
2-VD	12	30%
3-VD	24	60%

Values are mean ± SD. MI = myocardial infarction; PCI = percutaneous coronary intervention; CABG = coronary artery bypass surgery; NYHA = New York Heart Association; CAD = coronary artery disease; VD = vessel-disease

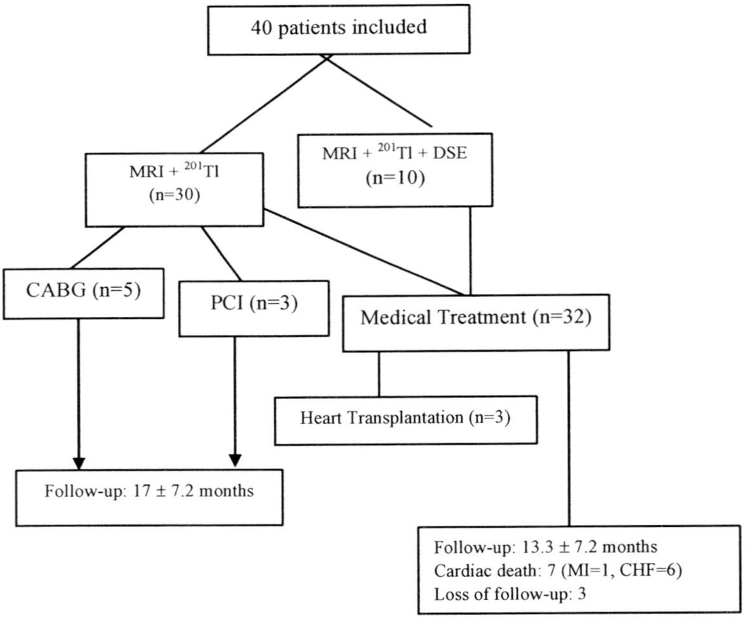

Figure 1. The flow chart of viability studies and treatments of patients included in this study. (DSE = dobutamine stress echocardiography; PCI = percutaneous coronary intervention; CABG = coronary artery bypass surgery; MI = myocardial infarction; CHF = congestive heart failure)

Echocardiography

M-mode and 2D echocardiography data were received at the echo lab using a Sonos-4500/5500 imaging system (Hewlett Packard, Palo Alto, CA) to assess contractile function and measure left atrial and LV dimensions according to standard criteria [16].

^{201}Tl SPECT Protocols

Eight patients were studied under exercise stress test. For the rest who were unable to exercise adequately, we used the pharmacological stress test: dipyridamole for 14 patients and simultaneous DSE and ^{201}Tl SPECT for the remaining 10 patents.

The exercise stress test was performed using a modified Bruce protocol [17]. The injection of ^{201}Tl (2-3 mCi) was timed at peak exercise. After the injection, exercise was continued for another minute.

For the dipyridamole stress test, intravenous dipyridamole (0.56 mg/kg in 4 minutes) was infused to induce coronary hyperemia and ^{201}Tl was injected 3 minutes after the completion of the infusion [18].

Simultaneous DSE and ^{201}Tl imaging was performed as described previously [5, 19]. In brief, dobutamine was intravenously infused at rates of 5, 10, 20, 30 and 40 μg/kg/min in 3-minute stages. Atropine was given if the patient's heart rate was lower than 85% of age-predicted maximum heart rate. ^{201}Tl was injected one minute before the termination of dobutamine infusion.

Stress SPECT imaging was started within 5 minutes after the injection of ^{201}Tl and the redistribution imaging was acquired 4 hours later. If images showed irreversible defects, additional 1 mCi ^{201}Tl was injected and a third set of images was obtained 15 minutes after the reinjection.

Rest-Redistribution ^{201}Tl SPECT (n=8)

Eight patients underwent rest-redistribution ^{201}Tl SPECT imaging because of their severe heart failure. The ^{201}Tl SPECT images were acquired 15 minutes and 4 hours after administration of 2-3 mCi ^{201}Tl. The post-processing and reconstruction of ^{201}Tl images was performed as described elsewhere [5, 17-20].

Cardiac MRI

Electrocardiographic-gated MRI was performed on a 1.5-T scanner (Sonata, Siemens, Erlangen, Germany) using a phased-array coil (CP Body Array Flex, Siemens, Erlangen, Germany) attached with respiratory and cardiac gating during repeated breath holds. Using steady-state free precession, MRI cine images were acquired as multiple short-axis views (every 1 cm throughout the entire LV) and 2 perpendicular long-axis planes. In another session, gadolinium contrast (Gd-DTPA, 0.15 mmol/kg) was administered intravenously, and contrast-enhanced images were acquired 10 minutes after administration using a segmented inversion-recovery prepared turbo gradient echo technique [15] in the identical planes. The imaging parameters were as follows: TR/TE/flip angle = 750 ms/4.18 ms/25°; FOV/matrix size/spatial resolution = 290×340 mm/216×256/0.75 mm; and the inversion time (TI) = 250 ms optimized to null the signal intensities of normal myocardium.

Image Processing and Analysis

The MRI images were interpreted by two independent blinded radiologists. If two interpretations did not agree with one another, the images were reviewed by the two physicians to reach a consensus. The LV myocardium was divided into 17 segments for analysis as AHA criteria recommendation [21].

Echocardiographic Analysis

Segmental wall motion and contractile reserve were defined by echocardiography before and after low-dose infusion of dobutamine as described earlier with accuracy of interobserver agreement 94% (κ=0.85) [17,22].

SPECT Image Analysis

SPECT images were normalized to peak myocardial activity as 100%. ^{201}Tl activity in each segment was scored as 0 = normal perfusion, 1 = mild decrease of photon counts, 2 = moderate decrease of photon counts, 3 = severe decrease of photon counts, and 4 = absent photon counts [23]. Each segment in SPECT images was scored for viability by perfusion photon counts normalized to peak myocardial activity as 100% based on the methods used previously [23, 24]. Our interobserver agreement for ^{201}Tl SPECT interpretations was 96% as previously reported [17].

MR Image Analysis

LV function parameters were assessed in a standard way using computing software (Matlab®, MathWorks Inc., MA, USA). The planimeter method was used to determine LV volumes, LVEF and cardiac mass and endocardial and epicardial borders on all short-axis cine images [25]. Wall thickening on cine MR images was measured as the percentage of systolic wall thickening (SWT) according to the following formula: (end-systolic wall thickness – end-diastolic wall thickness)/end-diastolic wall thickness × 100%. The delayed contrast enhancement (DC) in each segment was quantified using computing software (Mathematica®, Wolfram Research, Inc., IL, USA), following the criteria as described elsewhere [26]. The percentage of pixels showing hyperintensities out of the total myocardial pixels was determined by a 4-score grading: grade 0, no DC; grade 1, 1% to 25% DC; grade 2, 26% to 50% DC; grade 3, 51% to 75% DC; grade 4, > 75% DC. To compare MRI with SPECT and DSE data, grade 3 defined as non-viable myocardium. In the follow-up study, an increase of ≥ 15% SWT change was used to define improvement of post-revascularization contractile function [27].

Statistical Analysis

Data were collected as mean ± SD showing comparisons between groups by use of 2-sample *t* test and chi-square analysis for continuous and categorical variables, respectively. ANOVA (analysis of variance) with Bonferroni's post hoc test was performed to detect any associations between two or more variables. Agreement between the diagnostic tests was evaluated using κappa index. Correlations between the extent of extent of DC on MRI and ^{201}Tl uptake on SPECT were analyzed using linear regression analyses. Changes between baseline and follow-up measurements were assessed by paired *t* tests. ROC curves were used to compare predictive accuracy of both MRI and ^{201}Tl SPECT to predict an increase of ≥ 15% SWT change at follow-up. Areas under the ROC curves were compared by use of the z test. A p value < 0.05 (two-sided) was predetermined to be statistically significant. All statistical analyses were done using scientific statistical software packages (Stata 8, Texas, USA).

RESULTS

Forty patients with demography as shown in Table 1, were studied at baseline by MRI and ^{201}Tl SPECT. Ten of them underwent simultaneous DSE and ^{201}Tl studies. Of these patients, eight underwent revascularization after viability studies, including percutaneous coronary intervention (PCI) in three (left anterior descending artery in two patients and left circumflex artery in one patient) and coronary bypass surgery (CABG) in five patients. Follow-up MRI studies were performed 5.0 ± 4.3 months after the revascularization procedures. One patient had non-ST elevation myocardial infarction during PCI. No other patient had clinical events between two MRI studies.

Of patients who were treated medically, three received heart transplantation within one month after viability studies. Seven patients died during the follow-up periods, including acute MI in one and intractable heart failure in another six patients as shown in Figure 1.

Comparison of Viability Data

The results of myocardial viability assessed by MRI and ^{201}Tl SPECT are shown in Table 2 (A, B). Viable myocardium detected on MRI had positive relationship with ^{201}Tl activity. The concordant rate of viability was 80.5% between ^{201}Tl SPECT and MRI (κ=0.52), and overall concordant rate was 66.5% among DSE, ^{201}Tl SPECT and MRI tests (κ=0.51).

The contractile reserve detected by late enhancement on MRI showed higher proportion of transmural extent of DC on MRI (Table 2C). In some cases, contractile reserve was impaired resulting with invisible or minor scar detected on MRI (21/102, 21%). All segments with extensive scar on MRI and or SPECT showed no contractile function at rest (Figure 2), although almost all segments with > 50% DC showed marked impairment of resting function.

Table 2. Comparison of Myocardial Viability Using Different Diagnostic Modalities

(A) Relationship between viability detected by dobutamine stress echocardiography, MRI and ^{201}Tl SPECT

170 segments	DSE +		DSE -	
	Tl +	Tl -	Tl +	Tl -
MRI +	79	12	23	14
MRI -	3	2	3	34

(B) Concordance between viability detected by MRI and ^{201}Tl SPECT

680 segments		MRI	
		+	-
Tl	+	411	33
	-	93	109

(C) Relationship between transmural extent of DC on MRI and contractile reserve detected by dobutamine stress echocardiography

170 segments	Transmural Extent of DC on MRI			
	0 - 25%	26 - 50%	51 - 75%	76 - 100%
DSE +	81	10	5	0
DSE −	21	17	17	9

DSE = dobutamine stress echocardiography; Tl = ^{201}Tl SPECT; + = viable; - = scar, DC = delayed contrast enhancement

(A)

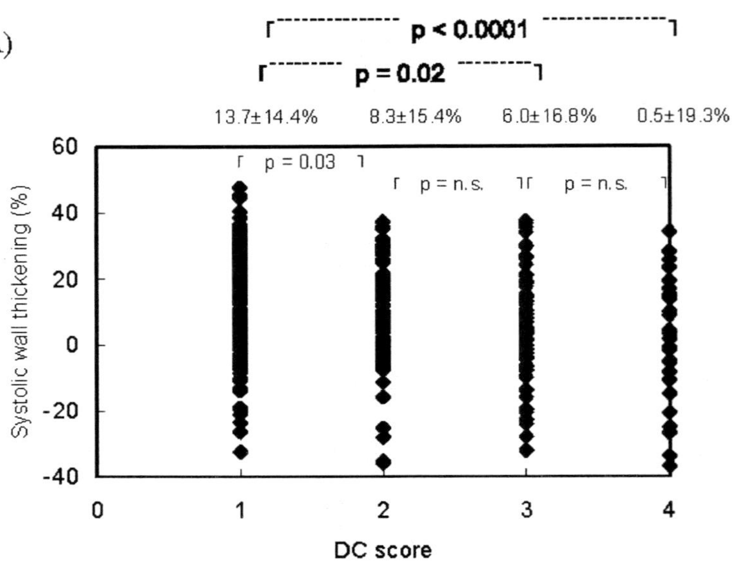

Figure 2. continued.

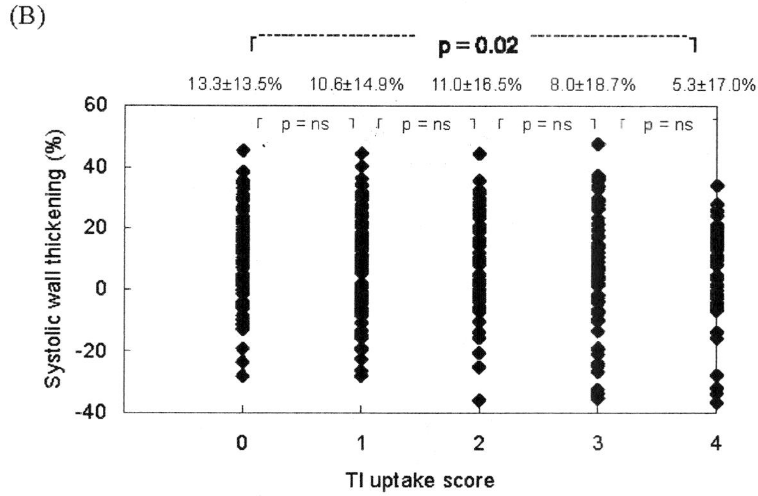

Figure 2. Relationship between (A) delayed contrast enhancement on MRI, (B) ^{201}Tl uptake on SPECT and percentage of systolic wall thickening on MRI (ns = non-significant, DC = delayed contrast enhancement)

In 680 segments from 40 patients, the amount of viable tissue on MRI correlated positively with ^{201}Tl uptake (^{201}Tl uptake score = 0.67 DC score - 0.69, r=0.61, p < 0.0001). The extent of DC enhancement on MRI and the reduction of ^{201}Tl uptake both showed agreement (κ=0.51, Figure 3). The MRI detected more myocardial viability than ^{201}Tl SPECT in the inferior wall (92/120 vs. 63/120, p < 0.0001), and apex (23/40 vs. 15/40, p < 0.0001). The discrepancy between viability determined by ^{201}Tl SPECT and MRI is shown in Table 3.

The representative examples of concordant and disconcordant myocardial viability detected by MRI and ^{201}Tl SPECT are shown in Figure 4 and 5.

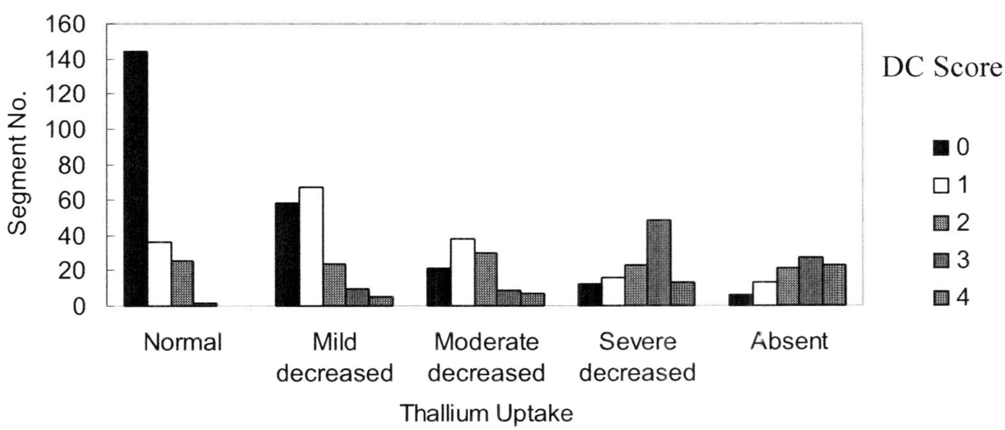

Figure 3. Relationship between thallium uptake and delayed contrast enhancement in MRI. (DC = delayed contrast enhancement)

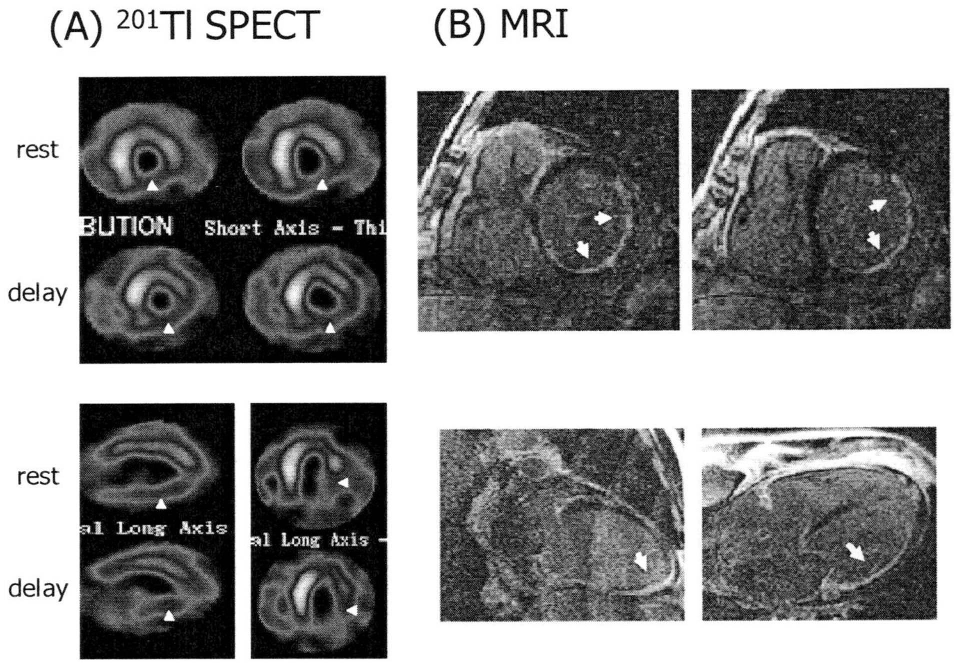

Figure 4. A 64-year-old patients with old inferior myocardial infarction (LVEF 17%) showed concordant scars in the inferior and inferolateral walls on the rest-redistribution ^{201}Tl SPECT (A, arrow heads) and delayed contrast-enhanced MRI (B, arrows)

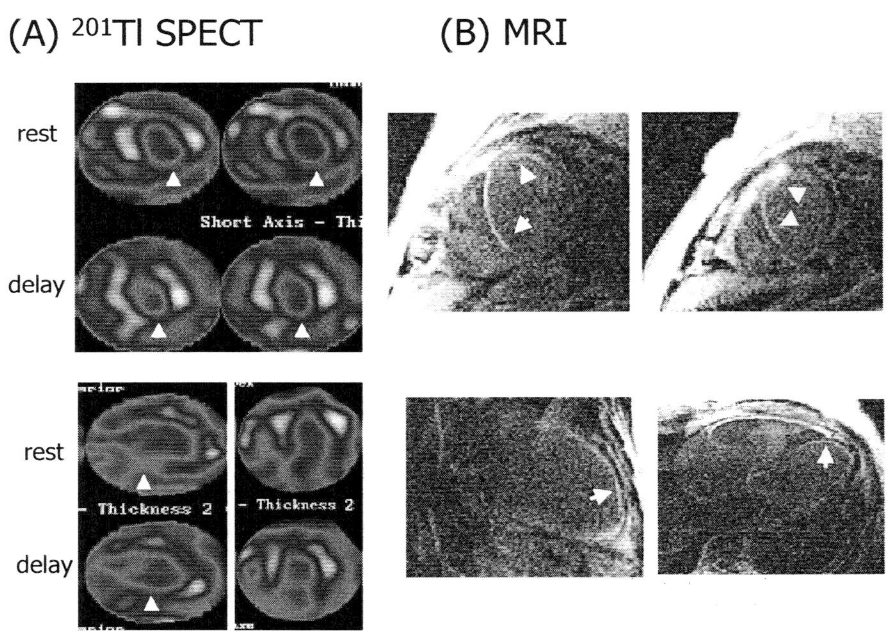

Figure 5. A 43-year-old man with 3-vessel disease (LVEF 8%) showed scar in the inferior wall (arrow heads) on the rest-redistribution ^{201}Tl SPECT (A), which is discordant with contrast-enhanced MRI (B) showing delayed enhancement in the anterior and septal walls (arrows)

Table 3. Distribution of Discrepancies in Identifying Myocardial Viability by 201Tl SPECT and MRI

(A) Scar detected by MRI but viable by ^{201}Tl SPECT (n = 33 segments)

	Anterior	Anteroseptal	Inferoseptal	Inferior	Inferolateral	Lateral	Apex
Basal	1	1	4	0	0	2	
Mid-ventricular	2	3	4	1	3	2	
Apical	1	4		2	2		2

(B) Scar detected by ^{201}Tl SPECT but viable by MRI (n = 93 segments)

	Anterior	Anteroseptal	Inferoseptal	Inferior	Inferolateral	Lateral	Apex
Basal	3	4	5	10	9	0	
Mid-ventricular	3	4	1	11	5	1	
Apical	6	6		11	5		9

Table 4. Influence of Transmural Extent of Delayed Contrast Enhancement on Recovery of Regional Function in 97 Dysfunctional Segments at Baseline

	Systolic Wall Thickening Ratio (%)			
Transmurality	**Baseline**	**Follow-Up**	**Difference**	***P***
0 - 25% (n=52)	9.7 ± 14.8	28.0 ± 12.9	17.9 ± 15.6	< 0.0001
26 - 50% (n=32)	6.2 ± 13.9	15.2 ± 15.3	9.0 ± 18.6	0.01
51 - 75% (n=9)	0.1 ± 6.0	3.7 ± 19.0	3.6 ± 17.9	0.56
76 -100% (n=4)	-11.9 ± 17.1%	-1.8 ± 22.8	10.2 ± 29.7	0.56

Follow-Up Data

A total of 106 segments (97 dysfunctional) in eight patients were revascularized after viability tests. Among 97 dysfunctional segments, 84 (87%) were viable on MRI and 71 (73%) were viable on ^{201}Tl SPECT. Two of the eight patients had evidence of new delayed enhanced segments in their post-revascularization scan (one patient in CABG group had three and the other patient in PCI group had two new delayed enhanced segments). The LVEF in the eight patients at baseline was 26.3 ± 8.1% and increased significantly to 38.6 ± 16.8% at follow-up (p=0.04). Total LV mass (217.5 ± 54.5 to 183.0 ± 47.9 g), LV end-diastolic volume index (110.5 ± 38.7 to 86.6 ± 36.0 mL/m^2), LV end-systolic volume index (82.3 ± 37.4 to 55.9 ± 36.9 mL/m^2) were also decreased postoperatively, but statistically insignificant.

In terms of regional function change, the SWT measured by MRI was used as the parameter of myocardial viability. Of the 97 dysfunctional segments, 55 (57%) showed functional recovery (increase of segmental SWT ≥ 15%). The overall diagnostic accuracy, sensitivity, specificity, positive predictive value and negative predictive value of viability detected by MRI were, respectively, 64%, 95%, 24%, 62% and 77%, whereas they were 55%, 75%, 29%, 58% and 54% by ^{201}Tl SPECT. Moreover, the SWT improvement after revascularization in dysfunctional segments was dependent on its transmural extent shown in Table 4. However, there was no significant difference in areas under the ROC curves by MRI and ^{201}Tl SPECT, respectively (0.59 ± 0.04 vs. 0.52 ± 0.05, p=0.07).

Of sixteen segments viable on MRI but nonviable on ^{201}Tl SPECT, twelve (75%) segments showed function recovery after revascularization, while only one of three segments classified as nonviable on MRI but viable on ^{201}Tl SPECT recovered function ($p < 0.05$). Out of ten segments classified as scar by both tests, no segment showed the function improvement after revascularization. Out of five new segments with hyperenhancement after the interventions, four segments indicated unrecovered regional wall function with transmural involvement (SWT change, –0.19 ± 8.9%). However, improvement was seen in the only segment with hyperenhancement confined to the subendocardial layer (SWT change, 33.75%).

Discussion

The identification of hibernating myocardium in patients with chronic heart failure is becoming state of the art in cardiovascular science. Previous studies have shown great potentials in terms of outcome and recovery of LV function after revascularization [1-5]. Myocardial viability assessment by ^{18}F-fluorodeoxyglucose (^{18}F-FDG) positron emission tomography (PET) is clinically important in these patients, but high costs and limited availability of PET cameras and radiotracers hamper the clinical applications. Recent advance in cardiac MRI allows imaging myocardial viability with excellent imaging quality [9-15]. However, reports on its value in predicting functional recovery after revascularization in patients with chronic severe LV dysfunction, in comparison with well-established ^{201}Tl SPECT and DSE, are still lacking.

Our results are in agreement with previous works [28,29] that dobutamine response depends on the transmural scar extent shown on DC. Our data corroborated with previous reports [1,6-8,29] and highlighted that DSE detected less viable myocardium in comparison with both ^{201}Tl SPECT and MRI imaging methods. However, the concordance between DSE and MRI (75.3%) or between DSE and ^{201}Tl SPECT (76.5%) was similar.

In present study, we observed that the amount of viable myocardial tissue on cardiac MRI was positively correlated with ^{201}Tl uptake. Similar findings were reported to assess by ^{18}F-FDG PET and MRI techniques [27,30]. Our data were consistent with previous findings that MRI identified subendocardial infarcts but missed by SPECT [14,29]. We also observed that ^{201}Tl SPECT might overestimate the scar tissue, especially in the inferior wall and apex. These discrepancies may be explained in part by the low-energy X-ray emission and soft tissue attenuation. The inferior wall is one of the most sensitive to ^{201}Tl attenuation region in the heart, thus greater attenuation of ^{201}Tl in the inferior segments could be anticipated. However, limited success was reported by using infarct location adjusted thresholds for viability assessment [31-34]. The regions of dysfunctional myocardium seen as viable on ^{201}Tl SPECT but MRI invisible can be attributed to the fact that ^{201}Tl scan could become positive in the presence of a thin rim of viable tissue as previously reported [35,36].

Earlier reports showed that in patients with LV dysfunction undergoing revascularization, the extent and severity of nonviable tissue defined by MRI correlates was well correlated with the likelihood of functional recovery assessed by LVEF [16,27]. Our study extends the information further showing relationship of chronic CAD and severe LV dysfunction in our research volunteers (most patients with LVEF ≤ 25%). Our results further suggest that the myocardial viability detected by MRI may be valuable on the clinical evaluation of potential benefits from high-risk revascularization procedures.

The functional recovery assessment shown in our study after intervention was not homogeneous. Several factors affect the functional recovery including different intervention procedures, completeness of revascularization, and peri- and post-operative MI events [37,38]. Furthermore, the degree and duration of pre-procedural cellular structure change may influence the functional recovery.

However, there are some recognized limitations. Our sample size was relatively small, and limited patients underwent revascularization. Neither of patients who received simultaneous DSE and ^{201}Tl imaging received the revascularization, so the comparison between DSE and MRI in predicting functional recovery is still lacking. The ^{201}Tl imaging method in this study reflected our routine clinical protocol, no additional correction algorithm or prone position imaging was applied, which has been proposed to decrease the false-positive rate [39,40].

Conclusion

Cardiovascular MRI provides a unique tool to assess cardiac structure and function in a single study session. The present study demonstrates the good correlations among DSE, ^{201}Tl SPECT and MRI in the detection of myocardial viability. MRI detects better viability than ^{201}Tl SPECT, especially in the inferior wall and apex. MRI has marginally higher predictive value in predicting functional recovery. For patients with severe ischemic cardiomyopathy, noninvasive MRI may provide better clinical decision on using high-risk revascularization procedures.

Acknowledgments

The work was supported in part by grant NSC-91-2314-B002-272 from the National Science Council, Taiwan.

References

[1] Allman KC, Shaw LJ, Hachamovitch R, et al. Myocardial viability testing and impact of revascularization on prognosis in patients with coronary artery disease and left ventricular dysfunction: a meta-analysis. *J Am Coll Cardiol* 2002; 39:151-158.

[2] Underwood SR, Bax JJ, vom Dahl J, et al. Imaging techniques for the assessment of myocardial hibernation: report of a study group of the European Society of Cardiology. *Eur Heart J* 2004; 25:815-836.

[3] Rahimtoola SH. A perspective on the three large multicenter randomized clinical trials of coronary bypass surgery for chronic stable angina. *Circulation* 1985; 72(6 pt 2) V-123-V-135.

[4] Van-den-Berg EK Jr, Popma JJ, Dehmer GJ, et al. Reversible segmental left ventricular dysfunction after coronary angioplasty. *Circulation* 1990; 81:1210-6.

[5] Huang PJ, Lin LC, Yen RF, et al. Accuracy of biphasic response, sustained improvement and worsening during dobutamine echocardiography in predicting recovery of myocardial dysfunction after revascularization: comparison with simultaneous thallium-201 reinjection SPECT. *Ultrasound Med Biol* 2001; 27:925-931.

[6] Shan K, Constatine G, Sivananthan M, Flamm S. Role of cardiac magnetic resonance imaging in the assessment of myocardial viability. *Circulation* 2004; 109:1328-1334.

[7] Dilsizian V, Rocco TP, Freedman NMT, Leon MB, Bonow RO. Enhanced detection ischemic but viable myocardium by the reinjection of thallium after stress-redistribution imaging. *N Engl J Med* 1990; 323:141-146.

[8] Cigarroa C, De Fillipi C, Brickner ME, Alvarez L, Wait MA, Grayburn PA. Dobutamine stress echocardiography identifies hibernating myocardium and predicts recovery of left ventricular function after coronary revascularization. *Circulation* 1993; 88:430-436.

[9] Mahrholdt H, Wagner A, Holly TA, et al. Reproducibility of chronic infarct size measurement by contrast-enhanced magnetic resonance imaging. *Circulation* 2002; 39:1151-1158.

[10] Al Saadi N, Nagel E, Gross M, et al. Noninvasive detection of myocardial ischemia perfusion reserve based on cardiovascular magnetic resonance. *Circulation* 2000; 101:1379-1383.

[11] Baer FM, Theissen P, Schneider CA, et al. Dobutamine magnetic resonance imaging predicts contractile recovery of chronically dysfunctional myocardium after successful revascularization. *J Am Coll Cardiol* 1998; 31:1040-1048.

[12] Ramani K, Judd RM, Holly TA, et al. Contrast magnetic resonance imaging in the assessment of myocardial viability in patients with stable coronary artery and left ventricular dysfunction. *Circulation* 1998; 98:2687-2694.

[13] Kim RJ, Fieno DS, Parrish TB, et al. Relationship of MRI delayed contrast enhancement to irreversible injury, infarct age, and contractile function. Circulation 1999; 100:1992-2002.

[14] Wagner A, Mahrholdt H, Regenfus M, et al. Contrast-enhanced MR and routine single photon emission computed tomography (SPECT) perfusion imaging for detection of subendocardial myocardial infarcts: an imaging study. *Lancet* 2003; 361:364-379.

[15] Kim RJ, Wu E, Rafael A, et al. The use of contrast-enhanced magnetic resonance imaging to identify reversible myocardial dysfunction. *N Engl J Med* 2000; 343:1445-1453.

[16] Oh JK, Seward JB, Tajik J. The echo manual. 2nd ed. Philadelphia, *Lippincott Williams and Wilkins*, 1999; 7-43.

[17] Huang PJ, Chieng PU, Lee YT,, et al. Exercise thallium-201 tomographic scintigraphy in the diagnosis of coronary artery disease: emphasis on the effect of exercise level. *J Formos Med Assoc* 1992; 91:1096-1101.

[18] Ho FM, Huang PJ, Liau CS, Lee FK, Chieng PU, Su CT. Dobutamine stress echocardiography compared with dipyridamole thallium-201 single-photon emission computed tomography in detecting coronary artery disease. *Eur Heart J* 1995; 16:570-575.

[19] Huang PJ, Ho YL, Wu CC, et al. Simultaneous dobutamine stress echocardiography and thallium-201 perfusion imaging for the detection of coronary artery disease. *Cardiology* 1997; 88:556-562.

[20] Lomboy CT, Schulman DS, Grill HP, et al. Rest-redistribution thallium-201 scintigraphy to determine myocardial viability early after myocardial infarction. *J Am Coll Cardiol* 1995; 25:210-217.

[21] Cerqueira MD, Weissman NJ, Dilsizian V, et al. Standardized myocardial segmentation and nomclature for tomographic imaging of the heart. *Circulation* 2002; 105:539-542.

[22] American Society of Echocardiography Committee on Standards: Recommendations for quantitation of the left ventricle by two-dimensional echocardiography. *J Am Soc Echocardiogr* 1989; 2:358-267.

[23] Kiat H, Maddahi J, Roy LT, Van Train K, Friedman J, Resser K, et al. Comparison of technetium-99m methoxy-isobutyteryle and thallium-201 evaluation of coronary artery disease by planar and tomographic methods. *Am Heart J* 1989; 117:1-11.

[24] Dilsizian V, Freedman NMT, Bacharach SL, Perrone-Filardi P, Bonow RO. Regional thallium uptake in irreversible defects: magnitude of change in thallium activity after reinjection distinguishes viable from nonviable myocardium. *Circulation* 1992; 85:627-634.

[25] Tseng WY, Liao TY, Wang JL. Normal systolic and diastolic functions of the left ventricle and left atrium by cine magnetic resonance imaging. *J Cardiovasc Magn Reson* 2002; 4:443-457.

[26] Mahrholdt H, Wagner A, Holly TA, et al. Reproducibility of chronic infarct size measurement by contrast-enhanced magnetic resonance imaging. *Circulation* 2002; 106:2322-2327.

[27] Knuesel PR, Nanz D, Wyss C, et al. Characterization of dysfunctional myocardium by positron emission tomography and magnetic resonance: relation to functional outcome after revascularization. *Circulation* 2003; 108:1095-1100.

[28] Shan K, Bick RJ, Poindexter BJ, et al. Altered adrenergic receptor density in myocardial hibernations in humans: a possible mechanism of depressed myocardial function. *J Am Coll Cardiol* 1996; 28:432-442.

[29] Nelson C, McCrohon J, Khafagi F, et al. Impact of scar thickness on the assessment of viability using dobutamine echocardiography and thallium single photon emission computed tomography: a comparison with contrast-enhancement magnetic resonance imaging. *J Am Coll Cardiol* 2004; 43: 1248-1256.

[30] Klein C, Nekolla SG, Bengel FM, et al. Assessment of myocardial viability with contrast-enhanced magnetic resonance imaging: comparison with positron emission tomography. *Circulation* 2002; 105:162-167.

[31] Vanoverschelde J-LJ, DeHondt A-M, Marwick T, et al. Head-to-head comparison of exercise-redistribution-reinjection thallium single photon emission computed tomography and low dose dobutamine echocardiography for prediction of reversibility of chronic left ventricular ischemic dysfunction. *J Am Coll Cardiol* 1996; 28:432-442.

[32] Gunnung MG, Anagnostopoulous C, Knight CJ, et al. Comparison of Tl-201, technetium-99m tetrafosmin and dobutamine magnetic resonance imaging in idenfying hibernating myocardium. *Circulation* 1998; 98:1869-1874.

[33] Udelson JE, Coleman PS, Metherall J, et al. Predicting recovery of severe regional ventricular dysfunction. Comparison of resting scintigraphy with 201 Tl and 99m-Tc-sestamibi. *Circulation* 1994; 89:2552-2561.

[34] Schneider CA, Voth E, Gawlich S, et al. Significance of rest technetium-99m sestamibi imaging for the prediction of improvement of left ventricular dysfunction after Q wave myocardial infarction: importance of infarct location adjusted thresholds. *J Am Coll Cardiol* 1998; 32:648-654.

[35] Zamorano J, Delgado J, Almeria C, et al. Reason for discrepancies in identifying myocardial viability by thallium-201 redistribution, magnetic resonance imaging and dobutamine echocardiography. *Am J Cardiol* 2002; 90:455-459.

[36] Baumgartner H, Porenta G, Lau YK, et al. Assessment of myocardial viability by dobutamine echocardiography, positron emission tomography and thallium-201 SPECT. Correlation with histopathology in explanted hearts. *J Am Coll Cardiol* 1998;32: 1701-1708.

[37] Ricciardi MJ, Wu E, Davidson CJ, et al. Visualization of discrete microinfarction after percutaneous coronary intervention associated with mild creatine kinase-MB elevation. *Circulation* 2001; 103:2780-2783.

[38] Selvanayagam JB, Petersen SE, Francis JM, et al. Effects of off-pump versus on-pump coronary surgery on reversible and irreversible myocardial injury. A randomized trail using cardiovascular magnetic resonance imaging and biochemical markers. *Circulation* 2004; 109:345-350.

[39] Esquerre JP, Coca FJ, Martinez SJ, et al. Prone decubitus: a solution to inferior wall attenuation in thallium-201 myocardial tomography. *J Nucl Med* 1989; 30:398-401.

[40] Hendel RC, Berman DS, Cullom SJ, et al. Multicenter clinical trial to evaluate the efficacy of correction for photon attenuation and scatter in SPECT myocardial perfusion imaging. *Circulation* 1999; 99:2742-2749.

In: Frontiers in Atherosclerosis Research
Editor: Karin F. Kepper, pp. 191-211

ISBN 1-60021-371-5

Chapter 10

ASPIRIN RESISTANCE: NEED FOR A SPECIFIC, RAPID, POINT-OF-CARE ASSAY

Gundu H. R. Rao[1]
Laboratory Medicine and Pathology
Lillehei Heart Institute

ABSTRACT

Background

Aspirin as a therapeutic drug has been in use for over hundred years. Its use as an anti-platelet drug was recognized in the early 70s. For secondary prophylaxis of vascular disease, it is the most useful and cost-effective drug. Large number of clinical trials using aspirin has concluded that at any given vascular risk, low to medium dose of aspirin (80-160mg), is as effective as any other drug of choice. However, in recent years, there are several studies, in which aspirin resistance in patients with various vascular diseases have been demonstrated. Furthermore, some studies have suggested worst outcome in aspirin non-responders.

Methods

Variety of methods has been used in these studies, to determine "non-responders" to the action of aspirin .The definition of "aspirin resistant" individuals is those whose platelet cyclooxygenase are not inhibitable by aspirin. Methods used for monitoring aspirin resistance in these studies are non-specific platelet function tests.

Results

Differences in the definition of aspirin resistance, variations in the methods used to detect "non-responders", inter-individual variations in the response of platelets to the action of different agonists, and lack of data from large clinical trials have hampered the advancement of knowledge in this area.

[1] MMC 609, University of Minnesota, Minneapolis
MN 55455; E mail: raoxx001@umn.edu
Phone: 612 626 2717

Conclusion

Therefore, there is a great need to develop specific and rapid Point-of-Care assays that could detect the prevalence of aspirin resistance in patient populations, so that those found to be non-responders to the action of aspirin might be provided alternate treatment regimen.

Keywords: aspirin resistance, non-responders, thrombosis, stroke.

INTRODUCTION

Role of platelets in the pathogenesis of atherosclerosis, thrombosis and stroke is well documented [1]. Therefore, there is a great need for developing specific and effective drugs for modulating platelet function. A thorough understanding of the signaling mechanisms involved in the regulation of platelet function will facilitate the development of better anti-platelet drugs. Agonists interact with the platelet at specific receptor sites on the plasma membrane and initiate a series of signaling events capable of modulating shape change, adhesion, aggregation, secretion of granule contents and expression of activation markers on the membrane [2-10]. Platelet aggregates are formed when the GP11b/111a receptors get activated and bind fibrinogen and recruit other platelets to form clumps. This phenomenon plays a significant role in the formation of effective haemostatic plug as well as growth of thrombus. Weak agonists such as epinephrine, ADP require the production of pro-aggregatory prostaglandin endoperoxides and thromboxane to cause platelet aggregation and secretion. Aspirin is a specific inhibitor of cyclooxygenase and prevents the formation of pro-aggregatory PG endoperoxides.

Data from large number of clinical studies have demonstrated that at any given risk, irrespective of the disease state, aspirin at low to medium concentration is as effective as any other drug [2-5]. Although ability of a plant bark (bark of willow, *Salix alba*) product to reduce fever was discovered two hundred years ago, the mechanism of action of aspirin remained elusive till late 1900 [6]. Nobel laureate Sir John R. Vane and his associates at the Royal College of Surgeons, in London, in 1971 proposed the first satisfactory mechanism as to how aspirin works [7, 8]. Within a short period of time extensive work was done by various groups to elucidate the mechanism of action of aspirin like compounds [8-20]. At the same period, another Nobel Laureate Dr. Bengt Samuelsson of the Karolinska Institute, Stockholm, Sweden, discovered that the prostaglandin synthase produces transient bioactive prostanoids like PGG_2 /PGH_2 and thromboxane A_2 from the substrate arachidonic acid [10]. These findings revolutionized the research in platelet physiology and pharmacology [2-21].

PLATELET PHYSIOLOGY

Blood platelets interact with a variety of soluble agonists such as epinephrine (EPI), adenosine diphosphate (ADP), thrombin and thromboxane (TXA_2); many cell matrix components, including collagen, laminin, fibronectin, and vonWillebrand factor and biomaterials used for construction of invasive medical devices [21-29]. These interactions stimulate specific receptors and glycoprotein-rich domains (integrin and non-integrin receptors) on the plasma membrane and lead to the activation of intracellular effector enzymes. Agonist–mediated activation of platelets stimulates phospholipase C (PLC) and it then triggers the hydrolysis of Phosphatidyl inositol 4, 5-bisphosphate, the formation of second messengers such as 1, 2-diacyl glycerol and inositol 1, 4, 5 trisphosphate. Diacylglycerol activates protein kinase and inositol trisphosphate facilitates the mobilization of free calcium from the storage sites. The majority of regulatory events appear to require free calcium. Ionized calcium is the primary bioregulator, and a variety of biochemical mechanisms modulate the availability of free calcium [27]. Elevation of cytosolic calcium stimulates phospholipase A_2 and liberates arachidonic acid (AA). Free AA is transformed to a novel metabolite thromboxane, a potent platelet agonist. This is the major metabolite of AA metabolism and plays an important role in platelet recruitment, granule mobilization, secretion of granule contents, and expression of activated GP11b/111a ($\acute{\alpha}_{11b}\,\beta_3$) receptors [22-30]. Up regulation of activation signaling pathways, will increase the risk for clinical complications associated with thromboembolic episodes.

Arachidonic Acid Metabolism

Arachidonic acid is a 20 carbon polyunsaturated fatty acid (20:4w6) found in membrane phospholipids. Cell activation stimulates Phospholipase A_2, which facilitates the release of this fatty acid from phospholipids. AA is converted to prostaglandin (PG) endoperoxides (PGG_2/PGH_2) by cyclooxygenase (Prostaglandin G/H synthase; COX1)). These transient metabolites are converted by thromboxane synthetase to thromboxane A_2, which is the major metabolite of this pathway in platelets [10]. Whereas, in vascular tissues, the endoperoxides generated by COX1 are transformed by prostacyclin synthetase to prostacyclin (PGI_2). Thromboxane is a potent platelet agonist and a vasoconstrictor. Prostacyclin is an antiplatelet compound and exerts vasodilatory effects on vascular tissues. Thus from a single substrate (AA), two pharmacologically opposing vasoactive prostanoids are generated by platelets and vascular tissues [3]. Aspirin selectively acetylates the hydroxyl groups of a single serine residue (position 529) in the prostaglandin G/H synthase and causes irreversible inhibition of the activity of this enzyme [12, 13]. Inhibition of PG synthase results in the decreased conversion of AA to PG endoperoxides, PGG_2/PGH_2. Molecular mechanisms involved in aspirin-mediated inhibition of prostaglandin G/H synthase are well documented [4-16].

However, little is known about how other non-steroidal anti-inflammatory drugs inhibit this enzyme [14]. To elucidate the mechanism by which this enzyme oxidizes AA, we developed a cell free assay system. This system used ferrous iron induced oxidation of AA. Oxidation of the fatty acids by iron was followed by nitrobluetetrazolium [31]. Several drugs known to be inhibitors of this enzyme were used in this system to evaluate the affinity of these compounds to ferrous iron. Results demonstrated these compounds could form a complex with ferrous iron and inhibit AA metabolism [32, 33]. Using a ferrous iron chelator, bypirydil, we demonstrated the ability of this compound to inhibit platelet prostaglandin synthesis and function [34]. In a separate study, we showed ibuprofen, a short acting drug, interacted with the active site of PG synthase and blocked the ability of aspirin to acetylate COX1 enzyme [35]. Based on these results and other studies, we concluded aspirin like compounds devoid of acetyl group interact with the heme part of the PG synthase and block

AA oxidation [31-33]. In platelets AA is converted by lipoxygenase to 12-hydroxyeicosatetraenoic acid. This pathway is not inhibited by aspirin.

Studies on the Use of Aspirin as an Inhibitor of Cox-1 Enzymes

Single oral doses of 10-100 mgs of aspirin can significantly inhibit the platelet PG synthase activity [36]. The inhibitory effect of aspirin on circulating platelets in the blood is fast and probably occurs in the portal circulation. The half-life of aspirin is very short (15-20 minutes) but sufficient to inhibit PG synthase of circulating platelets. Since these cells lack DNA and the ability to resynthesize the enzyme, the dysfunction caused by aspirin cannot be overcome. Therefore, platelets exposed to aspirin loose the ability to make the prostanoids completely. However, one should keep in mind that once the aspirin is hydrolyzed to salicylic acid, ability to inhibit prostaglandin synthase is lost. Hence the platelets produced from the marrow after the aspirin is hydrolyzed, will have active prostaglandin synthase. Approximately 10% of fresh platelets are added on to the circulating blood every day. Although aspirin treated blood platelets do not make prostaglandins, they respond with aggregation to the stimulation by prostaglandin endoperoxides and thromboxane. Fresh platelets formed after the hydrolysis of aspirin, can synthesize prostanoids and these newly formed metabolites of AA can cause aggregation of aspirin exposed platelets. In view of the fact that aspirin irreversibly inhibits prostaglandin synthase, it is possible to take advantage of repeated low-dose aspirin to achieve a cumulative effect [42-55]. Even doses as low as 30-50 mg aspirin taken daily will suppress platelet thromboxane synthesis significantly in 5 to 10 days.

Vascular tissues on the other hand have the ability to resynthesize prostaglandin G/H synthase [36]. Therefore, these cells can recover the enzyme activity following aspirin exposure. It is therefore, possible to develop a strategy to promote the biochemical selectivity of aspirin in terms of inhibition of platelet prostaglandin synthase. This is done by modification of the drug delivery, so the amount of drug delivered is just enough to inhibit platelet enzymes in the peripheral circulation and spare the systemic effect on vascular endothelium [37, 38]. Several studies have demonstrated the feasibility of this approach and various control release or timed release formulations have been developed for this novel therapy [37-39].

As mentioned earlier, aspirin is metabolized rapidly and the major metabolite, salicylic acid is a poor inhibitor of platelet prostaglandin synthase. Therefore, it is essential to develop appropriate strategies to maximize the beneficial effect of this novel drug. As low dose as 20 mg taken daily, reduces the platelet thromboxane formation by more than 90 percent. However, it is generally believed that higher doses are essential for preventing thromboxane dependent platelet activation. Studies by Wilson et al demonstrated that maximal plasma concentration of 12umol/L could be achieved by a single oral 50 mg dose of enteric-coated aspirin [17]. This dose was found sufficient to cause significant inhibition of platelet function and daily ingestion of low-dose aspirin demonstrated a cumulative effect. In a separate study, McLeod et al used doses ranging from 50-3900 mg of aspirin and monitored platelet function, bleeding time, and concluded that maximum dysfunction was obtained with daily doses of about 100 mg and no further changes were observed in these studies with higher doses [18]. Several workers have demonstrated the efficacy of low-dose oral aspirin in preventing platelet thromboxane production [2-4, 18, 44]. Indeed one of these studies has demonstrated beneficial effect of a dermal aspirin preparation on selective inhibition of platelet prostaglandin synthase, sparing the prostacyclin biosynthesis (38). It is very well established that 100 mg of aspirin per day is sufficient to significantly reduce the platelet thromboxane production [2-4, 20, 21, 40-42]. Furthermore, studies by McLeod et al have shown that dosages higher than 100 mg per day do not produce any greater inhibition of platelet function or enhance bleeding times [18]. Therefore, it is reasonable to conclude that 80-160 mgs aspirin per day should be the choice for an ideal preventive protocol [41]. However, there is considerable room for improvement to maximize the benefits by better understanding the pharmacology of aspirin and platelet physiology [2-4]. It is possible to customize the aspirin treatment based on the individual patient needs. One can monitor the platelet prostaglandin synthase activity following aspirin ingestion and recommend a dose that is appropriate [34, 41]. It is possible to monitor the platelet response to agonists such as ADP or arachidonate and determine the degree of inhibition by aspirin like compounds [18]. In order to get maximum inhibition of platelet COX1 enzymes, continuous release aspirin formulations can be developed and tested against currently available aspirin formulations. Platelets are produced and released constantly to the circulation. Therefore, a time release aspirin which would make available small amounts of aspirin into the circulation may be effective. For instance, a 100 mg formulation capable of releasing 10 mg acetyl salicylic acid per hour may be better than a preparation which releases all of its active principle in a short span of time. Using the strategy of slowing down the release of active principle, newer formulations could be used effectively, to provide needed amounts of the drug into circulating blood at regular intervals. These novel formulations may also provide selectivity of aspirin action by preventing platelet thromboxane production and sparing the endothelial prostacylcin synthesis. McLeod et al studied the effect of various doses of aspirin (50, 100, 325, 1000 mg) on platelet and vascular tissues [43]. They did not observe inhibition of urinary 6-keto-PGF1 alpha production at low doses of 50 and 100 mg. They attributed these findings to the differential and selective inhibition of platelet function and the sparring effect of vascular COX1 enzymes. Sullivan and associates studied the effect of two different doses of aspirin on platelet function and TXA_2 production [45]. Platelet function in healthy volunteers was inhibited by both the doses (75 and 300 mg). Low dose failed to inhibit completely TXB_2 production 24 hours later, whereas 300 mg aspirin did. Even alternate day regimen of these doses prevented platelet function and significantly inhibited the urinary levels of the 11-keto-TXB_2. In a separate study, in healthy volunteers, formation of thrombin (Fibrinopeptide A; FPA), alpha granule release (beta-thromboglobulin; beta TG), and thromboxane (TXB_2) were monitored in vivo, in blood emerging from a template bleeding incision [46]. At the site of plug formation significant platelet activation and thrombin generation was observed as indicated by 110 fold, 50 fold, and 30 fold increase in FPA, beta TG, and TXB_2, within the first minute. A low dose regimen (0.42m/kg/day for 7 days) caused greater than 90% inhibition of TXB_2 formation in both bleeding time and clotted blood in these studies, suggesting critical role of platelet activation at the site of haemostatic plug formation. In a study to evaluate the effect of low dose aspirin (0.5and 15 mg/kg/day) on platelet and renal prostanoids, Wilson et al monitored serum TXB_2 and urinary 6-keto PGF1 alpha [47]. Serum TXB_2 level was reduced to 3% of control by low dose and to 0.1% by the higher dose.

Urinary TXB_2 was reduced only to 68% by low dose aspirin and to 51% by high dose. Urinary 6-keto-PGF1 alpha was not reduced by either dose. Based on their observation, they concluded low dose aspirin could significantly affect platelet PG production without affecting stimulated release of PGI_2 production.

Clinical Studies on the Use of Aspirin

The two major clinical trials on aspirin concluded that ingestion of 160 mg per day or 325 mg alternative day provided significant benefit in preventing fatal events associated with CAD [20, 21]. Whereas, a 10 year trial involving nearly 40,000 women aged 45 and older with no evidence of cardiovascular disease found that a regular alternate day low-dose (100mg) aspirin was effective in reducing the incidence of stroke, but it did not have any effect on the incidence of heart attacks [48]. They concluded that the reasons for any sex-based differences in the efficacy of aspirin for primary prevention are unclear. According to Minnesota Heart Survey, about 6% of healthy women under age 65 and 30% of those over 65 take low-dose aspirin to prevent acute vascular events. Data from this primary prevention study dose not apply to women who already have had a heart attack or heart surgery or diagnosed with coronary artery disease. For such women, as found in men, regular daily low dose (80-160mg) of aspirin clearly reduces the risk of developing acute coronary events.

Several earlier studies evaluated the effect of low dose aspirin on normal healthy volunteers as well as patients with various vascular diseases [45-58]. However, earlier studies did not report prevalence of any aspirin resistance. Zucker et al evaluated the effect of low dose aspirin (0.45mg/kg/day) and a high dose (900mg/day) in type 11 hyper-lipoproteinemic subjects [49]. They found that low dose aspirin effectively inhibited platelet function in these patients. Increased platelet thromboxane production has been described in several disorders including type-2 diabetes and type 11a hypercholesterolemia. This increased production of TXB_2 in hyper-cholesterolemic patients is attributed to abnormal cholesterol levels in these patients. It has been shown that even a low dose of aspirin (50 mg/7 days) significantly reduces 11-dehydro-TXB_2, in these patients [50]. The effect of low dose aspirin has been evaluated in patients with diabetes, coronary heart disease, myocardial infarction (MI), cerebrovascular disease, peripheral artery disease and a variety of surgical procedures [45-58]. Diminno et al studied the effect of single doses of 100 and 1000 mg aspirin for 1 month in normal volunteers and patients with diabetic angiopathy [51]. They found a dose schedule of aspirin, which may suffice in normal volunteers, was not effective in patients with diabetic angiopathy. Contrary to this observation, Terres et al found a low dose of aspirin (100mg) caused significant inhibition of platelet function in both healthy subjects and patients with coronary heart disease [52]. Similarly, a low dose (0.45mg/kg/day) was found adequate for selective inhibition of TXA_2-related platelet function, in patients recovering from MI [53]. Looks like the results on the effect of low-dose aspirin vary considerably, depending upon the type and stage of disease, dose of aspirin, and severity of procedure. In a study evaluating the effect of low dose aspirin (100mg) on hematological activity of left ventricular (LV) thrombus in anterior wall acute MI (AMI), Kupper et al found that low-dose had no effect on the incidence of hematologic activity and embolic potential of LV thrombosis in anterior wall AMI [54]. On the other hand, a low dose aspirin (40mg/day) taken daily was found to be as effective as higher doses in preventing platelet functional responses in patients who had recent cerebral ischemia [55]. Uchiyama et al evaluated the effect of low dose aspirin, ticlopidine, and a combination of both these drugs in patients with cerebral ischemia [56]. Aspirin alone markedly inhibited platelet aggregation induced by AA, partially inhibited aggregation induced by ADP and did not inhibit aggregation by platelet activating factor. Combination of these drugs inhibited aggregation by all agonists. Rao et al demonstrated, in healthy volunteers, low doses of aspirin (40-80mg) had no inhibitory effect on the response of platelets to ADP, epinephrine and thrombin, but effectively inhibited the platelet response to threshold concentrations of AA [3, 4]. Epinephrine at concentrations too low to cause aggregation restored the sensitivity of aspirin-treated platelets to AA [59-61]. This phenomenon, in which weak agonists restore the sensitivity of drug-induced refractory platelets to the action of other agonists, was described from our laboratory as "mechanism of membrane modulation" [58-65].

ASPIRIN RESISTANCE

Studies from our laboratory for the first time demonstrated that one could induce drug-mediated resistance in platelets to the action of aspirin [66]. In this study, the subjects were given a short acting inhibitor of COX1, Ibuprofen. This was followed by administration of a full strength (325mg) aspirin. Ibuprofen-mediated inhibition of COX1 enzyme lasts for a short time, whereas, aspirin induced inhibition is irreversible. Ibuprofen treated platelets recovered their sensitivity to the action of AA by 24 hrs. Whereas, aspirin treated platelets failed to respond to the action of AA even after 24 hrs. In those subjects who had ingested aspirin after taking Ibuprofen first, aspirin failed to inhibit irreversibly the COX1; suggesting Ibuprofen molecules effectively prevented the acetylation of COX1enzyme by aspirin. One of the earliest work describing "non-responders" and "responders" evaluated the effect of low dose aspirin and a thromboxane synthetase inhibitor dazoxiben (UK3724B) in healthy subjects [57]. These studies demonstrated that low dose aspirin and ingestion of two dazoxiben tablets prevented the release of granules from platelets in response to AA in some individuals (responders) and not in others (non-responders). These subtle differences in response of platelets to various drugs as well as differences in response to various agonists may be critical when considering the outcome of acute vascular events. For instance, collagen seems to exert its effect by multiple mechanisms. In a study, using aspirin, monoclonal antibodies to 11b-111a receptor and fibrinogen, it was demonstrated that there exists at least three mechanisms by which collagen activates platelets; 1) GP11b-111a associated activation, 2) prostaglandin dependent pathway, 3) alternate pathway responsible for 20-30% platelet aggregation [67].

Although it is well known that there are individual differences in response to drugs as well as agonists, this subject has not been studied thoroughly. Studies from Harvard researchers have demonstrated that the onset of myocardial infarction and sudden death is frequently triggered in early hours of the day. Aspirin and beta adrenergic blocking agents have been shown to prevent morning onset of acute vascular events [68]. In a limited chronobiologic study (n=7) on the efficacy of low-dose aspirin, international womb-to-tomb chronome initiative group demonstrated, that aspirin was more effective in the early hours of the day than late in the afternoon or evening [69, 70] Influence of dietary components and supplements on the efficacy of anti-platelet drugs also is poorly understood. Vitamin E and its quinone are potent inhibitors of platelet function and interfere with the release of arachidonic acid by cell membranes [71, 72]. Studies from our laboratory have demonstrated that heme chelators, non-steroid anti-inflammatory drugs, antioxidants such as butylated hydorxytoulene, butyalted hydroxyanisole and fish lipids compete with arachidonic acid metabolism and prevent the formation of pro-aggregatory PG metabolites [71-74]. Docosahexaenoic acid (DHA) is poorly metabolized by Cox-1 enzymes. However, *in vitro* studies have demonstrated that DHA is a potent inhibitor of AA metabolism and platelet function [74]. Eicosapenaenoic acid, oleic acid, linoleic acid, linolenic acid competitively inhibit COX1 enzymes in in *vitro* studies. We do not know very much about the influence of dietary lipids on AA metabolism by platelets.

Several recent studies have demonstrated drug resistance in patients with a variety of vascular diseases [75-118]. This subject currently is a very hot topic and has made national headlines. Andrew Pollack published an article in July of 2004 in New York Times, on this subject titled, “For Some, Aspirin May Not Help Hearts” [75]. According to this article, 5-40% of aspirin users are “non-responders” or “resistant” to the drug. In the same article, he cites the opinion of Dr. Daniel I. Simon, the associate director of interventional cardiology at Brigham and Women’s Hospital, Boston, which reads as follows: “They are taking it for stroke and heart attack prevention and it’s not going to work”. He also reports the opinion of Dr. Michael J. Domanski; head of clinical trials unit at the NIH, in his opinion, the non-responders may represent a huge number of patients. According to Dr. Deepak L. Bhatt, director of interventional cardiology Cleveland Clinic, aspirin resistance is associated with worst outcome. Professor Eric Topol, Chairman, Cardiovascular Medicine Cleveland Clinic, USA states, “Aspirin resistance carries high risk, with over 20 million Americans taking aspirin to prevent heart attacks or strokes, it is important that further work to be done to confirm our findings and develop a rapid detection method. He also assures that for individuals with aspirin resistance, there are excellent alternatives”.

These observances from health care providers and researchers raise number of issues. Do we know enough about aspirin resistance? What is the prevalence of aspirin resistance in healthy population? What causes this resistance to develop in patient populations? Are there specific, rapid, cost-effective tests available? What alternative long-term treatments are available, if patients are resistant to common anti-platelet drugs such as aspirin and Clopidogrel? Should the doses of these drugs used for therapy be increased? Should we drop the use of these drugs in non-responders? We need to find answers to these and other emerging questions soon. In the next few paragraphs a brief overview of what is known about the prevalence of aspirin resistance, clinical findings, and methodologies available, will be provided.

The first and foremost need at this time is to standardize a definition of aspirin resistance. The mechanism of action of aspirin is very well documented [7-13]. The drug acetylates the platelet COX1 enzyme and irreversibly inhibits its ability to convert AA to PG endoperoxides [12, 13]. In the absence of COX1 enzyme activity, platelets do not respond to AA stimulation with aggregation. Weak agonists such as ADP, Epinephrine depend on the formation of PG endoperoxides to initiate secondary wave of aggregation and promote release of platelet granule contents [3]. Therefore, weak agonists fail to induce platelet aggregation and release granules from aspirin-treated platelets. Failure of AA, ADP and Epinephrine to cause aggregation of platelets more or less establishes drug-induced platelet dysfunction. If platelets obtained from individuals who have ingested a full strength aspirin, respond with aggregation to the action AA, ADP and EPI, and release their granule contents, then one can safely conclude that these platelets are resistant to aspirin action. Further proof for aspirin resistance of platelets can be provided by studying AA metabolism by such platelets, monitoring serum TXB_2 levels, or urinary levels of TXB_2 or its metabolite, 11-dehydro-TXB_2. Methods are available to monitor all these parameters. According to Cattaneo, "aspirin resistant" should be considered as description for those individuals whom aspirin fails to inhibit thromboxane A2 production, irrespective of the results of unspecific tests of platelet function [110].

PREVALENCE OF ASPIRIN RESISTANCE

Aspirin resistance has been poorly defined, variety of non-specific methods have been employed to monitor the "aspirin resistance" and conflicting reports have been published on the rates of prevalence and outcome of continuing this therapeutic modality [75-93]. Aspirin resistance has been reported in patients with cardiovascular, cerebrovascular, and peripheral vascular disease [75-93]. Because of the differences in methodologies used to monitor this phenomenon and lack of a specific assay to determine the true aspirin resistance, there is considerable confusion and the true significance of this observation remains obscure [76- 78]. It also raises the question, as to how we missed this phenomenon of drug resistance all these years? Large numbers of clinical trials have demonstrated the beneficial effects of aspirin therapy irrespective of the disease state [40]. Is it possible that these earlier trials missed aspirin non-responders? On the other hand, it is quite possible that only responders to the action of aspirin got the benefit of this therapy.

Studies in our laboratory over three decades, have failed to show any aspirin resistance in normal healthy subjects. The only subject whose platelets failed to aggregate in response to AA stimulation was found to be deficient in platelet COX1enzyme activity [60]. Platelets obtained from this subject responded with aggregation when stirred with epinephrine and arachidonate, suggesting PG endoperoxides and TAX_2 are not essential to cause irreversible aggregation of platelets. There is not much data on the prevalence of aspirin resistance in general healthy subjects. In patients with various vascular diseases, the rate of non-responders reported varies between less than 2% to over 60%. Since the methods used to monitor aspirin resistance in these reports are not specific, the prevalence rate published is debatable [75-93].

Hurlen et al used the method of Wu and Hoak to determine the platelet aggregation ratio as a marker for assessing platelet function and evaluated the effect of aspirin (160mg/day) in 143 patients who had survived myocardial infarction [80, 81]. Based on their definition of non-responders to the action of aspirin, they could only identify two subjects as primary non-responders. Gum et al from Cleveland Clinic studied 326 stable cardiovascular subjects on aspirin (325mg/day) and tested aspirin sensitivity by platelet response to aggregating agents such as ADP and AA. They found 5.5% as non-responders to aspirin and 24% as semi-responders [82]. Gum and associates used the PFA-100, a method that measures platelet function, to determine aspirin resistance in their patient population [83]. Based on the results of their studies with this methodology, they found 9.5% to be non-responders to aspirin action.

Some studies have reported as high as 30-40% non-responders of stroke or vascular disease patients and predicted >80% increase risk for a repeat event during a 2-year follow up period [84-88]. Eikelboom et al analyzed base line urinary levels of TXB2 metabolites 11-dehydro thromboxane B2 in 5529 patients enrolled in the Heart Outcomes Prevention Evaluation (HOPE) study [88]. Of these subjects 488 were on aspirin regimen. On the basis of their findings they concluded that in aspirin-treated patients, increased levels of urinary metabolite of TXB_2 predict future risk of myocardial infarction or cardiovascular death. The patients with the highest levels of urinary TXB_2 metabolite had 3-5 fold higher risk of cardiovascular death compared to those in the lowest quartile. Another study reporting clinical outcomes of aspirin resistance is from Austria [85, 87, 90]. In this study patients undergoing arterial angioplasty were on 100 mg aspirin per day. Platelet function was assessed by whole blood aggregometry. This study demonstrated that reocculsion at the sites of angioplasty occurred only in men for whom platelet dysfunction was evident by aggregometry [87]. Zimmerman et al identified aspirin non-responders as those who had >90% inhibition of TXB_2 formation in presence of 100umol/L aspirin and 1mmol/L arachidonate [91]. In patients who had undergone coronary bypass surgery (CABG), AA and Collagen stimulated formation of TXB_2 was same before and after CABG, indicating oral aspirin did not significantly inhibit platelet COX1. However, the *in vitro* studies with 100umol/L aspirin on blood obtained from these subjects showed decreased TXB_2 (>10%) in most samples studied. They concluded that platelet COX1 inhibition by aspirin is compromised for several days after CABG, probably due to an impaired interaction between aspirin and platelet COX1. This observation indicates how complex the issues are when evaluating the effect of anti-platelet drugs during and after interventional procedures. Sane et al evaluated the effect of aspirin (325 mg/day/month) in patients suffering from congestive heart failure [92]. These researchers used whole blood aggregometry (Chronolog Corp, PA., USA), Platelet receptor expression by flow cytometry and PFA-100. Patients were considered non-responders when 4 of the 5 parameters assayed were observed. Using this complex rating, persistent platelet activation was observed in 50 of the 88 patients (56.8%). These observations remind us of the inadequacy of the existing methods to detect what truly represents "aspirin resistance".

Clopidogrel Resistance

Muller et al have reported prevalence of Clopidogrel "non-responders" among patients with stable angina scheduled for coronary stent replacement [93]. They evaluated the effect of 100mg/day aspirin with a loading dose of 600mg of Clopidogrel. They defined Clopidogrel non-responders by an inhibition of ADP (5and 30umol/L) induced platelet aggregation to less than 10% of base line values after the ingestion of the drug. They found 5-11% of the patients as non-responders and 9-26% semi-responders. Lau et al studied both normal subjects and patients undergoing stent replacement to determine the prevalence of drug resistance [94]. Since Clopidogrel is activated by hepatic cytochrome P450 (CYP) 3A4, they monitored the activity of this enzyme in both the test subjects. They concluded that some patients are resistant to these drugs because of biological variability and drug-drug interactions. They also attributed the difference due to variations in (CYP) 3A4 activity. Angiolillo et al compared the effect of standard dose of 300mg with a high dose of 600mg Clopidogrel after coronary stenting [95]. They concluded that use of higher dose optimizes platelet inhibitory effects. Serebruany et al evaluated the effect of Clopidogrel in a large heterogenous population using ex vivo measurements of platelet aggregation [96], Prevalence of hypo-responsiveness and hyper-responsiveness to Clopidogrel in these patient population was 4.2% and 4.8% respectively. A Polish study with a small sample size (n=31) studied the effect of Clopidogrel (300) in patients with stable angina using a rapid whole blood platelet function assessment [97]. They conclude that the clinical importance of Clopidogrel resistance is still debatable. In view of the fact that data are not available on large number of clinical trials, their conclusion is reasonable.

METHODOLOGIES

Researchers have used a variety of methods to assess the aspirin and Clopidogrel resistance [81-98]. In spite of the inherent problems associated with platelet aggregometry, it still is the gold standard to detect aspirin sensitivity of platelets. Studies from our laboratory and that of others have shown even low doses (40-80 mg) of aspirin effectively inhibit arachidonate-mediated platelet aggregation. In the absence of any other specific rapid Point-of-Care assay system for detecting the sensitivity of platelets to aspirin or lack of aspirin sensitivity, it is preferable to use optical whole blood aggregometry to validate the results obtained by other methods. Hurlen et al used platelet aggregate ratio (PAR) to evaluate the effect of aspirin in post-MI patients [80]. Basically the method developed by Wu and Hoak uses a ratio of platelets obtained with EDTA/formalin as anti-coagulants and comparing the counts of platelets obtained with EDTA [80, 81]. In the presence of platelet aggregates the ratio is <1.0. Using this method they found two individuals as primary non-responders and 14 patients as secondary non-responders.

Several researchers have used Platelet Function Analyzer PFA-100 (Dade International Inc, Miami USA), to evaluate aspirin resistance in patients with various vascular diseases [83, 92, 101, 103, 104, 113, 119]. This analyzer measures platelet function as their ability to occlude a membrane coated with collagen and epinephrine (EPI) or collagen and ADP under high shear stress. Sambola et al evaluated the effect of low dose aspirin (100mg/day/1month, 6month) in 100 patients with acute coronary syndrome [101]. At one-month post-aspirin therapy, they found 49 patients to have sub-optimal response to aspirin (SASAR), whereas only 25 of them showed SASAR by conventional aggregometry. Anderson et al evaluated the effect of 75 mg aspirin in patients (n=202) with MI. In patients on aspirin alone they found 25/71 as non-responders with the epinephrine cartridge. They did not find a significant difference between EPI cartridge and ADP cartridge. Gum et al. evaluated the phenomenon of aspirin resistance in 325 stable cardiac patients [83]. They found 5 per cent were non-responders and 23 per cent semi-responders by optical aggregometry. Whereas, using PFA-100 they found 9.5% as aspirin resistant. This detection system does not seem to detect difference between the effects of low and high-dose aspirin on platelet function. Since it evaluates the synergistic effect of a combination of two agonists on platelet function, the results obtained or similar to that obtained in our aggregation studies [58-66]. In a series of studies we have demonstrated a combination of two agonists overcomes the inhibition by aspirin and other drugs [58-66].

Malinin et al used THE Ultegra RPFA-ASA (VerifyNow; Accumetrics, Inc., San Diego, California, USA) to monitor the effect of a single dose of aspirin (325 mg) in subjects with multiple risk factors [100]. This system uses turbidometric optical detection system. It uses a test cartridge that contains lyophilized preparation of human fibrinogen-coated beads, platelet agonist, and buffer. Fibrinogen-coated beads bind available receptor on platelet membrane. A cationic agonist, propyl gallate, is used to obtain complete activation of platelets. It uses citrated whole blood for assays. The results are expressed in aspirin response units (ARU). Of the 14 subjects studied, only one was found to be non-responsive by aggregometry, whereas they found 10 subjects as non-responders by RPFA-ASA. They concluded this system was a sensitive device for measuring anti-platelet responsiveness. Newly introduced "VerifyNow" kit includes arachidonic acid as an agonist for activating platelets. Inclusion of this agonist instead of propyl gallate has considerably improved the performance of this system. In our hands, this system is as good as whole blood aggregometry (Chronolog Corporation) in identifying aspirin non-responders.

Aspirin resistance could be monitored by a variety of assays, including platelet aggregometry, PAR, PFA100, RPFA-ASA; plasma, serum, urinary TXB_2 and urinary 11-dehryothromboxane-2 [46, 47, 80-84, 87, 88, 92, 95, 98, 100]. We use majority of these methods to validate data in our efforts to develop a rapid, specific Point-of-Care assay system, for monitoring platelet function. Majority of these methods are labor intensive, time consuming and expensive. Technologies are available to develop a rapid and specific assay system, which can monitor platelet function. Specific fluorescent antibodies can be used to detect platelet bound fibrinogen, P-selectin or released granule products such as beta-thromboglobulin, platelet factor 4 and soluble P-selectin. Furthermore, ATP release or thromboxane generated also could be easily monitored. All the available methods use large quantities of blood and take considerable amount of time. It is possible to device methods that use only small quantities of blood obtained from a finger stick. By using state-of-the-art detectors one could detect the luminescence (ATP) or fluorescence (specific antibodies) in minutes and develop needed software to standardize the results. If the assay uses AA as standard platelet agonist then specificity could be built into this system for monitoring aspirin sensitivity. Similarly by using ADP as agonist one can build the needed specificity to monitor non-responders to Clopidogrel. The limiting factors for non-availability of such a Point-of-Care assay system are lack of funds and the assumption that currently available methods detect platelet sensitivity or otherwise to anti-platelet drugs effectively.

Discussion

Aspirin is the most-effective, widely used, relatively inexpensive anti-platelet drug currently available. In the developing countries, aspirin is the most cost-effective drug for primary as well as secondary prophylaxis for platelet-mediated vascular complications [3-5]. The mechanism by which it inhibits platelet function is well documented [7-14]. Many large clinical trials have established beyond any doubt that aspirin therapy significantly reduces the incidence of acute events in a variety of vascular diseases [40]. Recent studies have provided evidence to suggest that some sub-population of patients on aspirin therapy may have developed resistance to the action of aspirin [75-98]. These observations have raised alarm in the public as to who is getting protection and who is not? Since there is no simple test that can be performed at the doctor's office to detect such a condition there is some panic in the patient population. Furthermore, there is still lack of awareness of this problem in the medical community at the time of this writing. There are only two major studies, which have described adverse outcome in those patients who are defined as non-responders to the action of aspirin [83, 88].

Based on methods, which still are not very specific, researchers have identified a sub-population of patients who are considered non-responders and another group as semi-responders to the action of aspirin [82-98]. Although the majority of methods used for monitoring this phenomenon lack specificity, it is important to recognize that this problem exists. If these patients for whatever reason are not getting appropriate protection from drug therapy, there is an immediate need to identify them and change their therapeutic regimen. It is equally important to recognize that even those who are considered responders, may need additional protection to prevent adverse out comes, if they have hyper-responsive platelets or hyper-responsive coagulation pathways. Basically, we need to identify aspirin non-responders, individuals with hyperactive platelets/coagulation pathways.

Subject of aspirin resistance has received lot of attention in the press and scientific publications (75-98). However, the practicing physicians and the pubic are not fully aware of the problem. Therefore, there is an immediate need for the development of awareness programs to educate the health care providers as well as the public who receive health care. Since there is considerable interest in this subject in the research community, a number of reviews have been published on this subject [75-98]. No attempt has been made in this article to extensively review this subject. Focus of this article has been to bring into discussion three specific areas of concern. First and foremost is the molecular mechanism involved in the initiation of thrombosis and stroke. Basically two major pathways (platelet activation dependent and coagulation cascade activation dependent) play a role in the pathophysiology of this process. Therefore, there is a need to identify the hyper-responsiveness of individuals to both these pathways and develop appropriate combination therapy. Secondly, arachidonic acid pathway blocks only one of the many mechanisms modulating platelet activation. Therefore, there is an immediate need to develop appropriate drugs or drug combinations to prevent the common pathway of platelet activation. Since fibrinogen binding to activated GP 11b/111a receptor promotes thrombus formation and growth, drugs should be designed and developed to modulate these mechanisms. Third, there is a need for better Point-of-Care assays, which can profile the coagulation pathway as well as platelet activation mechanisms. Such an assay system could be effective in identifying non-responders to commonly used anti-platelet drugs, semi responders or hyper responsive individuals and those with hyper coagulable states. Since there is no such detection system a lot of individuals at risk are not getting appropriate treatment or prophylaxis against acute vascular events.

In the early 80s, based on our extensive studies, we concluded that aspirin and other anti-platelet drugs do not prevent platelet activation under a variety of experimental conditions [58-66]. Aspirin only inhibits one of the many platelet activation mechanisms. Furthermore, it does not prevent platelet interaction with vessel wall [63]. However, in large number of clinical studies, aspirin has been shown to offer significant beneficial effect to patients with various vascular diseases [40]. Several recent studies have demonstrated that there exists some degree of non-responders to the action of aspirin [75-98]. Therefore, it is of great importance to thoroughly examine this issue of drug resistance and determine the prevalence of true “aspirin resistance” among the patients and provide them alternate therapies. Since our studies have clearly demonstrated epinephrine, nor-epinephrine, and ADP can potentiate the action of other agonists on platelets, we may as well screen those who are hyper responsive to various agonists, so that these individuals also could be provided appropriate therapeutic regimen. There are reports suggesting those who are non-responders to the action of aspirin may be more responsive to the action of agonists such as ADP or collagen. Studies should take into consideration that platelets can be stimulated by a variety of soluble agonists as well as cell matrix components and increased shear stress.

In spite of the fact that several attempts have been made to explain the mechanisms involved in aspirin resistance, there exists no clear explanation. Studies should be initiated immediately to explore the mechanism by which an individual develops resistance to these drugs. Since platelets lack DNA, it is highly unlikely that these cells re-synthesize COX1 enzyme. Since many of these patients are on long-term aspirin therapy the effect of aspirin on megakaryocytes should be further explored. Platelets are formed from megakaryocytes and these cells do have DNA, hence studies are warranted to explore the effect of aspirin on bone marrow megakaryocytes. Majority of patients with vascular disease also will be taking many other drugs. As such, some amount of drug-drug interaction cannot be ruled out. Whatever may be the mechanism by which individuals with vascular disease develop resistance to aspirin, a better understanding of the molecular mechanisms involved will facilitate the development of appropriate therapeutic regimen.

Now that anti-platelet drug resistance has surfaced out and created concern in the clinical community, there will be renewed interest in the devise development, for improving the available technologies for monitoring platelet and coagulation pathways [75-118] Chronolog corporation, one of the leaders in developing optical aggregometers, has already come up with a less expensive whole-blood aggregometer for monitoring aspirin resistance. Accumetric system has recently introduced arachidonic acid as a stimulant instead of propyl gallate, for monitoring aspirin resistance. Similarly research and development work is going to improve the PAF-100 system as well, for monitoring aspirin resistance. Currently available data on the use of PFA-100 to monitor aspirin resistance is inconclusive. A large study using 1000 patients is in progress to evaluate the applicability of PFA-100 to monitor drug resistance [119]. Results from this study may shed some light on the useful ness of this detection system. All the currently available methodologies require relatively large quantities of fresh blood. Platelet function assays are labor intensive, non-specific and time consuming. Future direction of research will focus on the development of rapid, specific, Point-of-Care assays using minimal amounts of blood from a finger stick, for monitoring platelet function as well as coagulation profile.

Conclusion

Platelets play a very important role in the pathogenesis of atherosclerosis, thrombosis and stroke. Aspirin, even at a low to medium dose (80-160mg/day) has been shown to offer significant protection to individuals from developing acute vascular events. Aspirin is the most cost-effective drug available for the secondary prophylaxis of cardiovascular diseases. From the available evidence both experimental and clinical, it is reasonable to conclude, that significant number of patients are not getting full protection from the use of aspirin. Even those who are considered responders to aspirin therapy may need additional protection, if their platelets are hypersensitive or have a hyper-responsive coagulation pathway. Since currently available methods to assess aspirin sensitivity are not specific, labor intensive and time consuming; efforts should be made to develop specific, rapid, detection methods. Serious attempts should be made to develop state-of-the-art Point-of-Care assay systems, which are capable of detecting not only individuals who develop resistance to currently available anti-platelet drugs but also those, who are hyper-responsive to both platelet and coagulation activation mechanisms.

REFERENCES

[1] Sherry S, Scriabine *A. Platelets and Thrombosis*. University Press, USA 1999. P.309

[2] Suldow C, Baigent C. Randomized Trials of Antiplatelet Therapy. *Handbook of Platelet Physiology and Pharmacology*. Rao GHR, (ed) Kluwer Academic Publishers, USA1999, p526-549.

[3] Rao GHR, Rao AT. Pharmacology of Platelet Inhibitory Drugs. *Ind. J. Physiol.*19994, 38:69-84.

[4] Rao GHR, Rao ASC, White JG. Aspirin in Ischemic Heart Disease-an overview. *Ind. Heart J.*1993, 45: 73-79.

[5] Rao GHR. Aspirin and Coronary Artery Disease: Coronary Artery Disease in South Asians: Epidemiology, Risk Factors and Prevention. Rao GHR, Kakkar VV(eds), *Jaypee Medical Publishers*, India, 2001, p263-278.

[6] Weisman G. Aspirin. *Sci Am.*1991, 264: 84-91.

[7] Vane JR. Inhibition of prostaglandin synthesis as a mechanism of action of aspirin-like drugs. *Nature* 1971, 231: 232-235.

[8] Vane JR, Flower RJ, Botting RM. History of aspirin and its mechanism of action. *Stroke* 1990, 21: IV-12.

[9] Ferreira SH, Vane JR. Newer aspects of the mode of action of non-steroidal anti-inflammatory drugs. *Ann. Rev. Pharmacol.* 1974, 14: 57-73.

[10] Hamberg M, Svensson J Samuelsson B. Thromboxanes: A new group of biologically active compounds derived from prostaglandin endoperoxides. *Proc. Natl. Acad. Sci.* 1975, 72:2994-2998.

[11] Marcus AJ. Aspirin as an anti-thrombotic medication. *N. Engl. J. Med.* 1983, 309: 1515-1517.

[12] Roth JG, Caverley DC. Aspirin, Platelets and Thrombosis: Theory and Practice. *Blood* 1994, 83: 885-898.

[13] Roth JG: Stanford N, Majerus PW. Acetylation of prostaglandin synthetase by aspirin. *Proc. Natl. Acad. Sci.* 1975, 72: 3073-3076.

[14] Meade EA, Smith WL, Dewitt DL: Differential inhibition of prostaglandin endoperoxide syhthase (cyclooxygenase) isoenzymes by aspirin and other non-steroidal anti-inflammatory drugs. *J. Biol. Chem.* 1993, 268: 6610-6614.

[15] Burch JW, Stanford N, Majerus PW. Inhibition of platelets prostaglandin synthetase by oral aspirin. *J. Clin. Invest* 1978: 61: 314-319.

[16] Reilly IA, FitzGerald GA. Aspirin in Cardiovascular Disease. *Drugs* 1988, 35: 154-176.

[17] Wilson KM, Siebert DM, Duncan EM. et al. Effect of aspirin infusions on platelet function in humans. *Clin. Sci.* 1990, 79: 37-42.

[18] McLeod LJ, Roberts MS, Cossum PA. et al. The effects of different doses of some acetyl salicylic acid formulations on platelet function and bleeding times in healthy subjects. *J. Haematol.* 1986, 36: 379-384.

[19] Masptti G, Galanti G, Pogessi L. Differential inhibition of prostacyclin production and platelet aggregation by aspirin. *Lancet* 1972, 2:11213-1216.

[20] Steering Committee of the Physicians Health Study Research Group. Preliminary Report: Findings from the aspirin component of the ongoing physicians' health study. *N. Engl. J. Med.* 1988, 318: 262-264.

[21] Steering Committee of the Physicians Health Study Research Group. Final Report. *N. Engl. J. Med.* 1989, 321: 129-135.

[22] Hallam TJ, Sanchez A, Rink TJ. Stimulus response coupling in Platelets. *Biochem J.* 1984, 218:819-827.

[23] Zucker MB Nachmias VT. Platelet Activation. *Arteriosclerosis*. 1985, 5:2-18.

[24] Edridge MJ. The molecular basis of communication within the cells. *Sci. Am* 1985, 253:142-152.

[25] Holmsen H. Platelet metabolism and activation. *Semin Hematol.* 1985, 22:219-240.

[26] Seiss W. Molecular mechanism of platelet activation. *Physiol. Rev.*1990, 70:115-164.

[27] Rao, GHR. Physiology of blood platelet activation. *Ind J Physiol Pharmacol.* 1993, 37:263-275.

[28] Rao, GHR. Signal transduction, second messengers and platelet function. *J Lab Clin Med.* 1993, 121:18-21.

[29] Rao, GHR. Signal transduction, second messengers and platelet pharmacology. *Pharmacol.* 1994,13:39-44.

[30] Packham MA. Role of platelets in thrombosis and hemostasis. *Can J Physiol. Pharmacol.* 1993, 72:278-284.

[31] Rao GHR, Gerrard JM, Eaton JW, White JG. The role of iron in prostaglandin synthesis: Ferrous iron mediated oxidation of arachidonic acid. *Prost and Med* 1978, 1: 55-70.

[32] Peterson DA, Gerrard JM, Rao GHR, Mills EL, White JG. Interaction of arachidonic acid and heme iron in the synthesis of prostaglandins. *Adv Prost and Thromb Res* 1980, 6; 157-161.

[33] Peterson DA, Gerrard JM, Rao GHR, White JG. Inhibition of ferrous iron induced oxidation of arachidonic acid by indomethacin. *Prost and Med* 1979, 2: 97-108.

[34] Rao GHR, Cox AC, Gerrard JM, White JG. Effects of 2,2' dipyrydil and related compounds on platelet prostaglandin synthesis and platelet function. *Biochem Biphys Acta* 1980, 628: 468-479.

[35] Rao GHR, Johnson GJ, Reddy KR. Ibuprofen protects cyclooxygenase from irreversible inhibition by aspirin. *Arteriosclerosis* 1983, 3: 384-388.

[36] Patrono C. Aspirin as an antiplatelet drug. *N Engl. J Med* 1994, 330: 1287-1294.

[37] Hanley SP, Cockbill SR, Bevan J. et al. Differential inhibition by low-dose aspirin of human venous prostacyclin synthesis and platelet thromboxane synthesis. *Lancet* 1981, 2: 969-971.

[38] Keimowitz RM, Pulvermacher G, Mayo G. et al. Transdermal modification of platelet function: A dermal aspirin preparation selectively inhibits platelet cyclooxygenase and preserves prostacyclin biosynthesis. *Circ* 1993, 88: 556-561.

[39] Clarke RJ, Mayo G, Price P. et al. Suppression of thromboxane A_2 but not systemic prostacyclin by controlled release aspirin. *N Engl. J Med* 1991, 325: 1137-1141.

[40] Antiplatelet Trialists' Collaboration. The Aspirin Papers. Brit. J. Med.1994, 308:71-72, 81-106.

[41] Fuster V. Dyken ML, Vokomas PS. Aspirin as a therapeutic agent in cardiovascular disease. *Circ.* 1993, 87:659-675.

[42] Rao GHR, Reddy KR, White JG. Low-dose aspirin, platelet function and prostaglandin synthesis: influence of epinephrine and alpha-adrenergic receptor blockade. *Prost. and Med.* 1981, 6:485-494.

[43] McLeod LJ, Roberts MS, Seville PR. Selective inhibition of platelet cyclooxygenase with controlled release low dose aspirin. *Aust. N Z J Med.*1990, 20: 652-656.

[44] Rao GHR, Radha E Johnson GJ. et al. Enteric coated aspirin, platelet cyclooxygenase activity and platelet function. *Prost. Leukot. Med.* 1984,13: 3-12.

[45] Sullivan MH, Zosmer A, Gleeson RP. et al. Equivalent inhibition of *in vivo* platelet function by low dose and high dose aspirin. *Prost. Leukot. Fatty Acids.* 1990,39:319-321.

[46] Kyrle PA, Eichler HG, Jager U. et al. Inhibition of prostacyclin and thromboxane A2 generation by low dose aspirin at the site of plug formation in man *in vivo*. *Circ.*1987, 75:1025-1029.

[47] Wilson TW, McCauley FA, Wells HD. Effects of low dose aspirin on responses to Furosamide. *J. Clin. Pharmacol.* 1986, 26:100-105.

[48] Ridker PM, Cook NR, Lee IM, et al. A randomized trial of low-dose aspirin in the primary prevention of cardiovascular disease in women. *N. Engl.J. Med.* 2005, 352, 1293-304.

[49] Zucker Ml, Trowbridge C, Woodroof J. et al. Low- vs high-dose aspirin. Effects on platelet function in hyper-lipoproteinemic and normal subjects. *Arch. Intern. Med.* 1986, 146: 921-925.

[50] Davi G, Averna M, Catalano I. et al. Increased thromboxane biosynthesis in type 11a hypercholesterolemia. *Circ.* 1992, 85: 1792-1798.

[51] Diminno G, Silver MJ, Cerbone AM et al. Trial of repeated low-dose aspirin in diabetic angiopathy. *Blood.*1986, 68: 886-891.

[52] Terres W, Schuster O, Kupper W. et al. Effects of low-dose acetylsalicylic acid on thrombocytes in healthy subjects and in patients with coronary heart disease. *Dtsh Med. Wochenschr* 1989, 18: 1231-1236.

[53] De Caterina R, Giannessi D Bernini W. et al. Low-dose aspirin in patients recovering from myocardial infarction. Evidence for a selective inhibition of thromboxane-related platelet function. *Eur. Heart J.* 1985, 6:409-417.

[54] Kupper AJ, Verheugt FW, Peels CH. et al. Effect of low dose acetylsalicylic acid on the frequency and hematologic activity of left ventricular thrombus in anterior wall acute myocardial infarction. *Am. J. Cardiol.* 1989, 63:917-920.

[55] Weksler BB, Kent JL, Rudolph D. et al. Effects of low dose aspirin on platelet function in patients with recent cerebral ischemia. *Stroke.* 1985, 16: 5-9.

[56] Uchiyama S, Sone R, Nagayama T et al. Combination therapy with low-dose aspirin and ticlopidine in cerebral ischemia. *Stroke.* 1989, 20: 1643-1647.

[57] Jones EW, Cockbill SR, Cowley AJ. et al. Effects of dazoxiben and low-dose aspirin on platelet behavior in man. *Brit. J. Pharmacol.* 1983, 15: 395-445.

[58] Rao GHR, White JG. Epinephrine-induced Platelet Membrane Modulation. The Platelet Amine Storage. Myers KM, Barnes CD (eds) *CRC Press*, Roca Baton, USA.1992, p117-149.

[59] Rao GHR, Johnson GJ, White JG. Influence of epinephrine on the aggregation response of aspirin-treated platelets. *Prost. Med.* 1980, 5:45-58.

[60] Rao GHR, White JG. Epinephrine potentiation of arachidonate-induced aggregation of cyclooxygenase deficient platelets. *Am. J. Hematol.* 1981, 11: 355-366.

[61] Rao GHR, White JG. Role of arachidonic acid in human platelet activation and irreversible aggregation. *Am. J. Hematol.* 1985, 19: 339-347.

[62] Rao GHR, White JG. Aspirin, PGE1 and Quin-2 AM induced platelet dysfunction. Restoration of function by nor-epinephrine. *Prost. Leukot. Essen. Fatty A*cids 1990, 39: 141-146.

[63] Rao GHR, Escolar G, White JG. Epinephrine reverses the inhibitory influence of aspirin on platelet vessel wall interaction. *Thromb. Res.* 1986, 44: 65-74.

[64] Rao GHR, Escolar G, Zavrol J. Influence of adrenergic receptor blockade on aspirin-induced inhibition of platelet function. *Platelets* 1990,1:145-150.

[65] Rao GHR, Reddy KR, White JG. Modification of human platelet response to sodium arachidonate by membrane modulation. *Prost. Med* 1981, 6: 75-90.

[66] Rao GHR, Johnson GJ, Reddy KR. Ibuprofen Protects Platelet Cyclooxygenase from Irreversible Inhibition by Aspirin. *Arteriosclerosis.* 1983, 3: 383-388.

[67] Connelan JM, Thurlow PJ, Barlow B. et al. Investigation of alternative mechanisms of collagen-induced platelet activation using monoclonal antibodies to glycoprotein 11b-111a and fibrinogen. *Thromb. Haemost.*1986, 55: 153-157.

[68] Muller JE, Tolfer GH. Triggering and hourly variation of onset of arterial thrombosis. *Ann Epideniol.* 1992, 2: 393-405.

[69] Rao GHR. Circadian Variations and coronary artery disease. *Chronobiol* 1994, 21: 63-64.

[70] Prikryl P, Siegelova J, Cornelissen G et al. Chronotherapeutic treatment daily low-dose aspirin. University of Minnesota *Medtronic Chronobiology Series* 1991.

[71] White JG, Rao GHR, Gerrard JM. Effects of nitroblue tetrazolium and Vitamin E on platelet ultrastructure, aggregation and secretion. *Am J. Pathol* 1978, 92:745-53.

[72] Rao GHR, Cox CA, Gerrard JM. Et al. Alpha tocopherol quinone: a potent inhibitor of platelet function. *Prog. Lipid Res.* 1981, 6: 51-64.

[73] Rao GHR, Tate MR, Murthy M. et al. Influence of antioxidants on arachidonic acid metabolism and platelet function. *Biocehm Med. and Met Biol.* 1994, 51:74-79.

[74] Rao GHR, Radha E, White JG. Effect of docosahexaenoic acid (DHA) on arachidonic acid metabolism and platelet function. *Biochem Biophs Res Comm.* 1983, 117: 549-556.

[75] Pollack A. For Some, Aspirin May Not Help Hearts. *New York Times.* 2004, July.

[76] Weber AA, Przytuski B, Schanz A. et al. Towards a definition of aspirin resistance: a typological approach. *Platelets.* 2002, 13: 37-40.

[77] Yilmaz MB, Balbay Y, Korkmaz S. Aspirin resistance. *Anadolu. Kardiyol. Derg* 2004, 4: 59-62.

[78] Patrono C, Coller B, FitzGerald GA. et al. Platelet-Active Drugs: The Relationships Among Dose, Effectiveness, and Side Effects. *CHEST* 2004, 126: 234S-264S.

[79] Howard PA. Aspirin resistance. *Ann Pharmacother*. 2002, 36: 1620-1624.

[80] Hurlen M, Seijeflot I, Arnesen. The Effect of Different Regimens on Platelet Aggregation After Myocardial Infarction. *Scand. Cardiovasc*. J. 1998, 32: 233-237.

[81] Wu KK, Hoak JC. A new method for the quantitative detection of platelet aggregation in patients with arterial insufficiency. *Lancet* 1974,11: 924-926.

[82] Gum PA, Kottke-Marchant K, Poggio ED. et al. Profile and prevalence of aspirin resistance in patients with cardiovascular disease. *Am. J. Cardiol*. 2001, 88: 230-235.

[83] Gum PA, Kottke-Marchant K, Welsh PA. et al. A prospective, blinded determination of the natural history of aspirin resistance among stable patients with cardiovascular disease. *J. Am. Coll. Cardiol*. 2003, 41: 961-967.

[84] Deliargyris E, Boudoulas H. Aspirin Resistance. *Hellenic J. Cardiol*. 2004, 45: 1-5.

[85] Grotemeyer KH. Effects of acetylsalicyclic acid in stroke patients; evidence of non-responders in a subpopulation of treated patients. *Thromb. Res*. 1991, 63: 587-593.

[86] Grotemeyer KH. Two-year follow-up of aspirin responder and aspirin non-responder. A pilot-study including 180 post-stroke patients. *Thromb. Res*. 1993, 71:397-403.

[87] Mueller MR, Salat A, Stangi P. et al. Variable platelet response to low-dose ASA and the risk of limb deterioration in patients submitted to peripheral arterial angioplasty. *Thromb. Haemost*. 1997, 78: 1003-1007.

[88] Eikelboom JW, Hirsh J, Weitz JI. et al. Aspirin-resistant thromboxane biosynthesis and the risk of myocardial infarction, stroke, or cardiovascular death in patients at high risk for cardiovascular events. *Circ* 2002, 105: 1650-1655.

[89] Smout J, Stansby G. Aspirin resistance. *Brit. J. Surgery* 2002, 89: 4-5.

[90] Helgason CM, Bolin KM, Hoff JA. et al. Development of aspirin resistance in persons with previous ischemic stroke. *Stroke* 1994, 25: 2331-2336.

[91] Zimmerman N, Wenk A, Kim U. et al. Functional and biochemical evaluation of platelet aspirin resistance after coronary artery bypass surgery. *Circ*. 2003, 108: 542-547.

[92] Sane DC, McKee SA, Malinin AI. Frequency of aspirin resistance in patients with congestive heart failure treated with antecedent aspirin. *Am. J. Cardiol*. 2002, 90: 893-895.

[93] Muller I, Besta F, Schulz C. et al. Prevalence of Clopidogrel non-responders among patients with stable angina pectoris scheduled for elective coronary stenting. *Thromb. Heamost*. 2003, 89: 783-787.

[94] Lau WC, Gubrel PA, Watkins PB. et al. Contribution of hepatic cytochrome P450 3A4 metabolic activity to the phenomenon of Clopidogrel resistance. *Circ*. 2004, 109: 166-171.

[95] Angiolilo DJ, Fernandez-Ortiz A, Bernardo E. et al. High Clopidogrel loading dose during coronary stenting: effect on drug response and inter-individual variability. *Eur. Heart J*. 2004, 25: 1903-1910.

[96] Serebruany VL, Steinhubl SR, Berger PB. et al. Variability in platelet responsiveness to Clopidogrel among 544 individuals. *J. Am Coll. Cardiol*. 2005, 45: 246-251.

[97] Dziewierz A, Dubek D, Heba G. et al. Inter-individual variability in responses to Clopidogrel with cardiac diseases. *Polis Heart J.* 2005, 62: 1-6.

[98] Altman R, Luciardi HL Muntaner J. et al. The anti-thrombotic profile of aspirin, aspirin resistance or simply failure? *Thromb. J.* 2004, 2: 1-8.

[99] De Gaetano G, Cerletti C. Aspirin resistance: a revival of platelet aggregation tests? *J. Thromb. Haemost.* 2004, 1: 2048-2061.

[100] Malinin A, Spergling M, Muhlestein B. et al. Assessing aspirin responsiveness in subjects with multiple risk factors for vascular disease with a rapid platelet function analyzer. *Blood Coag. Fibrinol.* 2004, 1%: 295-301.

[101] Sambola A. Heras M, Escolar G. et al. The PFA-100 detects sub-optimal antiplatelet responses in patients on aspirin. *Platelets.* 2004, 1-8.

[102] Coleman JL, Wang JC, Simon DI. Determination of individual responses to Aspirin therapy using the Accumetric Ultegra. *The J. Near-Patient Testing and Technol.* 2004, 3: 77-82.

[103] Feuring M, Hasseroth K, Janson CP. et al. Inhibition of platelet aggregation after intake of acetylsalicylic acid detected by a platelet function analyzer (PFA-100). *Int. J. Clin Pharmacol Ther.* 1999, 37: 584-548.

[104] Andersen K, Hurlen M, Arnesen H. et al. Aspirin-responsiveness as measured by a PFA-100 in patients with coronary artery disease. *Thromb. Res.* 2002, 108: 37-42.

[105] Singh S, Kothari SS, Bahl VK. Aspirin Resistance: Myth or Reality? *Ind. Heart J.* 2003, 55: 1-8

[106] McKee SA, Sane DC, Deliagyris. Aspirin resistance in cardiovascular disease: A review of prevalence, mechanisms, and clinical significance. *Thromb. Haemost.* 2002, 88: 711-715.

[107] Eikelboom JW, Hankey GJ. Aspirin resistance: a new independent predictor of vascular events? *J. Am. Coll.Cardiol.* 2003, 41: 966-968.

[108] Berger PB. Resistance to antiplatelet drugs: Is it real or relevant? *Cath. And Cardiovasc Interven.* 2004, 62: 43-45.

[109] Shemesh CG, zehavi M, Dinur I et al. Lack of aspirin effect: aspirin resistance or resistance to taking aspirin? *Am. Heart J.* 2004, 147: 293-300.

[110] Cattaneo M. Aspirin and Clopidogrel: efficacy, safety, and the issue of drug resistance. *Arterscler. Vasc. Biol.* 2004, 24: 1980-87.

[111] Nguyen TA, Diodati JG, Pharand C. Resistance Clopidogrel: a review of the evidence. *J. Am Coll Cardiol* 2005, 45: 1157-64.

[112] Sztritha LK Sas K, Vecsei L. *Aspirin resistance in stroke:* 2004. 2005, 230:163-69.

[113] Coma-Canella I, Velasco A, Castano S. Prevalence of aspirin resistance measured by PFA-100. *Int. J. Cardiol.* 2005, 101:71-76.

[114] Kuliczkowski W, Halawa B, Korolko B. Aspirin resistance in ischemic heart disease. *Kardiol Pol.* 2005, 62: 14-25.

[115] Schwartz KA, Schwartz DE, Ghosheh K et al. Compliance as a critical consideration in patients who appear to be resistant to aspirin after healing of myocardial infarction. *Am. J. Cardiol* 2005, 95: 973-75.

[116] Driewierz A, Dudek D, Heba G, Inter-individual variability in response to Clopidogrel in patients with coronary artery disease. *Kardiol Pol.* 2005, 62: 108-118.

[117] Serebruaany VL, Steinhubl SR, Berger PB. et al. Variability in platelet responsiveness to Clopidogrel among 544 individuals. *J Am Coll Cardiol.* 2005 45: 246-51.

[118] Rao GHR. Aspirin resistance: A fact or a myth? *Expt. and Clin. Cardiol.* 2005, 10: 17-20.

[119] Pettersen AA, Seljeflot I, Abdelnoor M et al. Unstable angina, stroke, myocardial infarction and death in aspirin non-responders. A Prospective, randomized trial. The ASCET (Aspirin non-responsiveness and Clopidogrel Endpoint Trial) design. *Scand Cardiovasc. J.* 2004, 38:353-56.

In: Frontiers in Atherosclerosis Research
Editor: Karin F. Kepper, pp. 213-219

ISBN 1-60021-371-5

Chapter 11

EFFECTS OF SILDENAFIL IN CARDIOVASCULAR DISEASE

Ram B. Singh[5], Dasa Dudova[2], Daniel Pella[2], Shashi B. Gupta[3] and Rakesh C. Kukreja[4]

[1]Halberg Hospital and Research Institute and
Subharti Medical College, Moradabad, India;
[2]Safaric University
[3]Kosice, Slovakia, Railway Hospital, Mumbai, India, [4]VCU Medical Centre, Richmond, VA, USA.

ABSTRACT

Recent studies indicate that sildenafil is cardioprotective by preconditioning of the myocardial and endothelial cells. In the present review, we examine the available evidence regarding this beneficial effect. Experimental studies indicate that sildenafil can provide beneficial effects to the myocardium and endothelium by enhancing preconditioning. There are a few clinical studies among healthy subjects and a few observational studies indicating that sildenafil is useful in patients with poor endothelial function and in those with myocardial ischaemia. We found among 6 volunteer patients with nonST-elevation myocardial infarction that treatment with sildenafil was protective in limiting infarct size. We also observed that sildenafil can decrease blood pressure among hypertensives and provide benefits against heart failure in patients with acute left ventricular failure.

Experimental and clinical experiences support the usefulness of sildenafil in patients with acute myocardial infarction, heart failure and hypertension. Randomized, controlled trials and long-term follow-up are necessary to confirm these observations.

Keywords: sildenafil,cardioprotective,hypertension,heart failure,nitric oxide.

[5] Correspondence: Dr R B Singh, Halberg Hospital and Research Institute, Civil Lines,Moradabad-10(UP)244001, India. Fax 0091 591 2411003,tel 0091 591 2417437; Email: icn2005@mickynline.com

INTRODUCTION

There is consistent evidence that sildenafil can protect against endothelial damage and myocardial injury by enhancing preconditioning [1, 2]. One study showed [2], that opening of mitochondrial ATP sensitive K channels by ischemic preconditioning or Diazoxide protected the endothelium by reducing the bursts of free radicals that occurred at reperfusion. Mitochonchria is rich in the coenzyme Q10 and carnitine, which are cytoprotective antioxidants and bioenergetic agents [3-5]. Both these agents are known to maintain ATP, which poses the possibility that endogenous levels of the agents or their supplementation may be protective against free radical-induced damage to ATP Sensitive K channels. It is also possible that these agents might enhance the capability of the myocardial and endothelial cells in preconditioning which is known to protect the cells against injury responsible for arrhythmias, and can modulate remodeling of the myocardium and endothelium against heart failure and atherogenesis.[4-6].It has been shown that this widely-used drug for treating erectile dysfunction reduces the apoptosis under heart attack-like conditions in a laboratory model. These findings may help researchers to develop a new treatment for patients with heart failure and acute myocardial infarction (AMI), where the loss of cells is primarily due to cell suicide or ischemic damage respectively [5, 6].

CLINICAL OBSERVATIONS

In our experience, 3 patients, aged 45-60years, (1 male and 2 females), presenting with congestive heart failure due to hypertension (systolic >200mmHg and diastolic >110mmHg) and ischemic heart disease, were given furosemide 40mg intravenously daily plus sildenafil 50mg twice daily, plus perindopril 4-8mg daily, there was a marked improvement in New York Heart Association(NYHA) class heart failure and quality of life including improvement in fatigue and dyspnea within 48hours of treatment. All the 3 patients were discharged by the end of one week. All these patients had radiological, electrocardiographic and echocardiographic manifestations of heart failure, including lower ejection fraction between 40-50%. There was a significant reduction in systolic and diastolic blood pressures in all the patients (>150/95mmHg).

In another clinical observation, among 6 patients with acute myocardial infarction(AMI),we noted that sildenafil (25mg 2-3 times, daily) can decrease anginal episodes, cause less increase in LDH and reduce electocardiographic QRS score(infarct size) when compared to another 6 age, sex and body mass index matched subjects not given this agent. There was a 20-25% increase in heart rate and decrease in blood pressures initially among patients receiving sildenafil compared to the baseline heart rate, which settled to baseline rates after about 5 days treatment. The patients in both groups also did not receive streptokinase because some of them presented beyond 20-24 hours of onset of chest pain and some had nonST-segment elevation AMI. Their age varied between 45-60 years and 5 were males and 1 female in each group. One patient with inferior wall infarction had hypotension, (80/50mmHg) where the dose of sildenafil was decreased to 25mg/day from 25mg thrice daily. There were no adverse effects of sildenafil in both of our observations and all patients gave written informed consent for the administration of sildenafil.

EXISTING CLINICAL EVIDENCE

In one study among healthy subjects [7], ischemia/reperfusion on endothelial and neutrophil function was studied, in which the forearm was made ischemic by inflating a blood pressure cuff to 200mmHg for 20 minutes. The dilator response to the endothelial dependent dilator, acetylecholine and the nonendothelial dependent dilator nitroglycerine was determined before and after ischemia/reperfusion. Neutrophil function was studied by determining the upregulation of the CD11b in the circulating blood. Ischemic preconditioning was developed by 3 five minute periods of ischemia/reperfusion prior to the 20 minute ischemic periods. There was a marked decline in radial artery dilation to acetylecholine but not to nitroglycerine and an upregulation of CD11b, due to ischemia/reperfusion in the control subjects. Ischemic preconditioning blunted these responses to ischemia/reperfusion. This study suggests possible pathways of pharmacological preconditioning of the vasculature causing better reflow in patients with endothelial injury. In another more recent study [8], the role of ATP sensitive K channels was studied in mediating the influence of ischemic preconditioning among healthy volunteers after ischemia/reperfusion of the forearm. Intraarterial administration of acetylecholine was used to determine vasodilator response, indicating endothelial function, before and at 15 minutes, after 20 minutes of forearm ischemia/reperfusion under the influence of various drugs. Ischemic preconditioning protected against induced endothelial dysfunction by ischemia/reperfusion and this protection was blunted by cotherapy with glibenclamide. However, pretreatment with diazoxide simulated the effects of preconditioning to protect against endothelial dysfunction, which was blocked by glibenclamide. Interestingly, in the absence of ischemia/reperfusion, diazoxide had no influence on vasodilator responses to acetylecholine. It is possible that ATP sensitive K channels have an important role in ischemia/reperfusion-induced endothelial damage in humans. It is also likely that modulation of channel pathways using certain agents by activation of K channels may have a therapeutic use in patients with AMI. Tomai et al [9], in one early study, reported that repeated episodes of angioplasty induced ischemia blocked by glibenclamide, had no beneficial influence on cardiomyocytes that was to be provided by preconditioning. These clinical studies and our observations in AMI indicate that activation of myocardial and and/or endothelial localized ATP sensitive K channels are useful in patients with coronary artery disease, which might decrease injury to endothelial cells as well as to cardiomyocytes. In a most recent observation, Gori et al [10] studied the effects of treatment with sildenafil (50mg/day) among 10 healthy male volunteers, 2 hours prior to 15 minutes of cuff-induced radial artery ischemia, followed by 15 minutes of reperfusion. In a double blind, randomized, crossover study, flow mediated vasodilation was determined prior to drug or placebo treatment as an indicator of endothelial function. Glibenclamide (5mg) was administered one hour prior to sildenafil administration in a randomized, double blind fashion, in a separate group of 7 healthy volunteers. There was a significant reduction in the endothelial function in placebo-treated controls and this decline was prevented by prior treatment with sildenafil. However, the beneficial effect of sildenafil was blunted by glibenclamide at a dose, which had no influence on endothelial function in the absence of sildenafil. This study has provided proof for the first time that sildenafil provides protection to the endothelium against ischemia/reperfusion in humans and this effect involves activation of vascular ATP sensitive K channels. One earlier study [11] also showed that treatment with sildenafil, acutely in patients with chronic heart failure enhances endothelium-dependent, flow mediated vasodilation in the brachial artery, one hour after sildenafil therapy compared to control subjects. In another study [12], 100mg/day of sildenafil was administered causing dilation of epicardial coronary arteries, and improvement in endothelial function in the brachial artery and it also inhibited platelet function in patients with coronary artery disease. There was a significant reduction in exercise-induced ischemia upon treatment with sildenafil, which showed moderate effects when compared to placebo and isosorbide dinitrate. It is clear that sildenafil was effective, both in healthy volunteers as well as in patients with chronic heart failure and coronary artery disease [11-13]. Our observations do not provide proof that sildenafil should be administered in the treatment of AMI. However, in view of the above studies, it indicates a need for randomized, controlled trials to determine its exact role in the prevention of complications in these patients, especially in those who have myocardial ischemia in the presence of coronary atherothrombosis and left ventricular dysfunction. There are no serious adverse effects of sildanafil, except hypotension, especially in those patients receiving nitrates and other nitric oxide donors [14, 15].

In one study [16] data were pooled regarding myocardial infarction (MI) and cardiovascular death from more than 120 clinical trials of sildenafil citrate (Viagra) conducted from 1993 to 2001. During placebo-controlled trials, the rate of MI or cardiovascular death was 0.91 (95% CI: 0.52-1.48) per 100 person-years (PY) of follow-up among sildenafil-treated patients compared with 0.84 (95% CI: 0.39-1.60) per 100 PY of follow-up among placebo-treated patients. The relative risk of MI or cardiovascular death was 1.08 (95% CI: 0.45-2.77) for sildenafil compared with placebo ($p = 0.88$). During open-label studies, the rate of MI or cardiovascular death was 0.56 (95% CI: 0.44-0.72) per 100 PY of follow-up. This analysis showed that the rates of MI and cardiovascular death were low and comparable between men treated with sildenafil and those treated with placebo. The use of sildenafil was not associated with an increase in the risk of MI or cardiovascular death.

Experimental Evidence

Several studies [17-21] have examined the cardioprotective effects of sildenafil on myocardial infarct size and arrhythmias. All the studies reported a beneficial influence except one [17] showing that slidenafil-nitric oxide donor combination promotes ventricular tachyarrhythmias in a swine right ventricle. In one study [18], both acute treatment with sildenafil given 30 minutes prior to ischemia, and chronic administration, given 24hours prior to the index ischemic period produced a marked preconditioning like effect in intact rabbits. After administration of the drug or the vehicle, rabbits were subjected to 30minutes of ischemia and 3 hours of reperfusion. The triphenyletetraz -olium histochemical staining technique was used to determine the infarct size and showed that delayed treatment with sildenafil decreased the infarct size by 41% and acute treatment by 68%, respectively. Treatment with 5-HD, a mitochondrial selective, ATP sensitive K channel antagonist, 10minutes prior to the index ischemic period, blocked these beneficial influences. Oral administration of sildenafil was associated with both acute and delayed cardiac protection.

Further studies [19, 20] showed that reduction of infarct size by sildenafil in acute administration was due to PKC and that an upregulation of both endothelial nitric oxide synthetase (eNOS) and iNOS occurred in a delayed preconditioning model in mouse hearts.

After 24 hours of sildenafil administration, treatment with a selective iNOS inhibitor, 1400W, antagonized the sildenafil-induced cardioprotection, if given 30 minutes prior to index ischemia. It is clear that PKC, nitric oxide and mitochondrial ATP sensitive K channels are involved in providing cardioprotective effects to reduce infarct size in experimental models.

Increased availability of coenzyme Q10 and carnitine may repair or strengthen these mechanisms, resulting in better protective effects.

Nagy et al [20] also showed that sildenafil decreased the severity of ventricular rhythm disturbances in experiments with dogs, 24 hours after oral treatment with this agent. However, when sildenafil was given in combination with nitric oxide donor nitroprusside or nitroglycerine, it became arrhythmogenic in nonischemic, buffer-perfused, isolated right ventricular walls of swine hearts. Myocardial tissue deficiency of coenzyme Q10 and carnitine, which were not available in this experiment, may be the cause of these adverse effects. We also observed a 20-25% increase in baseline heart rate among patients with AMI receiving sildenafil. Other factors responsible for this discrepancy, may be due to protocol differences, a drug interaction or due to species differences between dogs and pigs.

Mechanisms

Recently, it has been reported [2, 6] that treatment with sildenafil citrate at clinically relevant concentrations produced therapeutic levels of nitric oxide (NO) in the heart cells by increasing protein levels of two enzymes responsible for the synthesis of NO. Employing a cellular model where heart attack-like conditions are simulated in a Petri dish, it has been demonstrated that NO produced from sildenafil inhibits cell death by stabilizing mitochondria, thereby increasing the level of the anti-death protein, Bcl-2, and inhibiting caspase 3, the protein considered to be the ultimate weapon in cell suicide. This research has established a strong basis for the design of future studies targeted toward investigating the clinical effects of sildenafil on survival of the heart muscle following a major heart attack. In addition, these findings suggest that this drug may slow or possibly reverse the progressive loss of heart cells during chronic heart failure in patients with acute or chronic coronary artery disease. Researchers used heart cells prepared from genetically engineered mice that lack nitric oxide synthesizing enzymes. The model was particularly useful in studying the protective effect of sildenafil in heart muscle cells independent of any vascular effects or other types of cells. Sildenafil not only protected against necrosis, accidental cell death occurring due to oxygen deprivation, but also against apoptosis, cell death following DNA fragmentation. Furthermore, the researchers found the presence of phosphodiesterase-5 (PDE-5), an enzyme responsible for the destruction of the cGMP molecule, in the heart cells. The cGMP is an intracellular messenger molecule that plays an important role in the dilation of arteries in the body. Sildenafil is able to preserve cGMP, and therefore dilation of the arteries by inhibiting PDE-5.

Conclusions

These observations have far-reaching implications for the treatment of patients with heart failure where loss of cells is primarily due to apoptosis, and in patients with AMI and angina pectoris where the cell loss may be due to ischemic injury. In several other studies [6-21] and due to our observations, it is proposed that sildenafil has a powerful, protective effect in the heart during experimental and clinical heart attack in animal models, and in humans, respectively, indicting that it could be protective against AMI and hypertensive heart failure and also possibly in patients with hypertension for decreasing blood pressure. Randomized, controlled, clinical trials are necessary to demonstrate the role of sidenafil in cardiovascular disease.

Acknowledgements

We are grateful to Raj Chopra, President of the Tishcon Corporation, Westbury, NY, for support in writing this article.

References

[1] Gross GJ.Sildenafil and endothelial dysfunction in humans (Editorial). *Circulation* 2005 (in press).

[2] Beresewicz A, Maczewski M, Duda M. Effect of classical preconditioning and diazoxide on endothelial function and O2 and NO generation in the post-ischemic guinea-pig heart. *Cardiovas Res* 2004,63:118-129.

[3] Chiang CA, Pella D, Singh RB. Coenzyme Q10 and adverse effects of statins. *J Nutr Environ Med* 2004,14:17-28.

[4] Singh RB, Neki NS, Kartikey K, Niaz MA, Thakur AS. Effect of coenzyme Q10 on risk of atherosclerosis in patients with recent myocardial infarction. *Mol Cell Biochem* 2003,246:75-82.

[5] Singh RB, Niaz MA, Agarwal P, Begom R, Rastogi SS, Sachan DS.A randomized, double blind, placebo controlled trial of L-carnitine in suspected acute myocardial infarction. *Postgrad Med* 1996,72:45-50.

[6] Kukreja RC, Ockaili R, Salloum F and Xi, L. Cardioprotection with phosphodiesterase-5 inhibition-a novel preconditioning strategy. *J Mol Cell Cardiol* 2004,36:165-173.

[7] Kharbanda RK, Peters M,* Walton B, Kattenhorn M, Mullen M, Klein N, Vallance P, Deanfield J, MacAllister R.*Ischemic preconditioning prevents endothelial injury and systemic neutrophil activation during ischemia-repurfusion in humans in vivo. *Circulation* 2001, 103:1624-30.

[8] Broadhead MW, Kharbanda RK, Peters M *MacAllister RJ.* K-ATP channels activation induces ischemic preconditioning of the endothelium in humans in vivo. *Circulation* 2004, 110:2077-2082.

[9] Tomai F, Crea F, Gaspardone A, *Gaspardone A, Versaci F, De Paulis R, Penta de Peppo A, Chiariello L, Gioffre PA. *Ischemic preconditioning during coronary

angioplasty is prevented by glibenclamide, a selective ATP-sensitive K+ channel blocket. *Circulation* 1994,90:700-705.

[10] Gori T, Sicuro S, Dragoni S, *Donati G, Forconi S, Parker JD.* Sildenafil prevents endothelial disfunction induced by ischemia and reperfusion via opening of ATP sensitive K channels. A human invivo study. *Circulation* 2005, 111:742-6.

[11] Katz SD, Balidamaj K, Homma S *Wu H, Wang J, Maybaum S.*Acute type 5 phosphodiesterase inhibition with sildenafil enhances flow- mediated vasodilation in patients with chronic heart failure. *J Am Coll Cardiol* 2000,36:845-851.

[12] Halcox JPJ, Nour KRA, Seals G *Mincemoyer RA, Waclawiw M, Rivera CE, Willie G, Ellahham S, Quyyumi AA.*The effect of sildenafil on human vascular function, platelet activation and myocardial ischemia. *J Am Coll Cardiol* 2002,40:1232-1240.

[13] Yellon DM, Downey JM. Preconditioning the myocardium: from cellular physiology to clinical cardiology. *Physiol Rev* 2003,83:1113-1151.

[14] Kloner RA. Cardiovascular effects of the 3phosphodiesterase-5 inhibitors approved for the treatment of erectile dysfunction. *Circulation* 2004, 110:3149-3155.

[15] Reffelman T, Kloner RA. Effects of sildenafil on myocardial infarct size, microvascular function and acute ischemic left ventricular dilation. *Cardiovasc Res* 2003,59:441-449.

[16] Mittleman MA, Glasser DB, Orazem J Clinical trials of sildenafil citrate (Viagra) demonstrate no increase in risk of myocardial infarction and cardiovascular death compared with placebo. *Int J Clin Pract.* 2003 Sep;57 (7):597-600.

[17] Ockaili R, Salloum F, Hawkins J and Kukreja RC. Sildenafil(viagra) induces powerful cardioprotective effect via opening of mitochondrial K ATP channels in rabbits. *Am J Physiol* 2002, 283:H1263-H1269.

[18] Das A, Ockaili R, Salloum and Kukreja, R.C. Protein kinase C plays an essential role in sildenafil-induced cardioprotection in rabbits. *Am J Physiol* 2003, 286:H1455-H1460.

[19] Salloum F, Yin C, Xi L and Kukreja RC. Sildenafil induces delayed preconditioning through inducible nitric oxide synthase dependent pathway in mouse heart. *Circ Res* 2003,92:595-597.

[20] Nagi O, Hajnal A, Parratt JR and Vegh A. Sildenafil(viagra)reduces arrhythmias severity during ischemia 24h after oral administration. *Brit J Pharmacol* 2004,141:549-551.

[21] Swissa M, Ohara T, Lee MH, Kaul S, Shah PK, Hayashi H, Chen PS, Karagueuzian HS. Sildenafil-nitric oxide donor combination promotes ventricular tachyarrhythmias in the swine right ventricle. *Am J Physiol* 2001, 282:H1787-H1792.

INDEX

A

B

D

E

F

G

H

I

M

N

O

P

Q

R

S

T

U

V

W

Y